Textbook of
COLOR DOPPLER IMAGING

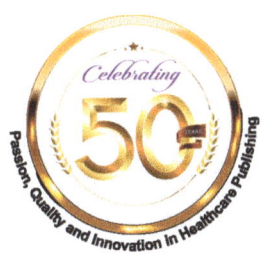

Textbook of
COLOR DOPPLER IMAGING

Third Edition

Editors

Sumeet Bhargava
MBBS DNB (Radiodiagnosis) FCGP FIAMS FICRI FIMSA MNAMS

Formerly Associate Professor
Department of Radiology and Imaging
Rama Medical College and Superspecialty Hospital
Ghaziabad, Uttar Pradesh, India

Satish Kumar Bhargava
MBBS MD (Radiodiagnosis)
MD (Radiotherapy) DMRD FICRI FIAMS FCCP FUSI FIMSA FAMS

Formerly Professor and Head
Department of Radiology and Imaging
University College of Medical Sciences (University of Delhi)
Guru Teg Bahadur (GTB) Hospital, New Delhi
Rama Medical College and Superspecialty Hospital, Ghaziabad
and
School of Medical Sciences and Research
Sharda Hospital, Greater Noida, Uttar Pradesh, India

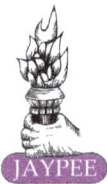

JAYPEE BROTHERS MEDICAL PUBLISHERS
The Health Sciences Publisher
New Delhi | London | Panama

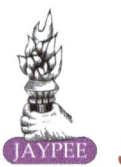 **Jaypee Brothers Medical Publishers (P) Ltd**

Headquarters
Jaypee Brothers Medical Publishers (P) Ltd
4838/24, Ansari Road, Daryaganj
New Delhi 110 002, India
Phone: +91-11-43574357
Fax: +91-11-43574314
Email: jaypee@jaypeebrothers.com

Overseas Offices

J.P. Medical Ltd
83 Victoria Street, London
SW1H 0HW (UK)
Phone: +44 20 3170 8910
Fax: +44 (0)20 3008 6180
Email: info@jpmedpub.com

Jaypee-Highlights Medical Publishers Inc
City of Knowledge, Bld. 235, 2nd Floor
Clayton, Panama City, Panama
Phone: +1 507-301-0496
Fax: +1 507-301-0499
Email: cservice@jphmedical.com

Jaypee Brothers Medical Publishers (P) Ltd
Bhotahity, Kathmandu, Nepal
Phone: +977-9741283608
Email: kathmandu@jaypeebrothers.com

Website: www.jaypeebrothers.com
Website: www.jaypeedigital.com

© 2019, Jaypee Brothers Medical Publishers

The views and opinions expressed in this book are solely those of the original contributor(s)/author(s) and do not necessarily represent those of editor(s) of the book.

All rights reserved. No part of this publication may be reproduced, stored or transmitted in any form or by any means, electronic, mechanical, photocopying, recording or otherwise, without the prior permission in writing of the publishers.

All brand names and product names used in this book are trade names, service marks, trademarks or registered trademarks of their respective owners. The publisher is not associated with any product or vendor mentioned in this book.

Medical knowledge and practice change constantly. This book is designed to provide accurate, authoritative information about the subject matter in question. However, readers are advised to check the most current information available on procedures included and check information from the manufacturer of each product to be administered, to verify the recommended dose, formula, method and duration of administration, adverse effects and contraindications. It is the responsibility of the practitioner to take all appropriate safety precautions. Neither the publisher nor the author(s)/editor(s) assume any liability for any injury and/or damage to persons or property arising from or related to use of material in this book.

This book is sold on the understanding that the publisher is not engaged in providing professional medical services. If such advice or services are required, the services of a competent medical professional should be sought.

Every effort has been made where necessary to contact holders of copyright to obtain permission to reproduce copyright material. If any have been inadvertently overlooked, the publisher will be pleased to make the necessary arrangements at the first opportunity. The **CD/DVD-ROM** (if any) provided in the sealed envelope with this book is complimentary and free of cost. **Not meant for sale.**

Inquiries for bulk sales may be solicited at: jaypee@jaypeebrothers.com

Textbook of Color Doppler Imaging

First Edition: 2003
Reprint: 2007
Third Edition: **2019**
ISBN: 978-93-5270-616-7

Dedicated to

*My Late Parents Shri Jagannath Bhargava and
Smt Brahama Devi Bhargava and
My loving Late Wife Kalpana Bhargava
Whose Inspiration and Motivation have made
possible to bring out this book*

—**Satish Kumar Bhargava**
Kalpana Bhargava Health Care Diagnostic Centre
Greater Noida (UP)

CONTRIBUTORS

AK SRIVASTVA
MSc PhD
Physicist
Department of Radiology and Imaging
University College of Medical Sciences (Delhi University) and GTB Hospital, New Delhi, India

AMIT SAHU
DNB (Radiodiagnosis)
Senior Consultant
Department of Radiogy and Imaging
Max Superspecialty Hospital
Saket, New Delhi, India

BHARAT PAREKH
MD (Radiodiagnosis) FICRI
Ex-Chairman, Inidian College of Radiology and Imaging and Consultant Radiologist, ECLAT Polyclinic
Mumbai, Maharashtra, India

DEEP N SRIVASTVA
MD (Radiodiagnosis)
Professor
Department of Radiodiagnosis
All India Institute of Medical Sciences
New Delhi, India

GP VASHIST
MD (Radiodiagnosis) FICRI
Director
Department of Radiology and Imaging
Batra Hospital and Medical Research Center
New Delhi, India

GOPESH MEHROTRA
MD (Radiodiagnosis)
Professor, Department of Radiology and Imaging
University College of Medical Sciences (Delhi University) and GTB Hospital, New Delhi, India

GURPREET GULATI
MD (Radiodiagnosis)
Professor
Department of Cardiac-Radiology
All India Institute of Medical Sciences
New Delhi, India

JAIDEEP MALHOTRA
MD FICOG FIAJAGO FICMCH FICMU
Malhotra Nursing and Maternity Home (P) Ltd
Agra, Uttar Pradesh, India

NARENDRA MALHOTRA
MD FICOG FIAJAGO FICMCH FICMU
Malhotra Nursing and Maternity Home (P)Ltd
Agra, Uttar Pradesh, India

OP SHARMA
MD (Radiodiagnosis) FICRI PHd (Radiology)
Ex-Professor and Head
Department of Radiology and Imaging
Institue of Medical Sciences, Banarus Hindu University
Varanasi, Uttar Pradesh, India

POONAM NARANG
MD (Radiodiagnosis)
Director Professor, Department of Radiology and Imaging
Maulana Azad Medical College and Associated GB Pant Hospital, New Delhi, India

RAJUL RASTOGI
MD (Radiodiagnosis) FIMSA
Associate Professor
Department of Radiology and Imaging
Teerthanker Mahaveer University
Moradabad, Uttar Pradesh, India

ROHINI GUPTA
MD (Radiodiagnosis)
Professor
Department of Radiology and Imaging
Vardhman Mahavir Medical College and Associated Safdarjung Hospital, New Delhi, India

SANJAY THULKAR
MD (Radiodiagnosis)
Professor
Department of Radiodiagnosis
All India Institute of Medical sciences
New Delhi, India

SANJEEV SHARMA
MD (Radiodiagnosis)
Professor and Head
Department of Cardiac-Radiology
All India Institute of Medical Sciences
New Delhi, India

SATISH KUMAR BHARGAVA
MD (Radiodiagnosis) MD (Radiotherapy)
DMRD FICRI FIAMS FIMSA FCCP FUSI FAMS
Formerly Professor and Head
Department of Radiology and Imaging
University College of Medical Sciences (University of Delhi)
Guru Teg Bahadur (GTB) Hospital, New Delhi
Rama Medical College and Superspecialty Hospital,
Ghaziabad and School of Medical Sciences and Research
Sharda Hospital, Greater Noida, Uttar Pradesh, India

SUCHI BHATT
MD (Radiodiagnosis) FICRI MNAMS
Associate Professor, Department of Radiology and Imaging
University College of Medical Sciences (Delhi University) and
GTB Hospital, New Delhi, India

SUMEET BHARGAVA
MBBS DNB (Radiodiagnosis) FCGP FIAMS FICRI FIMSA MNAMS
Formerly Associate Professor
Department of Radiology and Imaging
Rama Medical College and Superspecialty Hospital
Ghaziabad, Uttar Pradesh, India

VIPUL GUPTA
MD (Radiodiagnosis)
Head
Department of Neuro-Radiology
Max Superspecialty Hospital, Saket, Delhi, India

PREFACE TO THE THIRD EDITION

With the more and more extensive utilization of the color Doppler in various systems of the human body, more so in antenatal check up, fetal monitoring and cardiac evaluation by 3D and 4D technology and due to its accuracy and correct diagnosis, the book has been revised with addition of more chapter on 3D and 4D technology, replacement and addition of few important illustrations, we are sure that book will definitely be more useful to Radiologists, Obstetricians and Gynecologists, Physicians, and Residents.

Sumeet Bhargava
Satish Kumar Bhargava

PREFACE TO THE FIRST EDITION

Color Doppler sonography has been in use for more than three decades now and has constantly evolved to its present status of being the minatory of the vascular laboratory. It has unparalled application in assessing cerebral, abdominal and peripheral vasculature. Color Doppler is now widely applicable in intravascular, and interventional procedures. This added a new dimension of its role in therapeutic radiology. Its role in differentiating benign versus malignant lesions is increasing day-by-day. The extent and severity of the disease process and hemodynamic alteration caused by it can be confidently estimated. In fact all sonographers, must now be familiar with Doppler imaging, as blood flow assessment is used virtually every time an ultrasound examination is carried out.

Color Doppler sonography is a combination of Doppler ultrasound and gray scale ultrasound to provide simultaneous realtime visualization of soft tissues structures and blood flow over the entire scan field. Interpretation of this information required a sound knowledge of the basic technical principles of color Doppler imaging and the pathophysiology involved in the disease process. This book is a sincere effort to provide a clear scenario of the fascinating world of color Doppler sonography. It deals with the basic fundamentals of color Doppler sonography and its application in the specific body regions. The extensive text covered in this book itself portrays the burden borne by this aspect of imaging. An attempt has been made to provide an update knowledge of the subject. Use of contrast medium in vascular ultrasonography has been highlighted in this book. A satisfactory number of illustrations have been included in each chapter to provide an interesting insight into the subject.

This is the first Indian book on color Duplex sonography. I feel that this sincere effort will be critically analyzed, appreciated and appraised.

Satish K Bhargava

ACKNOWLEDGMENTS

We are grateful to our colleagues and friends who gave timely support and stood solidly behind us in our joint endeavor of bringing out this book which was required keeping in view of wide acceptability of ultrasound in developing countries.

We both would like to thank Shri Jitendar P Vij (Group Chairman), Mr Ankit Vij (Managing Director), Ms Chetna Malhotra Vohra (Associate Director–Content Strategy), Ms Madhuri Aggarwal (Development Editor), and all the staff of M/s Jaypee Brothers Medical Publishers (P) Ltd, New Delhi, India, for their efforts and input enabling timely publication of the book.

CONTENTS

Chapter 1. The Story of Doppler — 1
Sumeet Bhargava, AK Srivastva

Chapter 2. Basic Hemodynamics — 3
Sumeet Bhargava, AK Srivastva, Satish Kumar Bhargava
- Physical Aspects 3
- Venous Hemodynamics 10

Chapter 3. Doppler Principle and Instrumentation — 13
Sumeet Bhargava, Satish Kumar Bhargava, AK Srivastva
- Doppler Effect 13
- Instrumentation 16
- Multigated PW Doppler Systems 19

Chapter 4. Doppler Spectral Analysis — 21
Sumeet Bhargava, Satish Kumar Bhargava, AK Srivastva
- Sample Volume 21
- Direction of Flow 22
- Waveform 22
- Envelope Traces of the Doppler Spectrum 24
- Diagnosis of Arterial Obstruction 26

Chapter 5. Color Flow Imaging — 29
Sumeet Bhargava, AK Srivastva, Satish Kumar Bhargava
- Principles of Color Flow Imaging 29
- Problems in Color Flow Imaging 31
- Clinical Advantages of Color Flow Imaging and its Limitations 31
- Power Doppler Flow Imaging 34
- Harmonic Imaging 35

Chapter 6. Contrast Agents in Ultrasound — 36
Sumeet Bhargava, Satish Kumar Bhargava, Suchi Bhatt
- The Impact of Contrast Enhancement 37
- Clinical Applications 38
- Transcranial Doppler 39
- Carotid Doppler 40
- Renal Doppler 40
- Portal Vein Doppler 40
- Peripheral Arterial Doppler 40
- Inferior Vena Cava 40
- Peripheral Venous Doppler 41
- Functional Uses of Contrast Doppler 41

Chapter 7. Cerebrovascular Doppler Sonography 46
Satish Kumar Bhargava, Gopesh Mehrotra, Rajul Rastogi
- Technique 46
- Abnormal Findings 48
- Doppler Criteria 48
- Direct Stenotic Measurements 49
- Plaque Characteristics 50
- Vertebral Arteries 53

Chapter 8. Transcranial Doppler Sonography 57
Vipul Gupta
- Basic Instrumentation 57
- Technique and Normal Parameters 57
- Arterial Stenosis and Occlusion 62
- Middle Cerebral Artery Stenosis/Occlusion 63
- Carotid Siphon Stenosis 63
- Assessment of Effects of Extracranial Occlusive Disease 64
- Emboli Detection 66
- Intraoperative and Procedural Monitoring 66
- Functional Reserve Testing 69
- Other Uses 69

Chapter 9. Doppler in Liver 73
Suchi Bhatt, Poonam Narang, Sumeet Bhargava
- Liver 73
- Technique 73
- Normal Patterns 73
- Portal Hypertension 74
- Qualitative Findings 76
- Semiquantitative Findings 79
- Quantitative Findings 79
- Evaluation of Medical Treatment in Portal Hypertension 80
- Color Doppler in Hepatic Lesions 83
- Liver Transplantation 85

Chapter 10. Role of Color Doppler in Splenic Lesions 90
Sumeet Bhargava, Suchi Bhatt, Poonam Narang, Satish Kumar Bhargava
- Portal Hypertension 90
- Splenic Infarction 91
- Intrasplenic Pseudoaneurysm 91

Chapter 11. Color Doppler in Pancreas 93
Sumeet Bhargava, Suchi Bhatt, Poonam Narang, Satish Kumar Bhargava
- Pancreatic Transplantation 93

Chapter 12. Role of Color Doppler in Urinary System 96
Suchi Bhatt, Satish Kumar Bhargava, Rajul Rstogi, Sumeet Bhargava
- Kidneys 96
- Color Doppler Sonography in Detection of Vesicoureteric Reflux 109
- Doppler Evaluation of the Prostate 110

Chapter 13. The Retroperitoneum and Great Vessels — 115
Sumeet Bhargava, GP Vashisht, Suchi Bhatt, Satish Kumar Bhargava
- Aorta *115*
- Aortic Pathology *117*
- Aortic Grafts *122*
- Complications of Graft Implantation *122*
- Aortic Branches *123*
- Superior Mesenteric Artery *123*
- Renal Arteries *124*
- Inferior Vena Cava *126*
- IVC Branches and Tributaries *127*
- Intraoperative Applications of Doppler *128*

Chapter 14. Current Role of High Resolution Ultrasonography and Color Doppler in the Diagnosis of Scrotal Diseases — 130
Rajul Rastogi, Sumeet Bhargava, Bharat Parekh
- Normal Ultrasound Anatomy *130*
- Testicular Torsion *131*
- Inflammatory Diseases *132*
- Scrotal Trauma *133*
- Hydrocele *134*
- Undescended Testis *135*
- Scrotal Calcifications *136*
- Varicocele *136*
- Scrotal Hernias *136*
- Testicular Tumors *136*

Chapter 15. Duplex Ultrasonography of Erectile Dysfunction — 139
Sanjay Thulkar, Deep N Srivastva
- Anatomy and Physiology of Penile Erection *139*
- Evaluation of Erectile Dysfunction *139*
- Technique *140*
- Treatment of Complications *142*
- Peyronie's Disease *142*

Chapter 16. Color Doppler of Small Parts — 143
GP Vashist, Satish Kumar Bhargava, Rajul Rastogi, Sumeet Bhargava
- Musculoskeletal System *143*
- Skin and Subcutaneous Tissues *144*
- Vascular Lesions *145*
- Parathyroid Adenoma *151*
- Color Doppler Imaging in Orbit *152*

Chapter 17. Doppler Imaging of Peripheral Arteries — 156
Rajul Rastogi, Satish Kumar Bhargava
- Instrumentation *156*
- Normal Anatomy and Doppler Waveform *156*

Chapter 18. Venous System — 166
Satish Kumar Bhargava, Rohini Gupta, Sumeet Bhargava
- Lower Limb Veins 166
- Upper Limb Veins 166
- Instrumentation and Technique 166
- Characteristics of a Normal Vein 168
- Lower Extremity Deep Venous Thrombosis 169
- Chronic Deep Venous Thrombosis 171
- Upper Extremity Thrombosis 171

Chapter 19. Intravascular Ultrasound: Newer Advances, Current Applications and Future Directions — 174
Sanjeev Sharma, Gurpreet Gulati
- Rationale for Intravascular Ultrasound Imaging 174
- Appearance on IVUS in Various Disease States 176
- Clinical Applications 178
- Miscellaneous Applications 179
- Limitations of Intravascular Ultrasound 179
- Future Directions 180

Chapter 20. Role of Color Flow and Doppler in Obstetrics, Gynecology, and Infertility — 182
Narendra Malhotra, Jaideep Malhotra, Rajul Rastogi, Sumeet Bhargava
- Imaging Problems 182
- Clinical Uses 182
- Color Doppler in Gynecology 184
- Role of Color Doppler in Infertility 191
- Role of Transvaginal Color Doppler in Other Conditions Associated with Infertility 195
- Tubal Evaluation 197
- Color Doppler in Relation to Obstetrics 198

Chapter 21. Gray Scale Ultrasonography and Color Doppler Study in Fracture Healing — 211
OP Sharma
- Experimental Study 211
- Clinical Study 211

Chapter 22. 3D and 4D Ultrasound: Principles, Advantages, and Applications — 215
Amit Sahu, Sumeet Bhargava
- Applications in Clinical Practice 215
- Limitations of Volumetry USG 217

Index — 219

Chapter 1

The Story of Doppler

Doppler color flow mapping, a new and exciting advancement in cardiac ultrasound is a method whereby blood flow is imaged and displayed on 2D image.

The first description of the physical principle used in color flow devices is attributed to Johann Christian Doppler, an Austrian mathematician and scientist who lived in the first half of the 19th century. Doppler's first descriptions concerned changes in wavelength of light as applied to astronomical events. In 1842, he presented a paper entitled "on the colored light of double stars and some other heavenly bodies" in which he postulated that certain properties of light emitted from stars depend upon the relative motion of the observer and the wave source. He suggested that the colored appearance of certain stars was caused by their motion relative to the earth, the blue ones moving toward earth and the red ones moving away. He drew an analogy of a ship moving to meet or retreat from incoming ocean waves. The ship moving out to sea would meet the waves with more frequency than a ship moving towards the shoreline. Interestingly Doppler never extrapolated his postulates to sound waves.

There was immediate criticism of Doppler. Just like today, critics abounded. Among them was Buys Ballot who in 1844 stated he simply did not believe Doppler. There is rather amusing account of the difficulties Buys Ballot encountered in attempting to disclaim the Doppler Effect. In 1845, he borrowed a steam locomotive from Dutch Government and arranged for a trumpet player to ride a fiat car as it approached and then left a station. Two other trumpet players were positioned on the ground one to either side, where an observer with the ability to appreciate perfect pitch listed to all the trumpets playing the same note. Following a hail-storm and other delays, the experiment finally took place. The note was higher in pitch as it departed when compared with trumpets on the ground. Aside from verifying Doppler's observations, this experiment proved that "getting started in Doppler" was difficult to understand even then.

Even with this scientific verification, Buys Ballot and others continued to level strong criticism. Those struggling to understand the Doppler principle will be interested to know that while Doppler's postulate concerning frequency shift from moving objects was ultimately shown to be correct his extrapolation about color shift of light from stars was later proven to be wrong. He incorrectly assumed that all the stars emitted white light. In reality the colors and lines of the various stars are a function of thin surface temperature rather than their direction or velocity of movement.

We are familiar with the Doppler effect in everyday life. For example an observer stationed on a highways overpass easily notices that the pitch of the sound made from the engine of a passing automobile changes from high to low as the car approaches and then passes into the distance. The engine is emitting the same sound as it passes beneath, but the observer notices a change in pitch depending upon the speed of automobile and its direction.

Doppler effect is now employed in modern astronomy. It has practical application in radar detection of storm and is

KEY POINTS

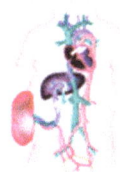

- ➡ Clinical Doppler ultrasound imaging is based on the Doppler principle and effect which was originally formulated by Austrian Mathematician and Scientist Christian Doppler in 1942.
- ➡ Doppler effect is observed in everyday life due to relative motion of sound waves between sound source and observer.

KEY POINTS

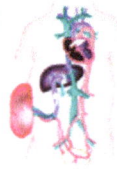

→ Doppler systems emit a short burst of ultrasound waves which are then reflected off the moving blood and then returned at transducer at a different frequency dependent on the speed and direction of moving blood. This information is displayed on color image together with gray scale image of stationary structure.

used in modern weather forecasting. It can help to form the "radar trap" used by police on modern highways to detect speeding automobiles in developed countries.

The medical applications of Doppler are dependent upon the use of ultrasound and have been in practice for sometime. Doppler systems emit a burst of very high frequency sound termed as ultrasound that is reflected off the moving red blood cells and then returned at a different frequency dependent upon the speed and direction of the moving blood. The result information is displayed as various waveforms on the velocity spectral analysis. The clinical uses of blood flow imaging systems have expanded immensely since the first measurement of flow in the heart that was performed by Satomura in 1956.

Despite its widespread use, Doppler methods and principle are difficult to understand and implement without considerable training and experience.

Chapter 2

Basic Hemodynamics

INTRODUCTION

Doppler ultrasound displays changes in sound frequency caused by moving blood. Consequently before discussing Doppler ultrasound and its application to imaging, it is necessary to describe the nature of blood flow.

Just as hydrodynamics describes the motion of fluids especially of water and interaction of fluid with its boundaries, hemodynamics is the term used to describe a collection of mechanism that influences the active and changing or dynamic circulation of blood. Circulation is of course a vital function. Blood is a mixture of plasma and cellular constituents mostly erythrocytes.

Hydrodynamic principles are applicable to blood vessels that are normally accessible to Duplex sonography (larger than 1 mm in diameter). But blood flow is influenced by many factors, which includes cardiac function, elasticity of vessels walls, vessel curvature and branching. Some of the factors can, however, be measured in reasonable simple term, but many other cannot be measured because they are difficult to quantify and generally are not well-understood.

With these limitations in mind, this chapter presents the basic principles of the dynamics of blood circulation and many factors that influence blood flow and the hemodynamics of occlusive disease. These considerations are helpful in understanding the normal physiology of blood circulation and the abnormalities that can occur in the presence of vascular obstruction.

PHYSICAL ASPECTS

Flow between two points which is the movement of a fluid in certain direction, can arise only when there is differences in energy level between these two points.

Usually, the difference in energy level is reflected by a difference in pressure, and circulatory system generally consists of a high pressure, high energy, arterial reservoir and a venous pool of low pressure and energy. These reservoirs are connected by a system of distributing vessels (smaller arteries) and by the resistance vessels of the microcirculation, which consists of arterioles, capillaries and venules.

During flow, energy is continuously lost from the blood because of the friction (viscosity) between its layers and particles. The viscosity of blood is determined mainly by its hematocrit.

Due to this internal friction both pressure and energy levels therefore decrease from arterial to the venous ends. The energy necessary for the flow is continuously restored by the pumping action of the heart which forces blood to move from the venous system into the arterial pressure and the energy difference needed for flow to occur. The high arterial energy level is result of the large volume of blood in the arterial reservoir. The function of the heart and blood vessel is normally required to maintain the volume and pressure in arteries within limit required for smooth function. This is achieved by maintaining a balance between the amount of blood that enters and leaves the arterial reservoir.

The amount that enters the arteries is the cardiac output. The amount that leaves depend upon the arterial pressure and on the total peripheral resistance, which is controlled in turn by the degree of vasoconstriction in the microcirculation.

Under normal condition, flow to all the body tissues is adjusted according to tissues particular needs at a given time.

This adjustment is accomplished by alteration in level of vasoconstriction of arterioles within the organ supplied. Maintenance of normal volume and pressure in arteries thus allows both for adjustment of blood flow to all parts of the body and for regulation of cardiac output.

Laminar Flow

In most vessels, blood moves in concentric layers or laminar hence, the flow is said to be laminar. Each infinitesimal layer flows with a different velocity (Figs. 2.1A and B).

In theory, a thin layer of blood is held stationary next to vessel wall at zero velocity because of an adhesive force between blood and the inner surface of vessel. The next layer flows with a certain velocity but its movement is delayed by the stationary layer because of friction between the layers generated by the viscous properties of the fluid. The second layer in turn delays the next layer which flows at a greater velocity. The layer in the middle of the vessel flow with highest velocity (Fig. 2.2) and the mean velocity across the vessel is half of the maximal velocity. Because rate of change of velocity is greatest near the wall and decreases towards the center of vessel, a velocity profile in the shape of a parabola exist along the vessel diameter.

Loss of energy during blood flow occurs because of friction, and the amount of friction and energy loss is determined in large part by the dimension of the vessels. In small vessels especially in the microcirculation even the layer in the middle of the lumen are relatively close to the wall and are thus delayed considerably, resulting in a significant opposition or resistance to flow.

In large vessels, by contrast a large central core of blood is far from the wall and the frictional energy loss are minimal but frictional and energy loss increases if laminar flow is disturbed.

The relation between flow volume per unit time q, viscosity η, length of vascular segment l, vessel radius r and pressure difference ($P_2 - P_1$) at proximal and distal end of tube is described by Hagen and Poiseuille's law as expressed in equation (1):

$$P_2 - P_1 = \frac{8l\eta q}{\pi r^4} \quad \ldots\ldots\ldots\ldots (1)$$

By analogy with Ohm's law

$$V = RI$$

$$R = \frac{8l\eta}{\pi r^4}$$

Where R is resistance to flow

This means even small changes in radius can result in large changes in flow.

For example a decrease in radius by one half would lead to increase in flow resistance by a factor of 16 or would lead to 95% decrease in flow.

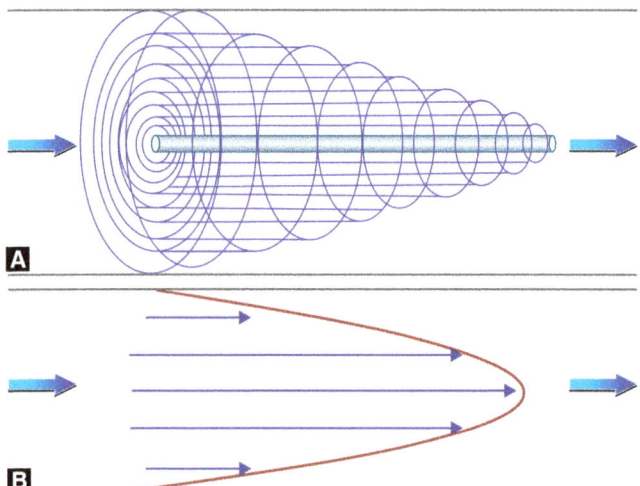

Figs. 2.1A and B: Principle of laminar flow in a vessel with a circular cross-section (A) the flow velocity within individual fluid layers (concentric cylinders) increases with distance from the vessel wall, and (B) laminar flow velocity profile in longitudinal section. The tips of the individual velocity vectors describe a parabola. Flow velocities are highest at the center of the vessel.

KEY POINTS

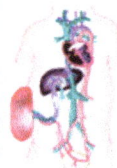

- Flow between two points in certain direction occurs only when there is difference in energy level (pressure) between these two points.
- In blood flow energy levels continuously decrease due to viscosity and this loss of energy inflow is continuously restarted by pumping action of heart.

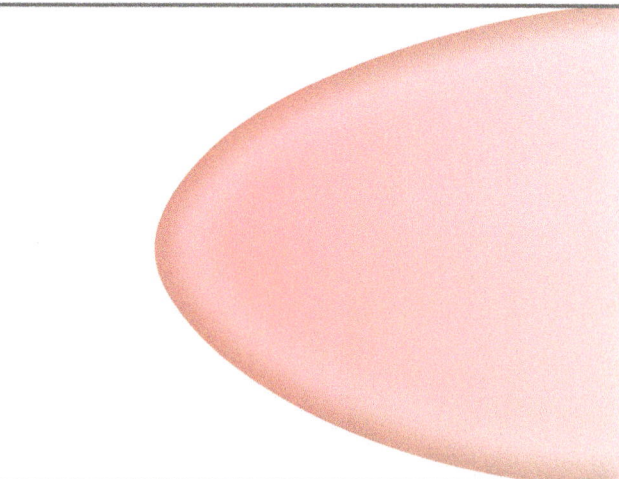

Fig. 2.2: Parabolic profile of laminar flow.

Because the length of the vessels and the viscosity of blood do not change much in the cardiovascular system, alteration in blood flow occur mainly as a result of changes in the radius of the vessels and in the difference in the pressure energy level available for flow.

Poiseuille's equation can be written as:

$$R = \frac{P_2 - P_1}{q}$$

Hence, by measuring pressure difference and blood flow (q) the resistance can thus be calculated.

The major part of the total resistance of vascular system originates from the arterioles—the part of arterial vascular tree with the largest capacity for vasomotor regulation.

Resistance can be thought of as the pressure difference needed to produce one unit of flow and can thus be considered as an index of the difficulties in forcing blood flow through vessel.

As discussed in earlier section regarding laminar flow, in color Doppler sonographic imaging, a laminar flow velocity profile is present when the lightest shades of a color are located along the center of a vessel, indicating central high velocity flow. At the same time, flow close to the vessel wall is coded in darker shades of same color representing lower flow velocity.

Poiseuille's law applicable with precision only to constant laminar flow of a simple fluid (such as water) in a rigid tube of uniform bore. In blood circulation, these conditions are not met.

Instead, the resistance is influenced by the presence of numerous interconnected vessels with a combined effect similar to that observed in electrical resistance.

In the case of vessels in series, the overall resistance is equal to the sum of the resistances of the individual vessels, whereas in the case of parallel vessels, the reciprocal of the total resistance equals the sum of the reciprocal of the individual vessel resistances.

Thus, the contribution of any single vessel to the total resistance of vascular bed or the effect of change in dimension of vessel, depend on the pressure and relative size of other vessel link in series or in parallel.

The mean flow velocity of a fluid originating from a reservoir or a vessel with a large diameter in comparison to the mean flow velocity in more distal segment with a reduced diameter will be lower than in distal segment due to the reduction in cross sectional area. This effect is based on the principle of continuity, i.e. there is no loss or gain of fluid volume (volumetric flow is independent of the vessel cross sectional area). The flow velocity profile in the initial portion of the segment is very flat (entrance effect, plug flow) except for a large velocity gradient in the boundary layer along the vessel walls, further along the distal segment the flow gradually reaches its steady-state parabolic velocity profile.

The opposite effect occurs when there is a sudden increase in the cross-section in vessel area (exist effect).

The flow velocity profile elongates as velocity gradient between the central and peripheral laminae increases. Eventually the parabolic flow velocity profile will be restored. The more drastic increase in lumen diameter, the greater the likelihood of flow separation near the vessel walls. This is characterized by localized zones of flow reversal.

This must be differentiated from turbulence. Thus type of physiological flow separation occurs for example in carotid bulb where the CCA bifurcates into the internal and external carotid arteries.

Flow separation is also commonly observed distal to a vascular stenosis especially when there is a sudden increase in the vessel diameter.

Disturbed Flow and Turbulence

Various degrees of deviation from orderly laminar flow occur in the circulation under both normal and abnormal conditions. Factors responsible for these deviations include the following:

1. The flow velocity, which changes throughout the cardiac cycle as a result of acceleration during systole and deceleration in diastole,
2. Alteration in the lines of flow, which occurs whenever a vessel changes dimension including variations in diameter associated with each pulse, and
3. The types of flow, which are distorted at curves, bifurcations and in the branches that take off at various angles.

Depending on the viscosity and density of fluid as well as the cross-sectional area of vessel lumen, the volume flow rate increases proportionally as predicted by the Poiseuille's law, when the pressure difference along the vascular segment increases. If the cross-sectional area of lumen remains constant, for example, the flow rate must increase. If the flow velocity is increased beyond a certain value, the initial laminar flow is destabilized. At first the fluid laminae are no longer continually directed parallel to vessel walls. Wave-like irregularities develop in the laminae creating a pattern known as "disturbed flow." As the flow velocity continues to increase, vortices may form near the vessel walls. Since the Doppler angles related to individual fluid, particles are no longer identical, an inhomogeneous distribution of different shades of color appear in CDS image across the vessel lumen. Same pixel may undergo a complete flips, even in disturbed flow, depending on the angle between the total vectors (vector sum of all the flow vectors) and the direction of the ultrasound beam. This will only occur if the angle between the total flow vector and ultrasound beam is closer to 90°.

When the flow velocity exceeds a critical value, the entire lumen is filled with fluid components where individual velocity vectors are randomly aimed in all the directions. This chaotic, flow pattern is the result of turbulence. Total velocity vector, however still points in the main flow direction. The flow velocity profile in a region with turbulent flow is very flat, resulting in a large velocity gradient near the vessel walls. Turbulent flow can be recognized in CDS by a mixture of different color pixels next to one another represents flow in different directions.

The existence of turbulent flow depend on the vessel diameter $d = 2r$ (r = radius) the average flow velocity v, across the lumen, the density of the fluid and viscosity of the fluid. The factor that affect the development of turbulence is expressed by the dimensionless Reynolds number (Re)

$$Re = \frac{qv2r}{\eta}$$

The Reynolds number is dimensionless. Because density and viscosity (η) of blood are relatively constant, the development of turbulence depends mainly on the size of the vessels and on the velocity of flow. In a tube model, laminar flow tends to be disturbed if Reynolds number exceeds 2000. However, in the circulatory system, disturbances and various degrees of turbulences are likely to occur at lower values because of body movements, pulsatile nature of blood flow, changes in vessel dimensions, roughness of the endothelial surface and other factors.

Turbulence develops more readily in large vessels under conditions of high flow and can be detected clinically by the findings of brutes or thrills. Bruits sometimes may be heard over the ascending aorta during systolic acceleration in normal individuals at rest and are frequently heard in state of high cardiac output and blood flow, even in more distal, such as femoral artery. Distortion of laminar flow velocity profile can be assessed using ultrasound flow detectors, and such assessments can be applied for diagnostic purpose. For example, in arteries with severe stenosis, pronounced turbulence is a diagnostic feature observed in post-stenotic zone. Turbulence occurs because a jet of blood with high velocity and high kinetic energy suddenly encounters a normal diameter lumen or lumen of increased diameter (because of post-stenotic dilatation) where both the velocity and energy level are lower than in stenotic zone.

During turbulent flow, the loss of pressure energy between two parts in a vessel is greater than that which would be expected from the factors in Poiseuille's equation and parabolic flow velocity profile is flattened.

Pulsatile Flow

Compared with continuous flow, the analysis of discontinuous pulsatile flow is considerably more complex.

With each heart beat, travel stroke volume of blood is injected into the arterial system, resulting in a pressure wave that travels throughout the arterial tree. The speed of propagation amplitude and slope of pressure wave change as it traverses the arterial system. These boundary conditions give rise to two basic Doppler system: (i) Low resistance and (ii) High resistance.

Pressure Change from Cardiac Activity

The pumping action of heart maintains a high volume of blood in the arterial end of the circulation as large pressure amplitude developed in the left ventricle during each cardiac cycle, the aorta and large vessel reduce the pressure amplitude that is transmitted to the arterial tree.

Because of the intermittent pumping action of the heart, the pressure and flow vary in a pulsatile manner.

During the rapid phase of ventricular ejection the volume of blood at the arterial end increases, raising the pressure to systolic peak. During the latter part of systole, when cardiac ejection decreases, the outflow through the peripheral resistance vessel exceeds the volume being ejected by the heart and pressure begins to decline. This decline continues to flow from the arterioles into the microcirculation. Part of the work of heart leads directly to forward flow, but a large portion of energy of each cardiac contraction results in distention of the arteries that serve as reservoir for storing the blood volume and energy supplied to the system. The storage of energy and blood volume provides for continuous flow to the tissue during diastole.

Arterial Pressure Wave

The pulsatile variation in blood volume and energy occurring with each cardiac cycle are manifested as a

---

KEY POINTS

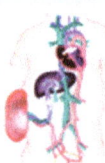

- Normal flow can be characterized as parabolic flow, however, due to presence of stenosis or drastic increase in diameter of lumen of vessel, flow profile may be disturbed or may be called as turbulent flow.
- Localized zones of flow reversal may also occur in normal flow near the bifurcation of arteries. Such flow separation occurs, for example, in carotid bulb where CCA bifurcate into internal and external carotid arteries. This normal flow must be differentiated from turbulence.

pressure wave that can be detected throughout the arterial system. The amplitude and shape of arterial pressure wave depend on a complex interplay of factors, which include the stroke volume and time course of ventricular ejection, the peripheral resistance, and the stiffness of the arterial walls. In general, an increase in any of these factors results in an increase in the pulse amplitude (i.e. pulse pressure, difference between systolic and diastolic pressures) and frequently in a concomitant increase in systolic pressure. For example, increased stiffness of the arteries with age tends to increase both the systolic and pulse pressures (Figs. 2.3A to C).

The arterial pressure wave is propagated along the arterial tree distally from the heart. The speed of propagation, or pulse wave velocity, increases with stiffness of arterial walls and with the ratio of the wall thickness and diameter.

In mammalian circulation, arteries become progressively stiffer from the aorta towards the periphery. Therefore, the special propagation of the wave increases as it moves peripherally. Also, the gradual increase in stiffness tend, to decrease wave reflection and has a beneficial effect in that the pulse and systolic pressure in the aorta and proximal arteries are relatively lower than in peripheral vessels.

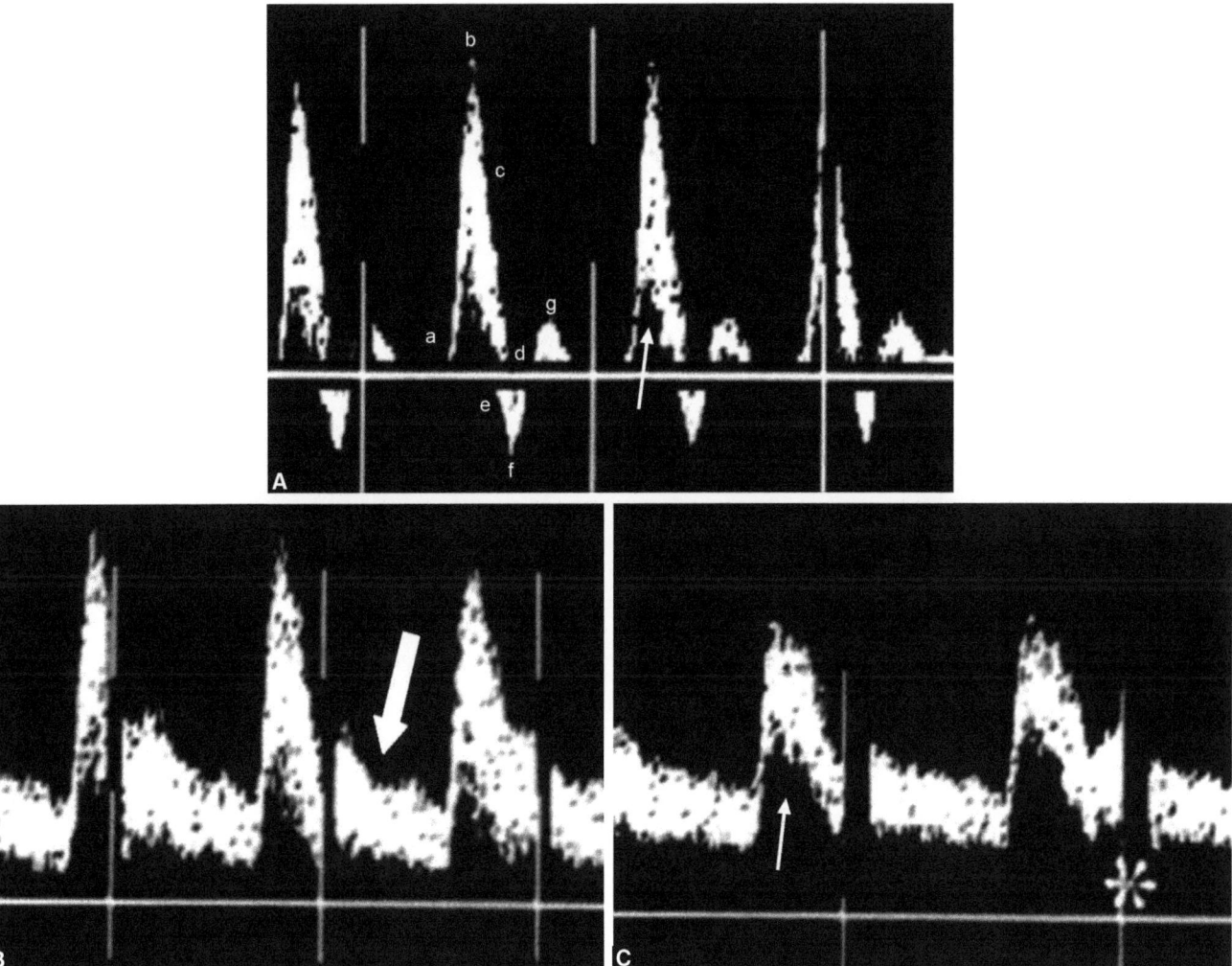

Figs. 2.3A to C: Influence of the peripheral flow resistance on Doppler spectra recorded from the brachial artery (A, B) and internal carotid artery (C) in a healthy subject. (A) Triphasic spectrum at rest. High peripheral vascular flow resistance (peripheral artery pattern) with a sharp systolic velocity increase (a-b), a rapid drop in velocity in late systole (c-d), diastolic flow reversal (e-f), and late diastolic forward flow (g). Note the spectral window below the systolic peak (white arrow), (B) after exercise, a pronounced forward-flow component appears in diastole (white arrow) due to the decrease in peripheral flow resistance. The spectral pattern is intermediate between A and C, and (C) low peripheral vascular flow resistance. The spectrum displays a high diastolic forward flow and less pulsatility than in A and B (parenchymal artery pattern). The empty systolic window (arrow) indicates undisturbed flow. Periodic refreshing of the colour Duplex image creates a brief, intermittent void in the spectral waveform (*).

The pressure against which the heart ejects the stroke volume associated cardiac walls are accordingly reduced.

Pulsatile Flow Pattern

Pulsatile changes in pressure are associated with corresponding acceleration of blood flow with systole and deceleration in diastole. Although energy stored in the arterial walls maintains a positive arteriovenous pressure gradient and overall forward flow in the microcirculation during systole, temporary cessation of forward flow or even diastolic reversal occurs frequently in position of human arterial system.

So in principle, pulsatile flow is laminar. However, the flow velocity profile of pulsatile blood flow is subjected to extensive changes during the cardiac study as discussed earlier.

The reason for this is that blood flow is opposing a resistance based on inertial forces which dump quick pulsatile change of motion. The flow velocity profile is flat during acceleration phase and approximates a parabolic shape only as long as same forward flow persists after the acceleration phase ends. If transient flow reversal occurs, it begins near the vessel wall where the lowest flow velocity prevails during antegrade flow and propagates towards the center of the vessel.

The flow is particularly unstable during this phase, and turbulence can develop even at very low Reynolds number.

Effect of Arterial Obstruction

As in continuous flow, the changes from laminar to turbulent flow are marked by transitional phenomena referred to as "disturbed flow". Unlike continuous flow, the Reynolds number in pulsatile flow varies over the cardiac cycle due to changes in flow velocity and vessel diameter.

Even in each physiologic condition, this can give rise to periodic turbulence during certain parts of the cardiac cycle. The development of turbulence in pulsatile flow is also influenced by the shape of the flow velocity profile and the heart rate.

Hemodynamics at Stenosis

Arterial obstruction can result in reduced pressure and flow distal to the site of blockage, but the effect on pressure and flow is greatly influenced by a number of factors proximal and especially distal to the lesion.

Encroachment on lumen of an artery by arteriosclerotic plaque can result in diminished pressure and flow distal to the lesion but this encroachment on the lumen has to be relatively little resistance to flow compared with the resistance vessels with which they are in series.

A basic understanding of flow dynamic is essential for the correct interpretation of most phenomena encountered in Doppler studies of arterial system—prestenotic, interstenotic, and poststenotic changes in absolute and relative flow velocities and flow pattern are the variables that lead to a correct diagnosis and permit a quantitative assessment of pathologic finding regardless of Doppler technology used.

Principle of Continuity in Assessing the Severity of Stenosis

Volume flow (flow rate/time) in a particular vessel remains constant in any given segment of the vessel except at sites where part of the flow volume is directed from the original channel at an arterial branching of the vessel.

Volume flow q is expressed by:
$$q = A \times v$$
Where, q = Volume flow/time
A = Cross-sectional area of vessel
v = Average flow velocity in a given cross-section of the vessel.

If the vessel has a circular cross-section the above equation changes to
$$\pi r^2 v$$
Where r = vessel radius

The principle of continuity is expressed (Fig. 2.4) by:
$$q_1 = q_2$$
$$q = A_1 v_1 = A_2 v_2$$
$$\frac{A_1}{A_2} = \frac{v_2}{v_1}$$

or

Where, $q_{1,2}$ = Volume flow/time at position 1 and 2
$A_{1,2}$ = Cross-sectional area of vessel with a position 1 and 2

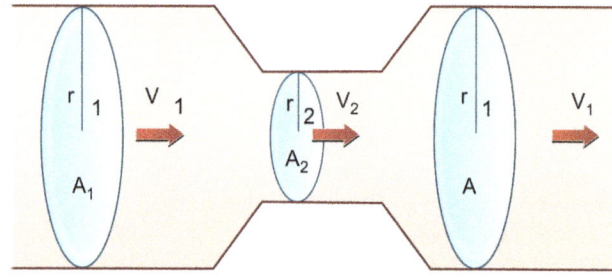

Volume flow = constant

Fig. 2.4: The principle of continuity. The flow velocity v_{1-2} changes according to the variations in the cross-sectional area A_{1-2} of the vessel. The flow volume in the vessel remains constant at all positions. Thus, the increase in flow velocity can be used in determining the reduction in luminal cross-section area and calculating the degree of stenosis (see text).

$v_{1,2}$ = Average flow velocity in a given cross-section of the vessel at position 1 and 2

A reduction in the lumen diameter necessarily leads to an increase in the flow velocity.

For example, 50% reduction in diameter corresponding to 75% reduction in area leads to an increase in flow velocity by a factor of 4. Based on the relative increase in flow velocity the degree of stenosis can be calculated as far as the continuity equation is valid.

$$X = 100\left(1 - \frac{(100)}{Y}\right)$$

Where, X = Degree of stenosis in %
Y = Relative velocity increase in %

or

$$X = 100\left(1 - \frac{v_1}{v_2}\right)$$

Where, v_1 is prestenotic velocity
v_2 Intrastenotic velocity.

Thus, detection and determination of the severity of vascular stenosis with Doppler ultrasound are based on recording the relative velocity increase or Doppler frequency shift that is produced by the stenosis. Very severe flow rate—limit lesion can also reduce intrastenotic flow velocity to such a degree that the absolute interstenotic flow velocity is less than that associated with a moderate, non-flow reducing stenosis.

As the degree of stenosis increases, the velocity measured by Doppler frequency analysis is lower than theoretically predicted as a consequence of intrastenotic energy losses due to friction that was neglected in the above equation.

During hemodynamic evaluation of severity of stenosis by Duplex sonography it is presumed that vascular segment of interest can be visualized in longitudinal section. The scan-plane must pass precisely through the center of prestenotic and intrastenotic areas to ensure that maximum flow velocities are obtained for use in the calculation. Prominent vascular calcification, entering gas or bone and obesity are physical obstacle that can prevent direct visualization of the stenotic area. In these cases Duplex ultrasound permits only an approximate indirect assessment of the severity of the vascular obstruction.

In vessels that do not show significant branching in the area near the stenosis, flow velocities should be measured at the interstenotic and immediate prestenotic levels for quantifying a stenosis.

Although continuity equation is still valid, the relative distribution of volume flow is unpredictable if the stenosis is located at a bifurcation or an arterial branching. The degree of stenosis can be determined from velocity measurements only by measuring both intrastenotic flow velocity and the flow velocity at a more distal site in a segment having normal lumen size, well away from stenotic jet or turbulence. Alternatively, the degree of proximal stenosis of internal carotid artery can be estimated from empirically derived ratios of the maximum systolic velocities at the prestenotic and intrastenotic levels.

There are two basic methods in Duplex sonography for determining the severity of stenosis on the basis of flow velocity (Figs. 2.5A to C).
1. By Doppler spectrum analysis
2. By evaluation of the color encoded flow velocities in CDS.

As a basic rule, the maximum flow velocity in a given vascular segment should be measured at the time of maximum systolic forward flow. The maximum flow velocity can be derived from Doppler spectrum or determined by using a special color in the color Duplex image to tag the highest flow velocities. The use of maximum systolic velocities permit the most accurate assessment of the degree of stenosis. If the time averaged velocities are used, the severity of the lesion will be underestimated due to

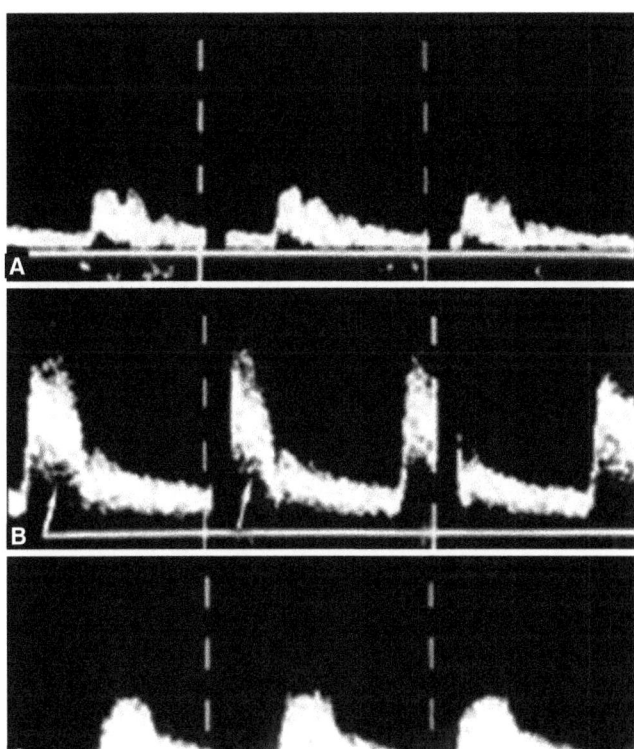

Figs. 2.5A to C: (A) Prestenotic spectrum from common carotid artery; (B) Intrastenotic spectrum shows a mark elevation of flow velocity; (C) Poststenotic spectrum shows filling in the systolic window.

entrance effects and changes in the flow velocity profile during pulse cycle.

It must be pointed out that it is absolutely mandatory to perform a Doppler angle correction when flow velocities are calculated from Doppler frequency shift. It is only possible to use the Doppler frequency shift in calculating the degree of stenosis if crossover angle between the longitudinal vessel axis and the individual ultrasound beam are same in both positions.

Interstenotic and Poststenotic Flow Changes

Due to increased flow velocity, the interstenotic Reynolds number can rise tremendously only in the case of severe lesion. This may lead to disturbed flow or even turbulent flow within stenosis (Fig. 2.6). Distal to stenosis, the maximum flow velocity continues to be elevated (Poststenotic jet) at least in certain zones of the vascular cross-section with exit effects playing a significant roles. Zone of retrograde inherently laminar flow can develop near the vessel wall distal to a stenosis (flow separation and flow reversal (Figs. 2.7A to E). These stationary Eddy current close to the vessel walls may propagate distally depending on the flow velocity and degree of stenosis.

The poststenotic Reynolds number may far exceed the intrastenotic Reynolds number as the flow enters the poststenotic lumen at elevated velocities. This may cause marked turbulence to develop in the poststenotic segments in addition to zones of flow reversal along the vessel walls. This may extend distally for a distance several times the normal vessel diameter. Besides the pressure drop across the stenosis, turbulence is partially responsible for the energy loss resulting in a volume flow reduction associated with severe stenosis.

Turbulence and flow reversal are easily recognized in color Duplex imaging using Doppler frequency analysis. Turbulent flow produces broadening of the Doppler spectrum that may completely fill in the systolic window beneath the spectrum envelope and simultaneous occurrence of positive and negative Doppler frequency shifts.

The location and extent of local flow reversal and turbulence depend in a complex way on the geometry of the stenosis, the degree of stenosis, the surface structure of vessel walls, the prestenotic flow velocity, the viscosity of the blood and pulsatility of the flow. There are no general rules for determining the severity of stenosis from the length and extent of flow reversal and turbulence.

The main value of a color coded presentation of these phenomena is that it permits the identification of a vascular stenosis when the lesion itself is obscured by vessel wall calcification or calcified plaque.

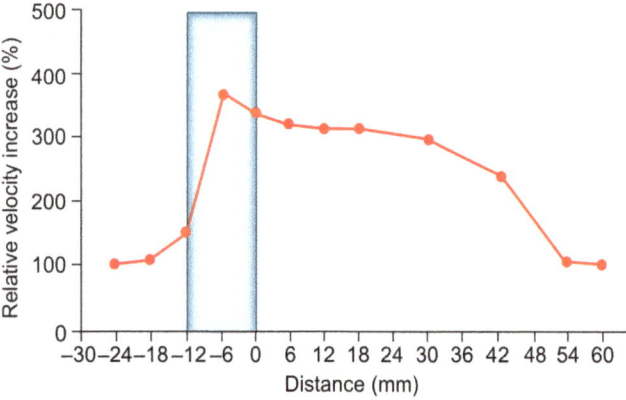

Fig. 2.6: Measurement of the flow velocities across a stenosis causing a 75% concentric area reduction (= 50% diameter reduction) in a vascular phantom. Luminal diameter is 6 mm proximal and distal to the stenosis. Length of the stenosis is 12 mm proximal and distal to the stenosis. Length of the stenosis is 12 mm. The shaded box indicates the vicinity of the stenosis (–12 to 0 mm). The Doppler sample volume was positioned mid-stream, and the velocities were calculated from the Doppler spectrum (maximum systolic velocity). The graph shows a typical progression of velocity changes across the stenosis (relative to the prestenotic value). The relative velocity increase does not quite reach the theoretically predicted value of 400% due to frictional losses. The poststenotic jet extends several centimeters distally past the stenosed segment.

VENOUS HEMODYNAMICS

The pressure remains in the vein, after the blood has reversed the arterioles and capillaries, is low when the subject is in the supine because their large diameters, medium and large veins, offer little resistance to flow and blood more readily flow from the small veins to right atrium where the pressure is close to atmospheric pressure.

Flow and pressure changes during the cardiac cycle. Figure 2.8 shows changes in the pressure and flow in large veins such as the vena cava that occurs during the phases of cardiac cycle. Such oscillations in pressure and flow at times may be transmitted to more peripheral vessels.

There are three positive pressure waves (Fig. 2.8). These can be distinguished in central nervous venous pressure and reflect corresponding changes in pressure in atria.

KEY POINTS

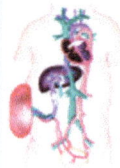

- Turbulence and flow reversal can be easily recognized in color Duplex imaging using Doppler frequency analysis.
- Turbulent flow produces spectral broadening and spectral window is completely filled with simultaneous occurrence of positive and negative Doppler frequency shift.

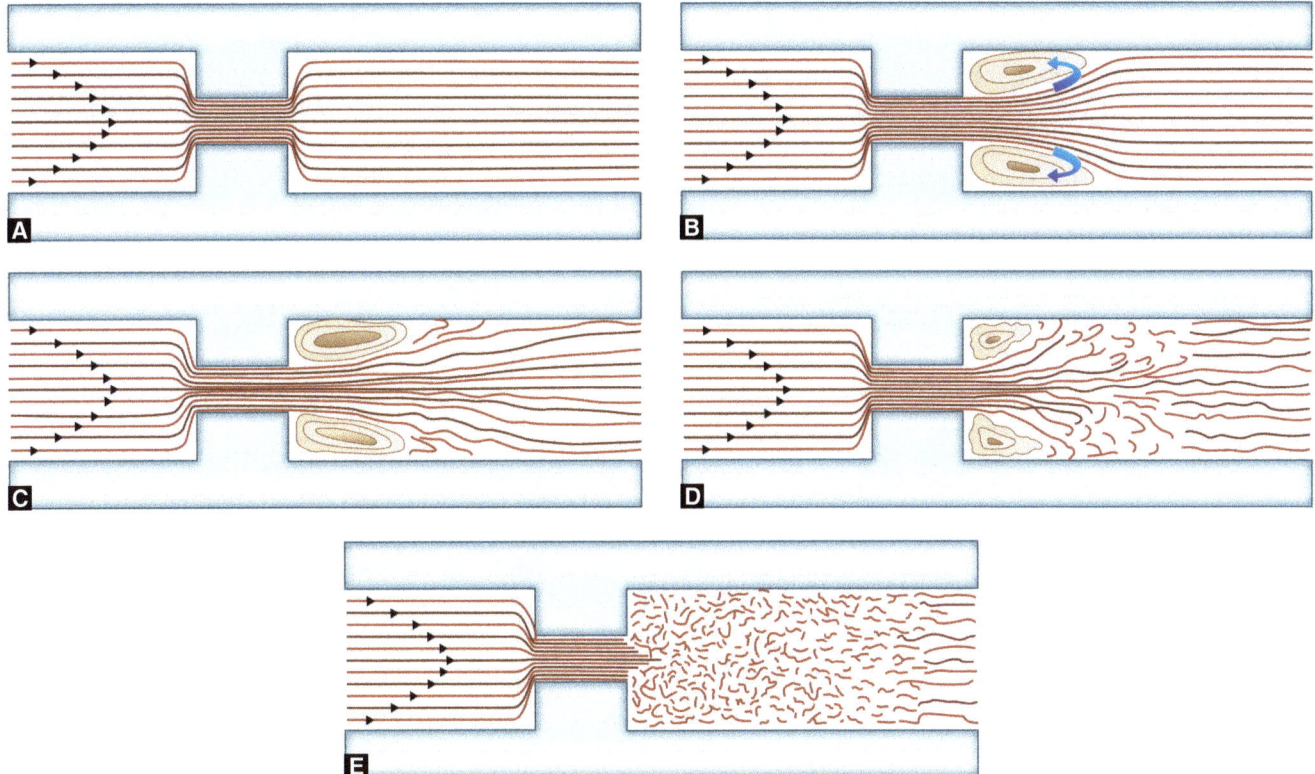

Figs. 2.7A to E: Schematic representation of poststenotic flow changes as a function of physical boundary conditions. The prestenotic flow velocity increases from A to E while the degree of stenosis remains constant. In principle, the progression of changes from A to E is characteristic of all factors that would produce an increase in the Reynolds number, (A) low prestenotic flow velocity. There are no poststenotic flow disturbances, (B) with a slight increase in prestenotic flow velocity, zones of flow reversal (curved arrows) develop near the vessel walls, but the flow remains generally laminar, and there is no turbulence, (C) when the prestenotic flow velocity is increased further, wave-like irregularities develop in the laminae (disturbed flow) in addition to flow reversal, (D) at a high prestenotic flow velocity, turbulence develops distal to the stenosis from the zones of flow reversal. Flow is still disturbed at some distance from the stenosis, and (E) a very high prestenotic flow velocity is associated with severe poststenotic turbulence.

One wave 'a' is caused by atrial contraction and relaxation. The upstroke of 'c' wave is related to the increase in pressure when the atrioventricular values are closed and bulge during isovolumetric ventricular contraction. The subsequent down stroke results from the fall in pressure caused by pulling the atrioventricular valve rings towards the apex of heart during ventricular contraction. The upstroke of 'v' wave results from a passive rise in atrial pressure during ventricular systole when the atrioventricular valve are closed and atria fill with blood from the peripheral veins. The 'v' wave downstroke is caused by fall in pressure that occurs where the blood leaves the atria rapidly and fills the ventricles soon after the opening of atrioventricular valve early in ventricular diastole.

In abnormal condition such as congestive heart failure or tricuspid insufficiency venous pressure is increased. This elevation of venous pressure may lead to the transmission and cardiac phase changes in pressure and flow to the

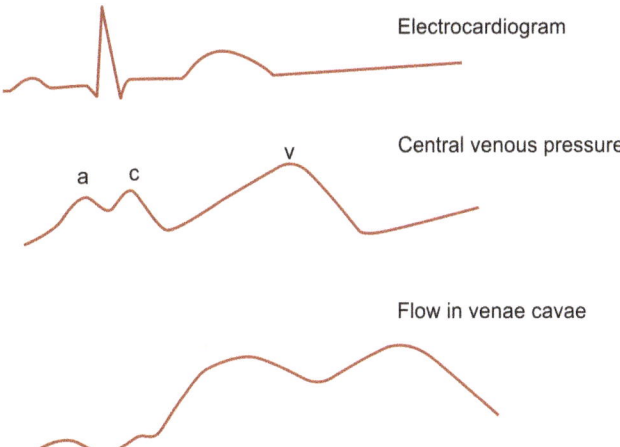

Fig. 2.8: Schematic representation of normal changes in pressure and flow in the central veins associated with the cardiac cycle. a = a wave; c = c wave; v = v wave.

peripheral vein of the upper and lower limb. Such phasic changes may occasionally be found in healthy well-hydrated individuals probably because a large blood volume distends the venous system.

Venous Effect of Respiration

Respiration has profound effect as venous pressure and flow during inspiration, the volume in the veins of thorax increases and the pressure decreases in response to reduced intrathoracic pressure. Expiration leads to the opposite effect, with decreased venous volume and increased pressure. The venous response to respiration is reversed in the abdomen where the pressure increases during inspiration because of the descent of diaphragm and decreases during expiration as the diaphragm ascends. Increased abdominal pressure during inspiration decreases pressure gradient between peripheral veins in the lower extremities and the abdomen thus reducing flow in the peripheral vessels.

During expiration, when extra-abdominal pressure is reduced, the pressure gradient from lower limb to abdomen is increased and flow in the peripheral veins rises correspondingly.

In the veins of the upper limbs, the changes in flow with respiration are opposite to those in the lower extremities because of reduced intrathoracic pressure inspiration. The pressure gradient from the veins of upper limb to right atrium increases when flow increases. During expiration flow decreases because of the resulting increase in intrathoracic pressure and the corresponding rise in the right atrial pressure. The respiratory changes in flow in upper limb may be influenced by changes in pressure. With the upper part of the body elevated venous flow tends to step at the height of inspiration and resumes with expiration, probably because of the compression of subclavian vein at the level of the first ribs during contraction of accessory muscles of respiration.

Venous Obstruction

Venous obstruction can be acute or chronic. In the case of severe chronic obstruction, edema may occur.

Acute obstruction, usually associated with thrombosis may lead to potentially fatal pulmonary embolism.

Doppler flow detection and Duplex scanner may be used for this purpose.

The presence or absence of obstruction is also gauged by increasing flow towards the examination in site by squeezing the limb distally or by activating the distal muscle group and thus increasing venous flow towards the flow detecting probe.

Absence of increased flow sound attenuation and increased flow is associated with obstruction between the probe location and the site from which the enhancement of venous flow is attempted.

When volumes are competent, flow in peripheral veins, is towards the heart.

When there are incompetent veins proximally, there may be retrograde filling in the peripheral veins such as these in ankle region from the more proximal veins in addition to normal filling from capillary beds.

The presence or absence of the retrograde flow may be detected by listening with a Doppler flow detector and squeezes the limb proximally.

Doppler Principle and Instrumentation

INTRODUCTION

Ultrasound imaging is especially useful in cardiovascular system because of its ability to produce images of cardiac anatomy and flowing blood through many points of vascular system. Approaches to the identification of the moving structure include relative pulse echo imaging, motion mode (M mode) display of reflected ultrasound pulse, and the Doppler's shift method.

The Doppler method has a number of applications in clinical medicine, including detection of fetal heartbeat, detection of air embolism, blood pressure monitoring, detection and characterization of blood flow, and localization of blood vessel occlusion.

Over 30 years, ultrasound scanner was exploited the Dopplers effect detection in above mentioned areas. The first measurement of flow in heart was performed by Satumora in 1956, currently available techniques include continuous wave Doppler, pulse wave Doppler, color flow imaging, and newest color amplitude imaging (power Doppler).

DOPPLER EFFECT

When there is relative motion between a source and a detector of ultrasound, the frequency of the detected ultrasound differs from that emitted by the source.

If the source and detector are moving away from each other, the frequency measured by the observer will be lower than the frequency detected by stationary observer. If they are moving towards each other, the frequency will be higher.

In daily life, everyone has probably noticed the Doppler shift effects (Fig. 3.1). The sound coming from the siren of a police car moving towards an observer is at higher pitch

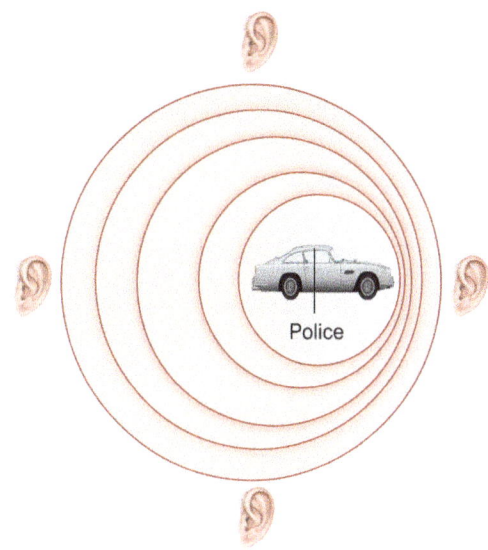

Fig. 3.1: Due to the movement of the source and the observer relative to one another, the frequency of the observed and transmitted signals differ.

than the sound measured by another observer when the police car is moving away from him. When the car is passing an observer, a sudden jump in the sound frequency can be clearly heard. Exactly same thing would be noticed in the opposite case, when an observer is moving towards a stationary sound source, passes it and then moves away from source. If the emitter and observer are moving towards one another, the perceived wavelength is shortened, resulting in the perception of a higher frequency. If the emitter and observer are moving away from one another, the perceived wavelength is longer than in stationary case, resulting in perception of a lower frequency.

The shift in frequency is illustrated in Figure 3.2. In Figure 3.2A, an ultrasound is moving with velocity vs, towards the detector. After some time following production of one particular wave front, the distance between the wave front and the source is $(C - v_s)/t$ where C is velocity of sound in the medium. The wavelength (λ) of the ultrasound in the direction of motion is shortened to:

$$\lambda = \frac{C - v_s}{f_o}$$

Where f_o is frequency of ultrasound from the source.

$$f_B = \frac{C}{\lambda} = \left(\frac{C}{C - v_s/f_o}\right)$$

f_B – frequency observed

$$f_B = f_o \left(\frac{C}{C - v_s}\right)$$

The shift in frequency f_D is then

$$f_D = f_B - f_o = f_o \left(\frac{v_s}{C - v_s}\right)$$

If the emitter and observer are moving away from each other this results in perception of lower frequency. In general,

$$f_B = f_o \frac{C + V_{observer}}{C - V_{source}}$$

f_B = Observed frequency
f_o = True frequency
C = Speed of sound
V_{obes} = Velocity of observer
v_s = Velocity of source

If the source and detector are at the same location and ultrasound is reflected from an object moving towards the location with a velocity V_{source} the object acts first as a moving receiver as it receives the ultrasound signal and then acts as a moving source as it reflects the signal. As a result, the ultrasound signal received by receiver exhibits a frequency shift.

$$F_D = 2f_o \frac{v}{c}$$

This is because

$$f_B = f_o \left(\frac{c + v}{c - v}\right)$$

$$f_B = f_o \left(1 + \frac{2v}{c}\right)$$

when v < c
using Taylor series ignoring the higher form

$$f_B - f_o = f_D = 2f_o \frac{v}{c}$$

hence

If an object is moving towards the source, shift in frequency is positive

i.e.

$$f_D = 2f_o \frac{v}{c}$$

If object is moving away from source and detector, the

$$f_D = -df_o \frac{v}{c}$$

or Doppler shift is negative.

Negative sign indicates that frequency of detected ultrasound is lower than that emitted by the source.

The above discussion assumes that ultrasound beam is parallel to the motion of an object. If the source and observer are not moving directly away from or towards each other but an angle θ the equation becomes,

$$f_D = 2f_o \frac{v \cos \theta}{c}$$

This technique is used to study motion, primarily that of circulatory system. Since RBCs are not continuous and act as rough surface and therefore, act as a scatter of US beam.

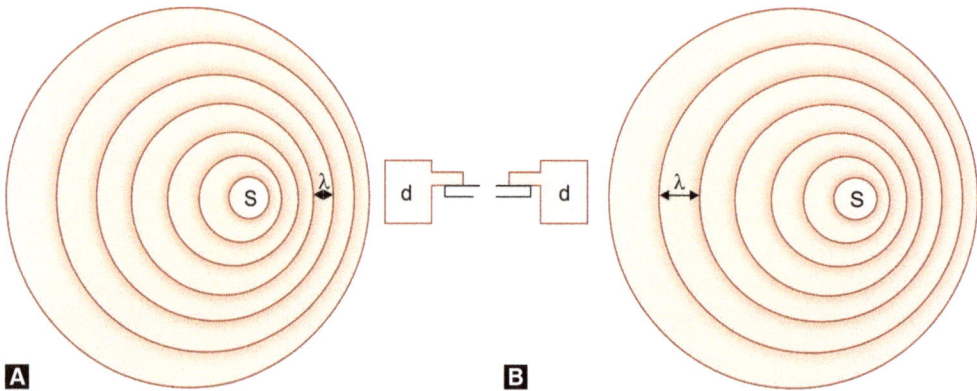

Figs. 3.2A and B: (A) Source moving towards a stationary detector; (B) Source moving away from a stationary detector.

This scattering is known as Rayleigh Tyndall scattering and caused by RBCs in blood.

The RBCs are particulate components of blood that interact with the ultrasound (Platelets are small in size and WBCs are very few in number).

A typical arrangement is illustrated in Figures 3.3A and B. An ultrasound transducer is placed in contact with the skin surface. It transmits a beam where frequency is f_o. The receiver frequency f_r will differ from f_o when echoes are picked up from moving scatter such as RBCs. The Doppler frequency f_D is defined as the difference between received and transmitted frequency and is given by:

$$F_D = f_r - f_o = \frac{2f_o n \cos\theta}{c}$$

where θ is called Doppler angle. This angle strangely influences Doppler shift for a given reflector velocity.

The reference frequency used is for clarity, always transducer central frequency, although this is by no means necessary. In most diagnostic ultrasound systems, a reference frequency about 25% lower than the central frequency is used in order to improve the penetration and the velocity range.

A factor of 2" occurs in the equation in the numerator because the sound must make two trips. One trip goes from transducer to receiver in motion (erythrocytes act as receiver) and ultrasound wave from transducer will be perceived as Doppler shifted. Second trip from moving reflector (erythrocytes will act as a transmitter in motion relative to stationary receiver transducer). Solving the equation for v results in

$$v = \frac{f_D c}{2f_o \cos\theta}$$

The actual determination of Doppler angle may be very difficult. However, when interpreting the measured shift it must never be forgotten that the effect is angle and reference frequency dependent. Only by measuring the Doppler angle, the reference frequency and Doppler shift, can the blood flow velocity be calculated.

Theoretically, no Doppler shift occur when probe is exactly perpendicular to the direction of motion, this is because θ = 90° and cos 90° = 0. In practice small Doppler shift may be detected when probe appears to be perpendicular to the direction of flow in vessel because some portion of beam is not perpendicular to the motion as a result of divergence of ultrasound beam.

When flow is directed toward the transducer θ = 0 and hence cos θ = 1. Hence, Doppler frequency detected for the orientation would be maximum.

As mentioned earlier absolute measurement of reflector velocity require that Doppler angle is accurately determined.

Uncertainty in the measurement of Doppler angle particularly at large angles, introduces error in velocity computation. A 5° error for 70° Doppler angle causes the velocity estimation to deviate by 25%. A decrease in the Doppler angle to 40° reduces this deviation to 8% for same uncertainty of 5° in the angle measurement.

As a general guideline, Doppler signals from superficial blood vessels (e.g. carotids) should be acquired at angle between 30° and 60° whenever possible.

The lower angular limit is recommended because total internal reflection occurs at the vessel wall-blood boundary for small angles and sound beam does not reach the moving blood. The accurate measurement of Doppler angle is difficult for tortuous vessels that radically change direction. Some Doppler instrument allow the operation to specify the direction of flow on an image and then instrument automatically calculate the Doppler angle.

Determining the volumetric flow of blood in the units of cubic centimeter per second requires an estimation of the

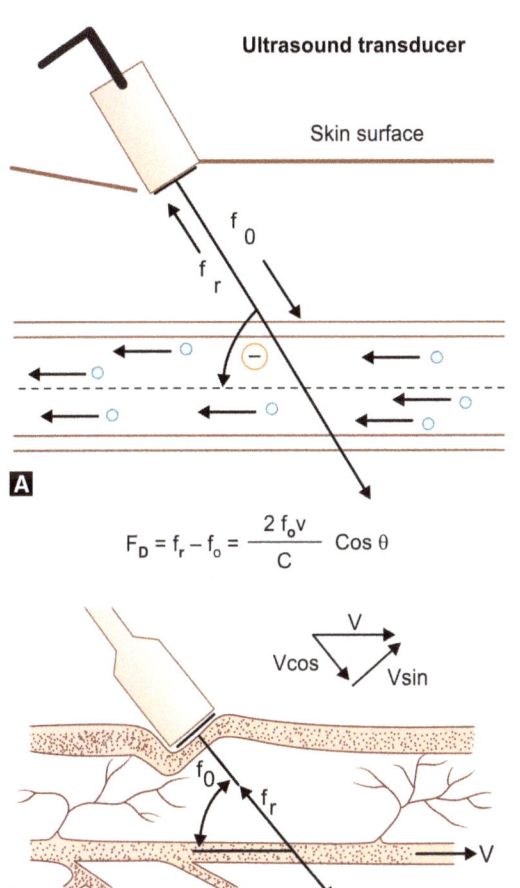

Figs. 3.3A and B: Arrangement for detecting Doppler signals from blood. The angle θ is the Doppler angle, which is the angle between the direction of motion and the beam axis, looking toward the transducer.

KEY POINTS

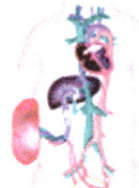

→ Doppler shift equation used in clinical imaging in

$$f_D = \frac{2f_o V \cos Q}{C}$$

Where f_o is frequency of sound source
V – Velocity of moving reflector
Q – Doppler angle
C – Velocity of sound source
f_D – Frequency of Doppler shift (in audible range)

→ As a general guideline Doppler signals from superficial blood vessels should be acquired at an angle between 30° and 60° whenever possible.

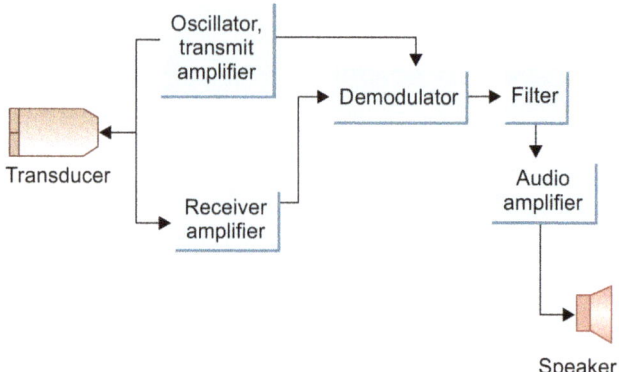

Fig. 3.4: Block diagram of CW Doppler instrument.

area of vessel as well as doppler angle. Volumetric flow Q is the product of average velocity v and cross section area of A of vessel

$$Q = vA$$

In clinical measurement of volumetric flow, several source of error reduces the accuracy below which what would be expected is based upon intrinsic precision of doppler shift measurements. The measurement of vessel area is typically based upon the measurement of vessel diameter in the image.

However, the angle at which the image plane cut through the vessel may cause either underestimation or overestimation of diameter. Also, the doppler unit may not sample the average velocity in a vessel. Flow in a vessel is not same throughout. It is usually greatest at the center and decreases to zero at the vessel wall. Complex flow profiles are possible, particularly if a stenosis, bifurcation or plaque formation is present. An accurate estimation of average velocity requires sampling of velocity at different radii within the vessel point across the stream. It is possible to make some simplifying assumption. For example, in laminar flow the average velocity is half the maximum value.

INSTRUMENTATION

The most basic Doppler system through which first Doppler blood velocity measurements were performed is continuous wave Doppler system. Continuous wave (CW) Doppler operation is used in a variety of instruments, ranging from simple, inexpensive hand-held Doppler unit to "high end" Duplex scanner in CW Doppler may be one of the several operating modes.

A simplified block diagram of the necessary component of CW Doppler system is presented in Figure 3.4.

Such a system requires a separate transmitter and receiver. For example, one can use two piezoelectric transducers mounted in same enclosure depicted in Figure 3.4. The transmitted sound wave and receiving pattern of receiver are very directional. To obtain maximum sensitivity for detecting returning echo signals the beam regions of the transmitter and receiver are caused to overlap. This overlap is achieved by inclining the transducer elements. The region of beam overlap defines the most sensitive region of the transducer. The transmitter continuously excites the ultrasonic transducer with a sinusoidal electric signal of frequency f_o producing incident ultrasound beam echo returning to the transducer have frequency f_r. These signals are amplified in the receiver and then sent to a demodulator to extract the Doppler signal. Here the signals are multiplied by reference signal from the transmitting, producing a mixture of signals, part having a frequency $(f_r + f_o)$ and part having a frequency $(f_r - f_o)$. The sum frequency $(f_r + f_o)$ is very high, twice the ultrasound frequency and easily removed by electronic filtering. This leaves signals with frequency $(f_r - f_o)$ at the output, which is the Doppler signal. It is possible to eliminate signal of certain frequency ranges that might be due to respiratory motion of the liver or another organ or due to pulsating, vessel wall. This is done in the instruments that have additional electronic filters in their circuitry. For example—by applying high pass filter.

The lower cut-off frequency of such wall filter is usually operator selectable.

Doppler frequency for blood flow lies within the audible range which is generally the case for most Doppler signals results from blood flow by using Doppler shift equation. This is because speed of interface for biological system are relatively small (0.5–200 cm/sec) compared with velocity of sound in tissue.

Basic CW Doppler units usually have only a few controls, but operators should be familiar with these on their own equipment.

Transmit power to vary the amplitude of signal from the transmitter to transducer thus changing the sensitivity to weak echoes, some simple units omit this control, keeping the transmit level constant.

Directional Doppler

A basic CW Doppler instrument allows detection of magnitude of Doppler frequency, but it provide, no information of whether flow is towards or away from the transducer that is, whether Doppler shift is positive or negative.

A common technique for determining flow direction is to use Phase V quadrature detection technique in the Doppler device which allows forward and reverse flow to be separated.

After the received echo signals are amplified, they are split into two identical channels for demodulation. The channels differ only in that the reference signals from the transmitter sent to the demodulators are 90° out of phase. Two separate Doppler signal are produced. They are identical except for a small phase difference occur between them, and thus phase difference can be used to determine whether the Doppler shift is positive or negative.

Since the frequencies used in medical ultrasound and velocity encountered in the human body, combine to produce Doppler frequency shift in audible range, it is customary to send the Doppler signal directly to loudspeakers. An experienced sonographer can gain significant diagnostic information from the audio output.

Another way of processing the Doppler signal is to digitize it in an analogue to digital converter (ADC) and then use, for example, fast fourier transform (FFT) to extract the spectral information (See in next chapter).

Continuous wave instruments such as carotid are good for superficial vessel. They are also very sensitive to weak, e.g. signal might be found in digital artery of a finger. CW system has no limit on the maximum velocity measures and can therefore measure any velocity correctly (lack of aliasing). Another advantage includes the high accuracy of Doppler shift estimate with the narrow frequency band width that is used.

However, system suffers from one major constraint. Since the information is received from entire ultrasound beam, it is impossible to determine the depth of specific blood vessel. Hence, an errorsome velocity measurement may result if several vessels are insonated simultaneously in the same area since any motion within the sample path of transmit and receive transducer will result in a Doppler shift. This sample volume starts near the transducer face and usually extends into the tissues as the beam will penetrate. In addition to this, technique is prone to object motion within the beam path.

Pulsed Wave Doppler

Pulsed wave (PW) Doppler unit use the echo ranging principle to provide quantitative depth information of the Doppler signals from different depth, allowing for detection of moving interface and scatter only from within a well-defined sample volume (Fig. 3.5). This sample volume can be positioned anywhere along the axis of the ultrasound beam.

The principal components of pulsed wave Doppler instrument are shown in Figure 3.5. One transducer is used in pulse echo format similar to imaging technique with the exception that spatial pulse length is usually longer to minimum of 5 cycle/pulse to 25 cycle/pulse is used to achieve better narrow band frequency characteristic for a more accurate determination of frequency shift. In conventional B-mode images no. of cycle/pulse is 2-3 cycle/pulse with this system same transducer element both sends and receives sound, similar to non-Doppler systems.

Depth selection is achieved with use of electronic gating. Here, transducer is excited with a short duration burst and then no sound sents for brief period of time, i.e. transducer is silent for a period of time to listen for echoes before another burst of ultrasound is generated. This differs from continuous wave Doppler where one transducer is continuously excited.

Here in PW, scattered and reflected echo signal are detected by same transducer as mentioned earlier. Detected signal is amplified by receiver and applied to demodulator. The output of demodulator is then applied to a sample and hold circuit, which integrates a portion of the signal selected by range gate. This means received signal is electronically gated for processing so that only those echoes detected in a narrow time interval after pulse, corresponds to a specific depth that contribute to the Doppler signal all other echoes are rejected by the electronics.

The delay time before the gate is turned on to determine the axial location of the sample volume or depth, the amount of time the gate is activated establishes the axial length of

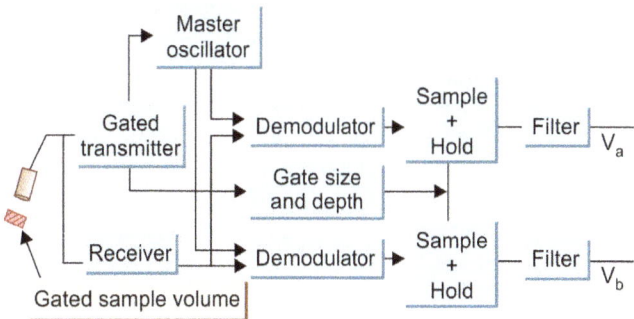

Fig. 3.5: Principal components of a pulsed Doppler instrument. The transducer is excited by a brief pulse; echo signals are amplified in the receiver and sent to the quadrature demodulators. A portion of the demodulated waveform is held in the sample and hold unit, which forms the Doppler signal by using several pulse-echo sequences. V_a and V_b are signals representing flow towards and away from the transducer.

sample volume. The depth of tissue being examined for flow is determined by varying the length of time after sound is transmitted before gate is turned on. Gate parameter such as position and duration are controlled by operator and can be adjusted. The sample length is between 1-15 mm. The lateral dimensions of sampling volume are dictated by beam width which is influenced by transducer frequency and focusing characteristics. The received echo must be evaluated to determine if the reflector is moving. This is accompanied by comparing the phase of the echo with a reference signal for which phase is synchronized with the transmitter pulse. Two waves are described as being in phase if their maximum, minimum, and zero point occur concurrently.

The echo from stationary reflector has the same phase as the reference signal where as the echoes from moving structure undergoes a phase shift via the Doppler effect.

The system is repeatedly pulsed. The pulse repetition frequency (PRF) is the frequency at which sound pulses are transmitted.

Hence, in pulsed wave mode, range discrimination is obtained, since the time of flight of a received echo can be converted into a specific depth. This assures propagational velocity of ultrasound in tissue to be known and received signal sampled accordingly.

One sample per period is acquired until enough data for an accurate estimation of Doppler shift have been collected, (typically 64-128 samples). The technique is known as range gating.

A comparison of CW and PW methods is given in Table 3.1.

Limitations of Doppler Systems

The use of CW and PW Doppler ultrasound raises a number of problems and ambiguities all of which influence the performance of color flow images (CFI) system as well.

Even when only one vessel is studied and only one frequency is emitted a range of Doppler frequencies will be received. This phenomenon is known as spectral broadening. It is due to either flow profile variation within the vessel (i.e. many different velocities are detected) or to transit time effect. The latter is a fundamental uncertainty inherent in Doppler measurement.

KEY POINTS

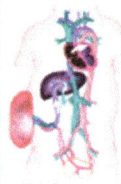

Basic Doppler systems used in Doppler sonography is:
- Continuous wave Doppler
- Single gated pulsed wave Doppler
- Multigated pulsed wave Doppler
- Duplex Doppler
- Color flow imaging
- Power Doppler imaging

It is due to the finite period of time that each erythrocyte contributes to the back scattered signal, when it passes through the beam. Thus, even a single scatterer moving at constant velocity will give rise to a spread of frequencies.

An echo must have returned to the receiver before the next pulse is transmitted, if the depth of origin is to be unambiguously determined. The maximum depth accessible is therefore limited by the propagation or velocity and the inter-pulse duration of the system (i.e. 1/PRF).

Further more there is a limit to the maximum velocity measurable. This is due to digitization applied. If the Doppler signal changes too rapidly then it is impossible to reconstruct the correct Doppler shift frequency.

This is known as aliasing.

A common way that aliasing is manifested on a Doppler spectral display is displayed in Figure 3.6.

The Doppler spectrum wraps around the display with high velocities being converted to reversed flow immediately at the point of aliasing and still high velocities in the flow signal appearing as progressively lower velocities.

TABLE 3.1: CW versus PW Doppler ultrasound.

CW Doppler	PW Doppler
+ sensitive	+ range resolution
+ inexpensive	+ variable sample volume size
+high signal/noise ratio	+ stepping stone to more advanced modalities
+ low acoustic output	– lower signal/noise ratio
– no range resolution	– high output power
– prone to object motion within beam path	– range velocity ambiguity

(CW: continuous wave; PW: pulsed wave)

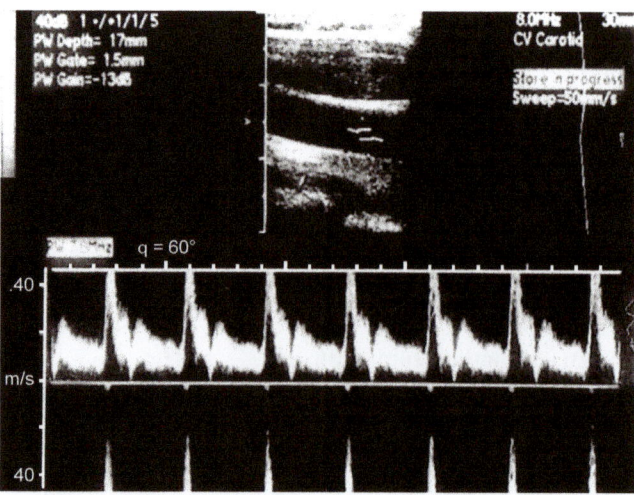

Fig. 3.6: Manifestation of aliasing on a spectral display.

To avoid aliasing the Nyquist sampling rate theorem must be fulfilled. This theorem states that

$$f_D \leq \frac{f_s}{2} = \frac{PRF}{2}$$

Where f_s is system's sampling frequency (equal to PRF). Hence, at a minimum the PRF must be at least two times the frequency of Doppler signal to construct the signal successfully.

When PRF equals $2 \times f_D$ this is known as Nyquist limit. Hence PRF $\geq 2 \, |f_D|$.

If the frequency of Doppler shift is above Nyquist limit then aliasing occur. An analogy would be a person who is trying to count a train of moving boxcars. This person keeps his eyes closed and opens them periodically for a brief look at the boxcars. He must open his eyes with a high enough frequency so that he sees each boxcars otherwise he may arrive at a count that is too low. The PRF must be high enough to sample the vessel adequately so that Doppler information is accurate.

To measure reflector moving with high velocity and producing large Doppler shift a high PRF is necessary.

But a high PRF limits the depth that can be sampled because a certain time is required to collect the echoes arising from that depth before the next pulse is sent out.

So while the maximum velocity measurable, v_{max} increases with increasing PRF, the maximum depth measurable, d_{max} decreases.

The ambiguities in maximum depth and velocity measurable are often combined into one expression.

$$v_{max} < \frac{C^2}{8 f_o \, d_{max}}$$

If the flow to be studied is known to be unidirectional, then relationship would be $C^2/4df_o$.

The maximum depth and velocity are inversely related and this equation is therefore independent of PRF. As sample volume depth increases, the maximum detectable Doppler signal frequencies increases and hence the maximum reflector velocity that can be detected decreases. At any depth lower ultrasound frequencies permit detection of greater velocities than high frequencies.

The trade off between maximum velocity and depth measurement constitute an important compromise inherent in PW Doppler system.

In practice, aliasing can be avoided or at least limited by changing a number of parameters as shown in Table 3.2.

One such example is shown in Figure 3.8 wherein base line has been increased to correct aliasing which is shown in Figure 3.5.

An additional problem which affects all Doppler scanner is the angular dependence when converting the Doppler shift from a frequency (in Hz) to a velocity in (m/s). The correct angle of incidence may not be known. Suppose as an example the true angle is 50° but it is estimated to be 45°. The error in velocity is 10%. At 70° the same uncertainly results in a 25% error, while at angle less than 20°, these errors are insignificant.

MULTIGATED PW DOPPLER SYSTEMS

A single gated PW Doppler system limits the information to one particular location or depth along the scan line. In order to obtain data from several depths simultaneously a so called multigated (MG) PW Doppler system must be employed. Multigated PW system typically contains 64–128 gates with a minimum axial length of 1 mm for each sample volume.

Basically, after demodulation the received signal is directed to a number of parallel processing channels. Each has a slightly different range gate setting. This allows number of adjacent sample volumes to be positioned across a vessel in Figure 3.7. The problem of locating a vessel is greatly reduced.

Since the assessment of the blood flow velocity is performed simultaneously in each sample volume, the velocity distribution along the vessel cross section can be determined as a function of time. The velocity profile will be influenced by the presence of for example plaques or stenosis and can be therefore a useful diagnostic tool.

TABLE 3.2: Technique for avoiding aliasing.

- Increase PRF
- Increase the beam/vessel angle
- Reduce the depth
- Reduce the transducer frequency
- Change the base-line
- Use CW instead

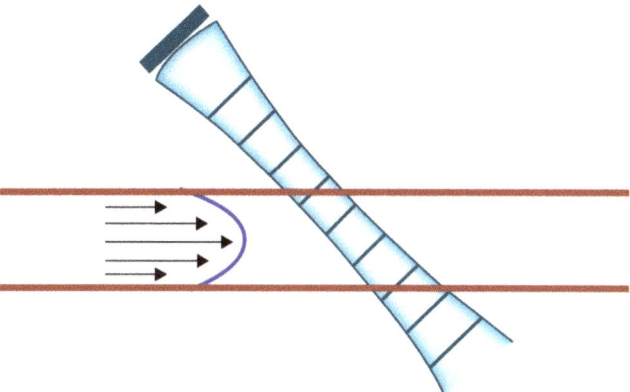

Fig. 3.7: Velocity profile measurement using a multigated (MG) Doppler system.

Duplex Doppler Systems

In spite of the advantage afforded by MG Doppler system, orientation and locating the desired vessel remain a problem. One way to overcome this is to combine 2D B-mode scan with flow information from Pulsed wave Doppler data.

The first such combined system was referred to as Duplex Doppler scanner.

This is because without some visual guidance to the vessel of interest, PW Doppler would be of little use.

In Duplex system a PW Doppler beam is visualized across the B-mode image with a sample volume position indicated by a cursor. This permits vessels to be easily selected for further evaluation. For example, as shown in Figure 3.8 with the Duplex image at the top and spectral data in the form of sonogram at the bottom. Notice how the location of the sample volume alters the measured spectra (low velocity at the vessel wall and higher flow in the center).

An advantage of a Duplex system is that the angle of incidence can be estimated from the B-mode. Thus Doppler frequency shift can be transferred to flow velocity estimates. The assessment of the angle of incidence rests on the number of assumptions such as flow parallel to the vessel wall and no curvature of the vessel in the scan plane. These assumptions are however rarely fulfilled. Due to error, one should always have a beam flow angle ranging from 30–60 degree. Other errors include vessel being off axis or curving compared to the scan plane. This problem also occurs in CFI system. The error in velocity measurement due to z plane misalignment or slice thickness have been found to be less than 5% at optimal setting but up to 20% error has been measured in nonoptimal circumstances.

In spite of the name "Duplex" the B-mode and Doppler scanning do not occur simultaneously. It takes significantly longer time to acquire Doppler data than B-mode data, and early Duplex scanner often "froze" the B-mode completely when obtaining flow information.

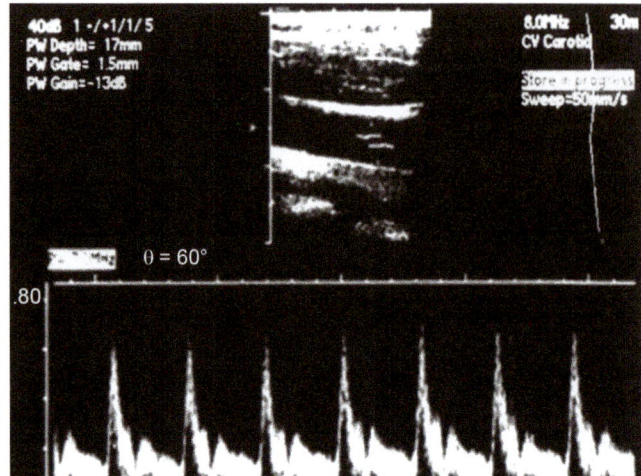

Fig. 3.8: Correction of aliasing by increasing the velocity scale on the machine.

The loss of real time imaging was a major drawback. More recently Duplex system employed mechanical transducer that might lower the frame rate but will not freeze the image. It is however relatively straight forward to employ different frequencies for imaging and Doppler.

Currently real time Duplex imaging is achieved with an electronically controlled transducer which can switch between imaging and Doppler fast enough to maintain an acceptable frame rate. Even though it is more complicated to obtain different transmit frequencies for Doppler and B-mode (it requires employing very broad band transducer). Such systems have many advantages when compared to their mechanical counterpart.

Chapter 4

Doppler Spectral Analysis

For many structures of interest, Doppler signal is in the audible range. For same applications, adequate clinical analysis may be made simply by listening to the signals. The listener then characterizes the flow according to the qualities of audible signal. However, great deal of information may be obtained by analysing the signal quantitatively, which is done by using digital technique called FFT (Fast Fourier Transformation).

If blood flow was continuous rather than pulsatile, if blood vessel followed straight lines and was uniform in caliber, if the blood following at the same velocity at the periphery and in the center of the lumen, and if the vessels were disease free, then each blood vessel would produce a single Doppler ultrasound frequency shift, and frequency spectrum is not needed.

But in case of blood flow, Doppler signal is fairly complex because flow is pulsatile and vessels are not always straight moreover flow is slower at the periphery than in the center of the vessels and vessel lumen may be distorted by other sclerosis and other pathology. This is why, blood flow produces a mixture of Doppler frequency shift that changes from moment to moment and from place to place within lumen. Spectrum shows the mixture of Doppler frequency present from vessel at that moment of time.

Separate a complicated signal into its individual frequency components so that relative contribution of each frequency components to the original signal can be determined (Fig. 4.1A).

The Doppler frequency spectrum is somewhat called power spectrum because the power or strength of each frequency is shown (Fig. 4.1B) by brightness of pixels. The power of given frequency shift in turns, proportional to number of RBCs produced at that particular frequency shift. If RBCs are large at a particular velocity then corresponding Doppler frequency shift is displayed as brighter on display on the other hand if small number of RBCs moving at a particular velocity then frequency shift corresponding to that velocity will be darker.

The Doppler frequency/velocity spectrum information can be presented in both frequency (kHz) and velocity. Velocity information is computed by assessing Doppler angle as shown (Fig. 4.1A) and then instrument automatically calculate velocity via Doppler equation (as discussed in Chapter 3).

As discussed in earlier section, Doppler angle between 60–30° is required because above 60°, any error in estimating Doppler angle may lead to large error in estimation velocity whereas less than 30° may cause total internal reflection.

When operating, Duplex instrument always use velocity mode rather than frequency mode for two reasons. First, velocity measurement compensates for variation in vessel alignment relative to skin surface as shown in Figure 4.1A.

Secondly Doppler frequency shift is inherently linked to output frequency of transducer but velocity is independent of transducer frequency.

SAMPLE VOLUME

The frequency spectrum shows blood flow information from a specific location called the Doppler sample volume. Three characteristics of sample volume must be known, first since it is a value which is 3-dimensional but displaced on two-dimension, thickness of sample volume cannot be shown which can lead to error of localization. Doppler signals may be obtained from vessel that are originally within the sample volume but are not shown on 2D display.

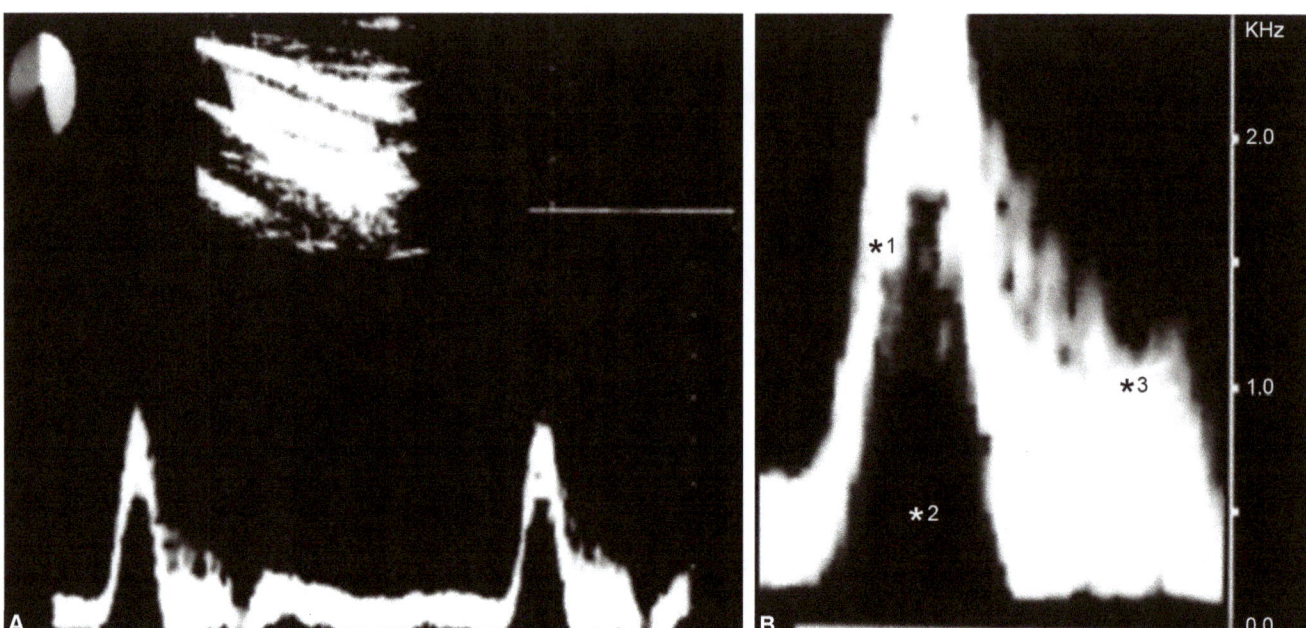

Figs. 4.1A and B: The Doppler spectrum display. The following information is presented on the display screen [(A) entire display; (B) magnified Doppler spectrum]. B-mode image The image of the vessel, the sample volume, and the Doppler line of sight are shown at the top of the display screen. Time: The time is represented on the horizontal (x) axis of the Doppler spectrum in divisions of a second. Frequency shift and velocity: The Doppler frequency shift (kHz) and the velocity (cm/sec) are shown on the vertical (y-axis) scales of the spectrum. Flow direction: The direction of flow is shown in relation to the spectrum baseline. For peripheral vascular work, flow away from the transducer is shown above the baseline, and flow towards the transducer is shown below the baseline. This relationship may be reversed by the operator. The distribution of velocities within the sample volume is illustrated by the brightness of the spectral display (z-axis). To better understand the z-axis concept, examine the magnified spectrum shown in B and imagine that the spectral display is made up of tiny squares called pixels (for picture elements). You cannot see the pixels in this image, because they are purposely blurred together to smooth the picture. The pixels are there, however, and each corresponds to a specific moment in time and a specific frequency shift and velocity. The brightness of a pixel (z-axis) is proportionate to the number of blood cells causing that frequency shift at that specific point in time. In this example, the pixels at asterisk 1 are bright white, meaning that at that movement, a large number of blood cells have a velocity corresponding to a frequency shift of +1.5 kHz. The pixels at asterisk 2 are black, meaning that at that movement, no (or very few) blood cells have a velocity corresponding to a frequency shift of +0.5 kHz. The pixels at asterisk 3 are gray, meaning that at that a moderate number of blood cells have a velocity corresponding to a +0.5 kHz frequency shift at that moment.

KEY POINTS

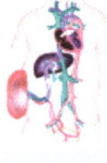

Doppler spectrum is a quantitative representation of Doppler Shift information obtaining using fast fourier transformation (FFT) technique. A great deal of information is obtained by analysing the spectra such as nature of spectra to sham normal flow and disturbed flow, spectral broadening or spectral window.

Secondly the actual shape or size of sample volume may be somewhat different from the linear representation shown on Duplex information.

Third, the Doppler spectrum displays flow information only within the sample volume and does not provide information about flow in other portion of the blood vessel that is visible on the ultrasound image.

DIRECTION OF FLOW

Direction is displayed relative to the direction of transducer. Flow in one direction is displayed above the baseline and flow in other direction is displayed below the baseline. The apparent direction may be reversed either by moving the transducer around and by pressing the button on the instruments. The arbitrary choice of this may lead to significant diagnostic error. If accurate flow direction is necessary comparison must be made in direction of known vessel in which direction of flow is already known by the operator.

WAVEFORM

In arteries each cycle of cardiac activity produces a distinct "wave" on the Doppler frequency spectrum.

The shape of Doppler frequency spectrum defines the flow property. These wave forms are illustrated in Figures 4.2A to C.

In case of low pulsatility Figure 4.2A, waveform shows broad systolic peaks and forward flow throughout diastole. The carotid, vertebral, renal, and coeliac arteries all have low pulsatile waveform in normal individuals because these vessels feed circulatory systems with low resistance to flow. Here, flow is always forward and therefore waveform is always displaced in one direction either positive or negative.

Moderate pulsatility as shown in Figure 4.2B, waveform shows tall and sharp systolic peak but forward flow throughout diastole. Examples of moderate pulsatility are few in carotid and superior, mesenteric artery (during fasting).

High pulsatility flow the waveform as shown in Figure 4.2C has tall, narrow and sharp systolic peaks and reverse or absent diastolic flow. The example of high pulsatility is the triphasic flow pattern seen in an extremity artery of a resting individual. Since only a low flow rate is required at rest in these vessels is the arterioles are most vasoconstricted.

A sharp systolic peak (first phase) is followed by brief flow reversal (second phase) and then by brief forward flow (third phase). These show that circulatory system with high resistance to blood flow, when body is at rest.

In most clinical situation qualitative assessment of pulsatility is sufficient but in some situation we may need it. For example, CDS greatly simplifies the identification of blood vessels and vascular pathology. Stenosing plaques are easily identified by the narrowing of the perfused vessel luman and typical stenotic flow abnormalities. The total occlusion of a vessel is manifested by the complete absence of color flow signal. The quantification of vascular stenosis can be accomplished with the help of color coded images alone by noting the relative interstenotic velocity increase. But when the conditions are less than ideal, their qualitative information is must.

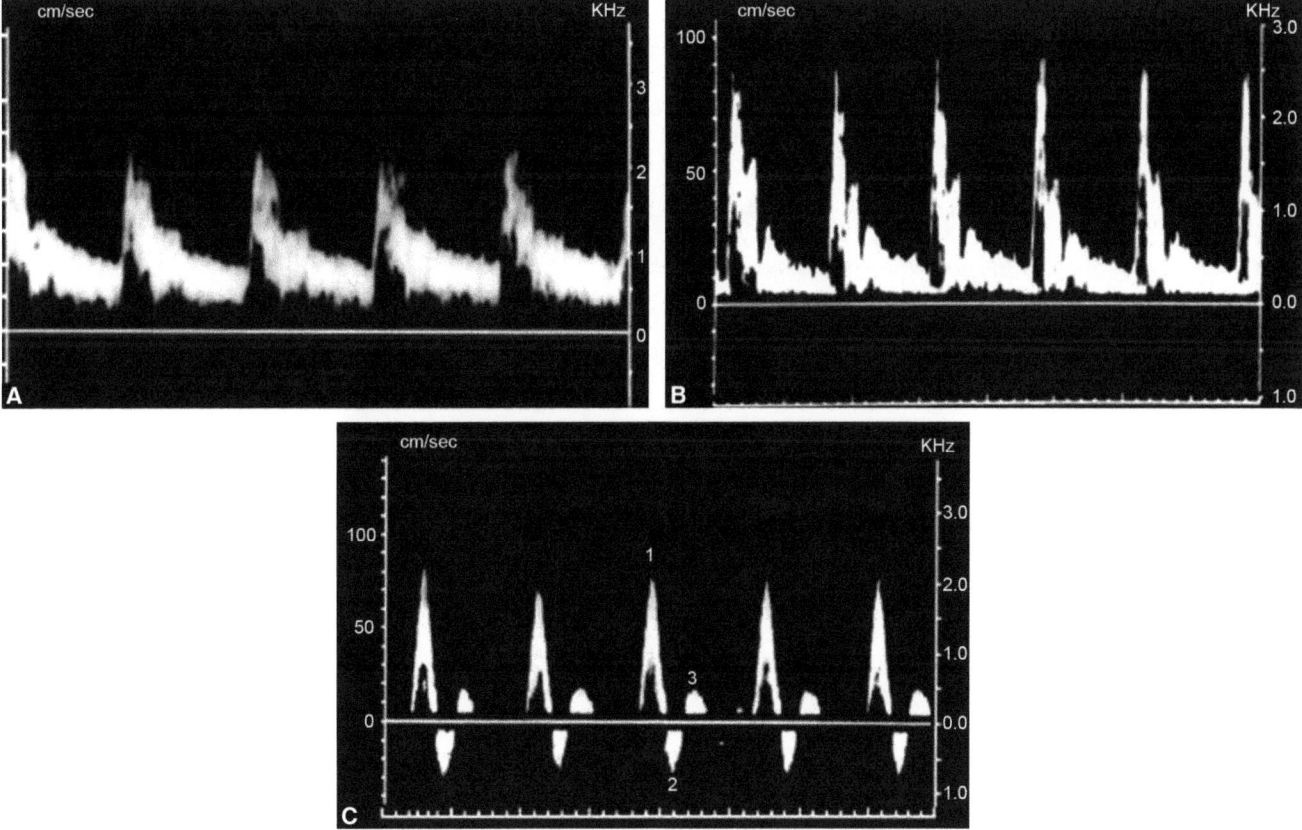

Figs. 4.2A to C: Pulsatility: (A) Low pulsatility is indicated by a broad systolic peak and persistent forward flow throughout diastole (e.g. Internal carotid artery); (B) Moderate pulsatility is indicated by a tall, sharp and narrow systolic peak, and flow reversal earlier diastole and absence of flow late in diastole; (C) In this classic triphasic example: the first phase (1) is systole, and the second phase (2) is brief diastolic flow reversal and the third phase (3) is diastolic forward flow and relatively little diastolic flow, high pulsatility is characterized by a narrow systolic peak flow reversal.

ENVELOPE TRACES OF THE DOPPLER SPECTRUM

So-called envelopes are commonly used in a simplified description of spectral waveforms and in the measurement of flow velocities.

The traces or curve may be drawn by machine itself or traced manually. An envelope is obtained by drawing a trace along the time axis in connection to the selected displayed Doppler frequency shift. The most common used envelopes trace to the maximum and mean frequency over time.

Various envelopes in Doppler spectrum analysis are showed in Figures 4.3A to C.
1. *Maximum frequency shift (A):* This is the highest Doppler frequency shift at each moment in time in the Doppler spectrum. In order to eliminate noise generally, the frequency below which a certain percentage (e.g. 95%) of all measure frequency shift tall is selected.
2. *Minimum frequency (B):* The lowest Doppler frequency shift at each moment in time in Doppler spectrum.
3. *Mean frequency shift:* Arithmetic mean of all Doppler frequency shifts at each moment in time.

Normal values for pulsatility measurement vary from one location in the body to other. In addition to this pathological and physiological process may alter arterial pulsatility patterns seen in extremity arteries during rest converted to a low-resistance, monophasic pattern after vigorous exercise, this pattern is distinctly abnormal in a resting patient and in that circumstances indicate arterial insufficiency in addition to this slowed ventricular emptying valvular reflex, valvular stenosis and other factor may significantly affect arterial pulsatility.

Acceleration is another important flow feature evident in Doppler arterial waveforms. In most normal situation flow velocity in an artery accelerate very rapidly during systole and flow peak reached within few microsecond after ventricular contraction begin.

Rapid flow acceleration produces an almost vertical deflection of the Doppler waveform at the start of systole. If however, severe arterial obstruction is present, proximal to the point of Doppler examination, systolic flow acceleration may be slowed substantially as shown in Figures 4.4A and B.

Quantitative measurement of acceleration is achieved by measuring the acceleration time and acceleration index as shown in Figures 4.4A and B.
1. Systolic acceleration time
2. Systolic acceleration rate = $\dfrac{\Delta V}{\Delta t}$

Vessel Identity

Doppler waveforms are particularly helpful in identifying the internal and external carotid arteries which have low and moderate pulsatility, respectively. Pulsatility is also of value for differentiating among portal veins, hepatic veins, and hepatic arteries within the liver.

Systolic Window

When in Doppler spectral analysis no frequency shift is detected within a certain range of frequencies this region remains black in conventional gray scale display when flow

KEY POINTS

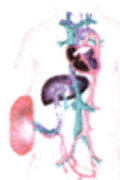

Y axis of Doppler spectra displays either frequency shift which is in audible range or flow velocity in CM/s. At a given time one can get numeric value of frequency or speed and distribution of frequency or velocity to show if range of frequency or velocity is narrow (such as a normal flow) or range of frequency or velocity is broad at that point of time (such as indisturbed flow). The shape of Doppler frequency spectrum defines the flow property.

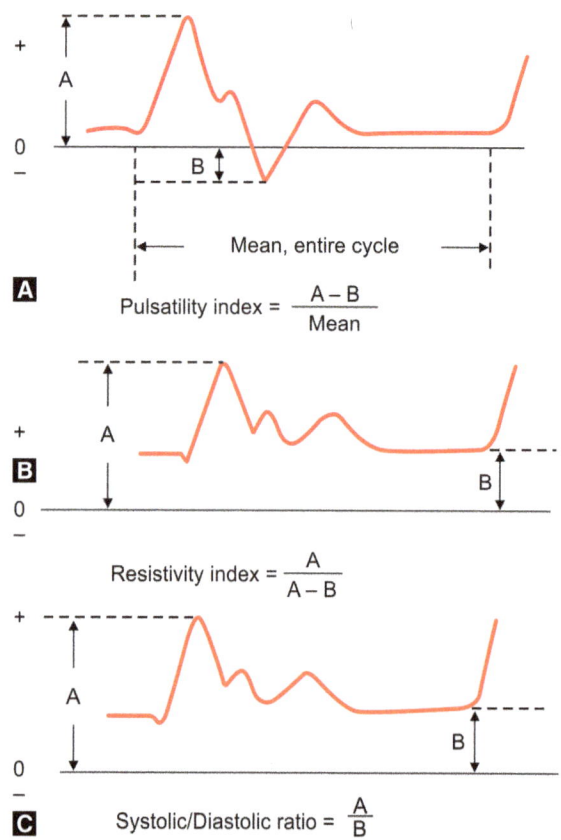

Figs. 4.3A to C: Pulsatility measurements. (A) The pulsatility index; (B) The resistivity index (Pourcelot); (C) The systolic/diastolic ratio.

Doppler Spectral Analysis | 25

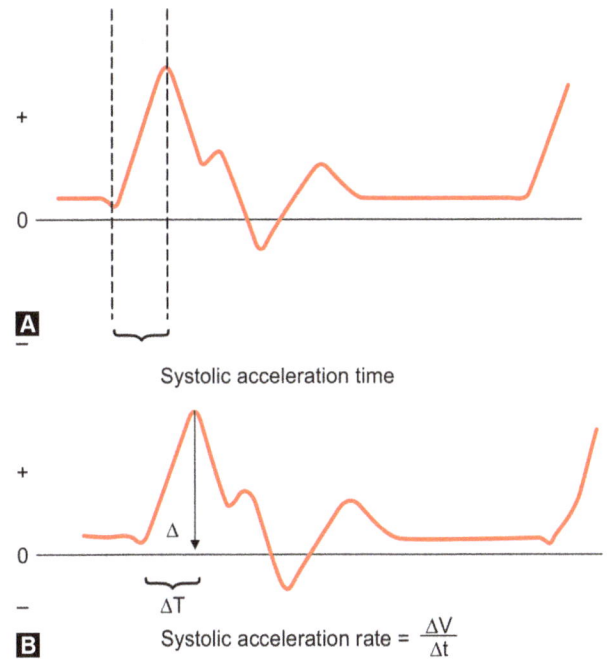

Figs. 4.4A and B: Acceleration measurements: (A) Acceleration time; (B) Acceleration index.

KEY POINTS

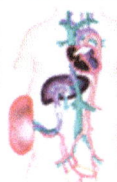

To analyze Doppler traces, Doppler indices are used which reflect the main characteristic of Doppler wave form. These are usually incorporated into the softwave of the ultrasound machine.

Pulsatility index $= \dfrac{A - B}{Mean}$

$= \dfrac{Peak\ systolic - End\ diastolic}{Mean\ velocity}$

Resistivity index $= \dfrac{A}{A - B}$

Systolic/diastolic ratio = A/B
A/B ratio is simple to use and calculate but it cannot account for reverse flow. It is commonly used in obstetrics for fetal and umbilical vessel evaluation.
RI: High diastolic flow leads to low value of RI. This does not handle reverse diastolic flow. Commonly used to evaluate renal transplant.
PI: Can reflect both reverse diastolic flow and a wide range of velocities. Commonly used to evaluate the extremities and carotids.

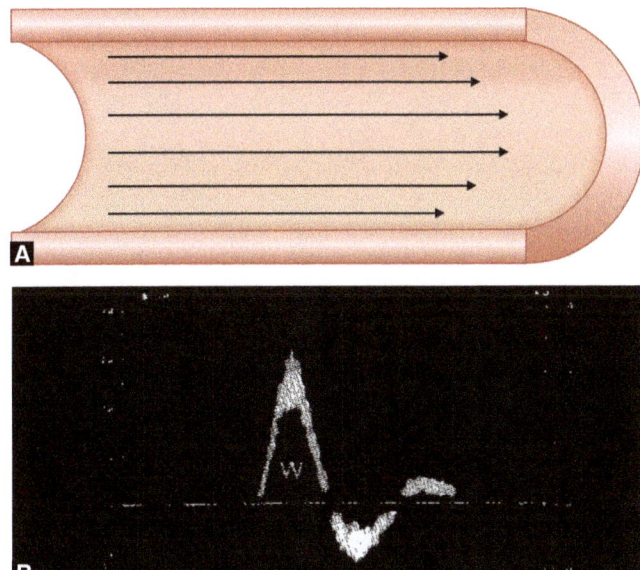

Figs. 4.5A and B: Laminar flow. (A) illustration of parallel lines of blood cell movement; (B) Doppler spectrum during laminar flow. At all times, the blood cells are moving at similar velocities. As a result, the spectrum is a thin line that encloses a well-defined black "window" (W)

is laminar for example the great majority of blood cells are moving at a uniform speed and spectrum displays a thin line that outlines a clear space which is known as spectral window (Figs. 4.5A and B).

Thus, systolic window is said to be empty or clear. The systolic window represents the frequency below the minimum detected Doppler frequency shift within each time increment. When a small volume is used the size of systolic window indicates the degree of laminar flow present.

The larger the bandwidth of measured Doppler frequency shifts, the smaller the systolic window becomes.

An increased bandwidth of measured Doppler shift represents the increased degree of flow disturbance based on non-uniform orientation of velocity vector of individual flow element in sample volume.

Especially in poststenotic spectra, the window may be completely filled in Figures 4.6A to D.

In disturbed flow, blood cell is less uniform as discussed which is manifested by spectral broadening or widening.

The degree of spectral widening is proportional to severity of flow disturbances as shown in Figures 4.6A and D.

26 | Textbook of Color Doppler Imaging

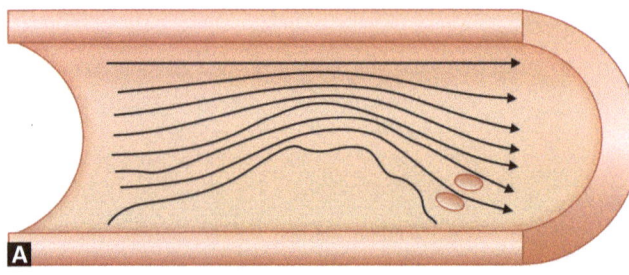

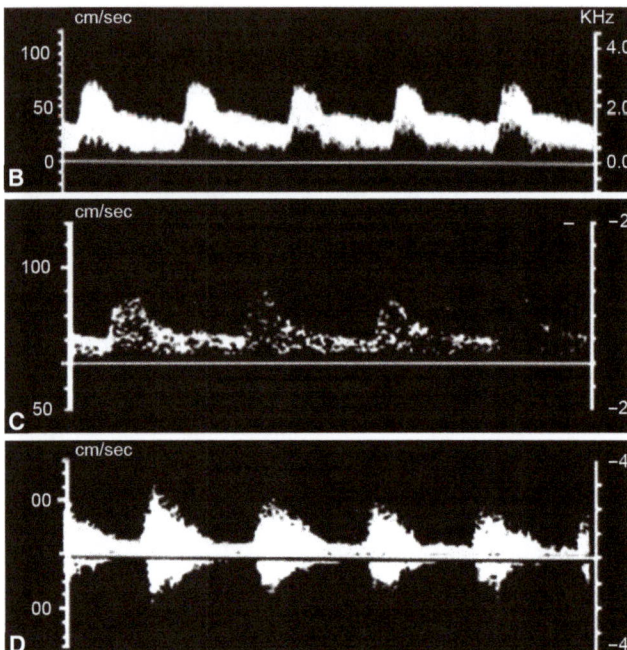

Figs. 4.6A to D: Disturbed flow. (A) disturbed flow illustration, (B) minor flow disturbance is indicated by spectral broadening at peak systole and through diastole, (C) moderate flow disturbance causes fill-in of the spectral window, and (D) severe flow disturbance is characterized by spectral fill-in, poor definition of spectral borders, and simultaneous forward and reversed flow. The audible Doppler signal has a loud, gruff character when flow is severely disturbed.

Although disturbed blood flow often indicates vascular disease but flow disturbances also occur in normal vessel.

Kinks, curves, and arterial branching may produce normal flow disturbance as shown in carotid flow where prominent area of reversed flow is normal occurrence (Figs. 4.7A and B).

DIAGNOSIS OF ARTERIAL OBSTRUCTION

Five main categories of information are used in this process:
1. Increased stenotic zone velocity.
2. Disturbed flow in poststenotic zone.
3. Proximal pulsatility changes.
4. Distal pulsatility changes.
5. Indirect effects of the obstruction such as collateralization.

The term stenotic zone refers to narrow portion of the arterial lumen. For determining the severity of arterial stenosis, the single most valuable Doppler finding is increased velocity in the stenotic zone (Fig. 4.8). This is because blood must move more quickly if the same volume is to flow through the narrow lumen as through the larger, normal lumen.

Amount of increased velocity is directly proportional to the severity of luminal narrowing.

Three stenotic zone velocity measures are commonly used to determine the severity of arterial stenosis.
1. Peak systolic velocity which is the highest systolic velocity within stenosis A.
2. End diastolic velocity which is the highest end diastolic velocity B
3. Systolic velocity ratio which compares peak systole in stenosis with peak systole proximal to the stenosis (normal portion vessel).

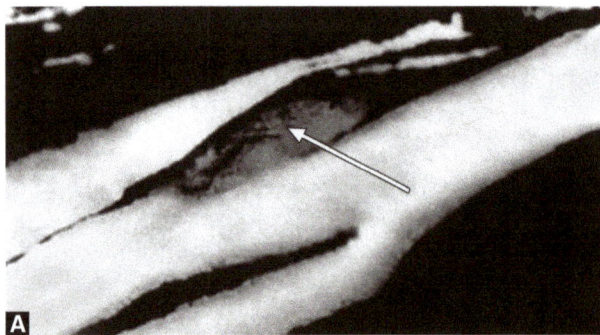
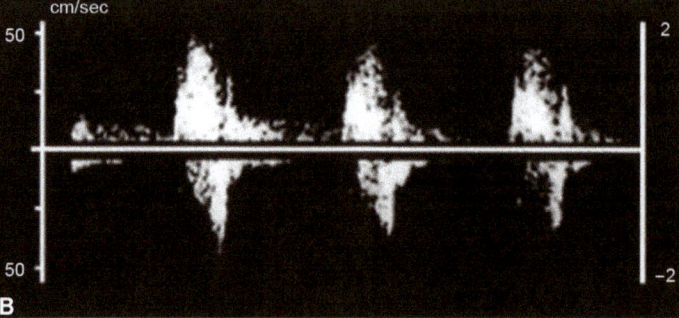

Figs. 4.7A and B: Normal bifurcation flow disturbance. (A) Flow reversal in the bulbous portion of the common and internal carotid arteries causes localized flow reversal (arrow); (B) Simultaneous forward and reverse flow is evident in the bulbous region on the Doppler spectrum.

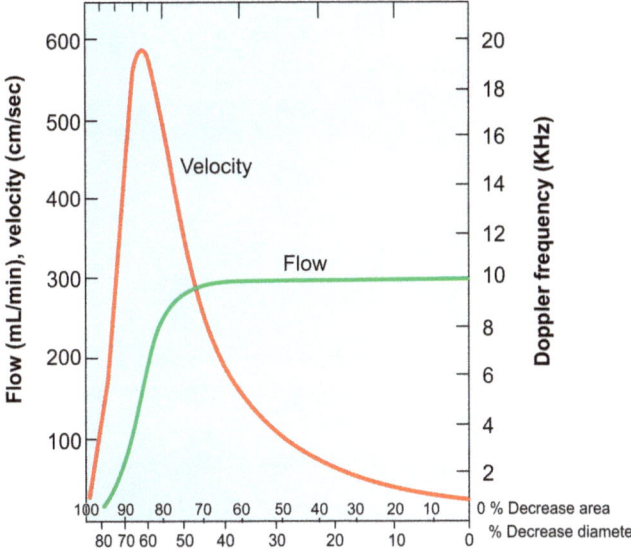

Fig. 4.8: Relationship among velocity, flow, and lumen size. This graph refers specifically to internal carotid artery stenosis, but the principles illustrated apply to stenosis in other arteries throughout the body. Note that peak systolic velocity in the stenotic internal carotid lumen (labeled velocity) increases exponentially as the lumen diameter decreases (from right to left). The highest velocities correspond to approximately 70% diameter reduction. With greater stenosis severity, peak systolic velocity falls off rapidly to zero (because of rapidly increasing flow resistance). In contrast to velocity, volume flow (labeled flow) remains stable until the lumen diameter is reduced by about 50%. With further reduction in lumen size, volume flow falls off very rapidly to zero. Finally, note the relationship of per cent diameter and area reduction, as shown at the base of the figure. Fifty percent diameter reduction equals about 70% area reduction, and 70% diameter reduction equals about 90% area reduction!

Peak systole in the stenotic zone is the first Doppler parameter to become abnormal as an arterial lumen becomes narrowed.

Shown in Figure 4.8, peak systole rises steadily with progressive narrowing but ultimately, the flow resistance becomes so high that peak systole falls to normal or even subnormal levels. This drop in velocity can cause under estimation of degree of stenosis.

Low flow velocity may also lead to false diagnosis of arterial occlusion, if the flow velocity is so low that Doppler signal cannot be detected with ultrasound.

The region of maximum velocity within stenotic zones may be quite small and due to this reason, the sonographer must search the stenotic lumen with the sample to locate the highest flow velocity. If highest flow velocity is overlooked then degree of stenosis may be underestimated.

End diastolic velocity also increase in proportion. So the degree of stenosis narrow is less than 50%. Then, this velocity may remain largely normal.

With moderate stenosis (50-70%) diameter reduction end diastolic velocity is above normal.

End diastolic velocity is particularly good marker for severe stenosis because the parameter is not elevated.

The systolic velocity ratio, as defined is an additional important parameter for the diagnosis of arterial stenosis. This ratio is used clinically for measurement of internal carotid renal and extremity artery stenosis as discussed earlier.

Poststenotic Flow Disturbance

The poststenotic zone is the region immediately beyond arterial stenosis where flow disturbances are commonly present.

As the flow stream from the stenotic lumen spread out in the poststenotic zone, the laminar flow pattern is lost and flow become disorganized which generate disturbed Doppler spectral pattern (Figs. 4.9A to D) with forward and reversal flow.

The maximum flow disturbance occurs with one cm beyond the stenosis and in very severe stenosis, soft tissue adjacent to this position of artery may vibrate causing a visible bruit on CDI.

About two cm beyond the stenosis the flow disturbance becomes less visible and spectral broadening diminishes. Normally laminar flow pattern usually is re-established with three cm beyond the stenosis. Severe flow disturbance however with simultaneous forward and reverse flow does not occur in normal vessel and therefore an important sign of high grade stenosis.

In some cases, stenosis may be obscured by plaque calcification and in such instances poststenotic disturbed flow may be the only sign of severe arterial stenosis.

Proximal Pulsatility Changes

Arterial obstruction causes increased pulsatility in portion of the artery proximal to the stenosis. For example with severe internal carotid artery obstruction the Doppler spectrum in the common carotid artery has high pulsatility feature rather than normal low pulsatility pattern (Figs. 4.10A and B).

Distal Pulsatility Changes

Doppler waveform abnormalities seen distal to stenosis also have considerable value in the diagnosis of arterial stenosis.

Doppler waveform distal to severe arterial obstruction has the damped appearance (Figs. 4.11A and B).

This means the systolic acceleration is slowed, the systolic peak is rounded, the maximum systolic velocity is lower than normal and the diastolic flow is increased.

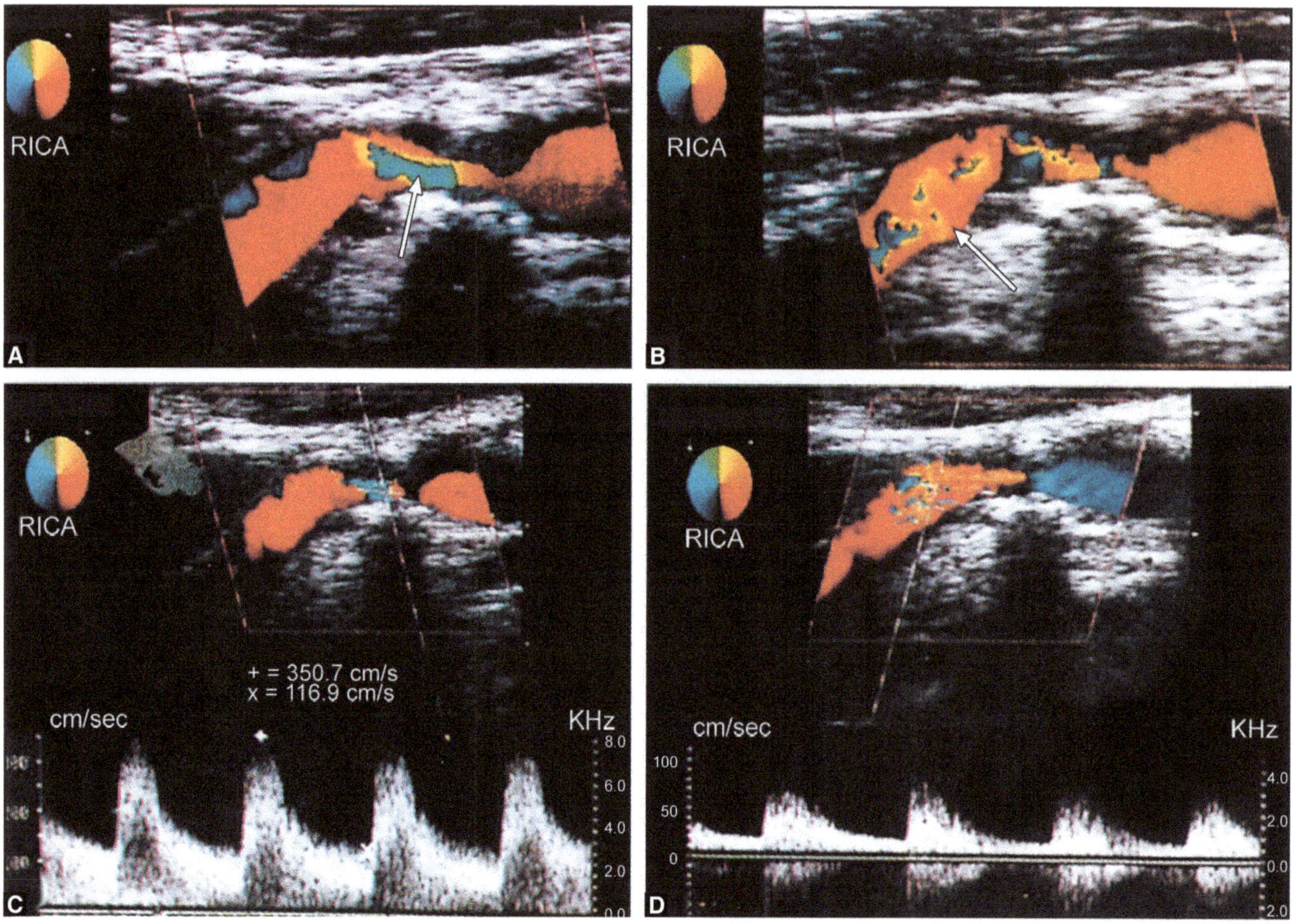

Figs. 4.9A to D: Local effects of arterial stenosis. (A) High velocities present in the narrowed portion of the arterial lumen generate an area of aliasing (arrow) within the stenotic lumen; (B) disturbed flow in the poststenotic area generates a mixture of colors (arrow); (C) Doppler spectral analysis shows markedly elevated velocity at peak systole (350.7 cm/sec) and end diastole (116.9 cm/sec); (D) Severe flow disturbance is evident in the poststenotic region, as indicated by simultaneous forward and reverse flow, spectrum fill-in, and poor definition of the spectrum margins.

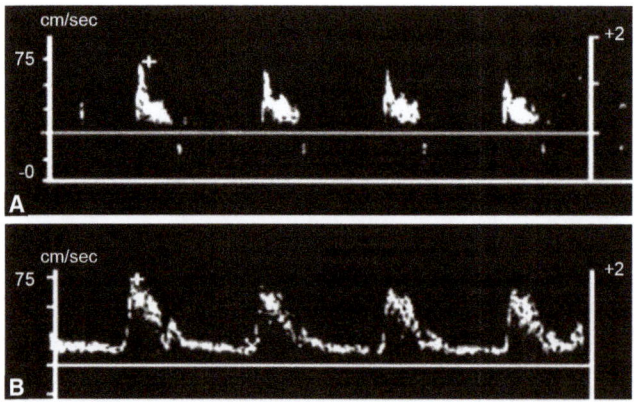

Figs. 4.10A and B: Increased common carotid artery pulsatility due to internal carotid artery occlusion.

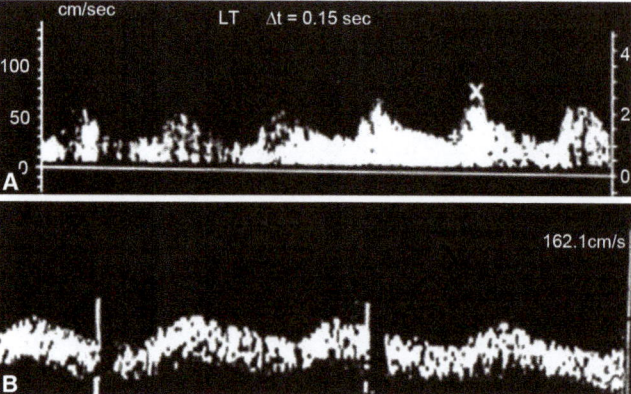

Figs. 4.11A and B: (A) The acceleration time is prolonged (0.15 sec) in the left kidney due to severe proximal renal artery stenosis; (B) severely damped dorsalis pedis artery waveform is distal to femoral/popliteal artery occlusion. Normally, this waveform is distal to femoral/popliteal artery occlusion.

Color Flow Imaging

After devising multigated Doppler systems (*See* Chapter 3) that acquire flow data along an entire scan line, and Duplex system which overlaps a Doppler beam on a B-mode image, the next step seems logical overlay a B-scan with flow information from all depths, i.e. along the entire A line and expand the number of A lines to cover a region of interest. This is the principle of all color flow imaging (CFI) systems. This imaging is one of most important development in ultrasound imaging. This imaging method superimposes a blood flow image on a standard gray scale, ultrasound image, permitting instantaneous visual assessment of blood flow. The estimated velocity of each sample volume is mapped in a color representing the direction of flow as well as its magnitude (via the color and hue).

Typically shades of red and blue are used for flow towards and away respectively, from the transducer. There are however, numerous other color maps available from different manufacture. The variance of velocity estimate, i.e. spectral broadening of the Doppler signal can be included as a third color which is often green (Figs. 5.1A and B).

PRINCIPLES OF COLOR FLOW IMAGING

Gray scale ultrasound instrument use only two pieces of information from each echo that returns from the patient's body: the distance from echo to the transducer and strength of echo.

The echo signal typically contains other information such as a Doppler frequency shift, but this information is disregarded. Color Doppler instruments are different from gray scale instrument because they use the Doppler shift information in addition to time of flight and amplitude information. For each echo show on color Doppler image, the instrument makes fine determination.

1. How long has it taken for the sound beam to travel to and from the site of the echo? This indicates the distance of echo reflector from the transducer.

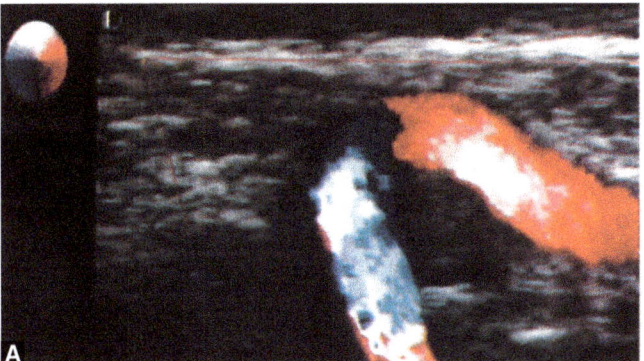 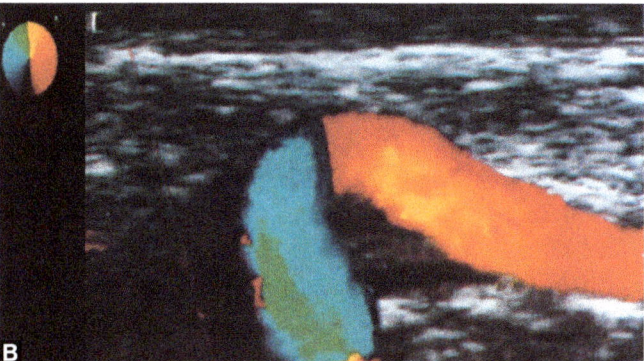

Figs. 5.1A and B: Color flow schemes. A variety of color schemes are used in color-Doppler instruments. (A) With this scheme, progressive increase in the frequency shift changes the image color from red to pink to white, or from dark blue to light blue to white, depending on the flow direction; (B) With this scheme, the color changes from red to yellow or from blue to green, as the frequency shift increases.

KEY POINTS

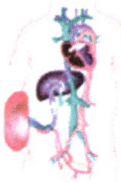

Color flow imaging (CFI) technique superimposes blood flow Doppler data on a standard gray scale US image. It is customary to show flow in one direction as red and flow in other direction as blue. Magnitude of velocities is displayed in different shades of color. In case of increased velocity, shades of color are shown from darker shades of red or blue toward lighter shades of red or blue.

2. How strong is the echo? The strength or amplitude of ultrasound signal determines how brightly the echo is displayed as the image (for both gray scale and color Doppler components).
3. Is a Doppler frequency shift present? If so, the echo is represented in shades of color.
4. What is magnitude of the Doppler frequency shift? The magnitude of the Doppler shift is proportionate to the blood flow velocity and the Doppler angle. Different frequency levels are shown as the image as different color shades or hues.
5. What is the direction of the Doppler shift?

The instrument determines whether flow is towards or away from the transducer by noting whether the echo has a higher or lower frequency than the ultrasound beam sent from the transducer. A higher Doppler frequency means flow is towards the transducer and low Doppler frequency means flow is away from transducer. It is customary to show flow in one direction in blue and flow in the other direction in red. However, the operator can select other color schemes if desired.

The way to show color has two different ways:
1. *Shifting line method:* Different colors are used to represent different frequency levels (e.g. blue, green, yellow, and white with increasing frequency).
2. *Changing shades method:* Here, same color is used but the color gets lighter as frequency increases (e.g. dark red, light red, pink, and white).

These color images are shown in Figure 5.1B.

Even though CFI systems may appear to constitute a logical extension of PW Doppler and Duplex Doppler, they do in fact represent a fundamentally different hardware structure. The reason for this is the time! In a PW system 64–128 samples are acquired per Doppler waveform over approximately 10 msec.

Even if each A line was processed enough in parallel channel to cover all depth along the scan line, there would not be sufficient time to record 128 Doppler A line and B-mode image in real time.

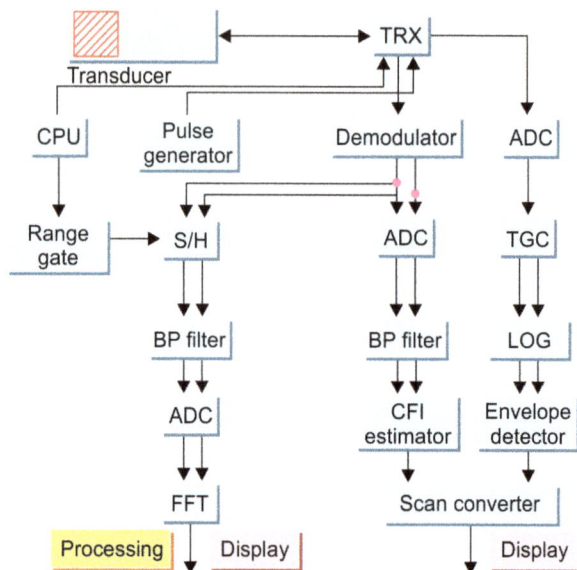

Fig. 5.2: Block diagram of integrated CFI scanner. The second column from the left represents the PW Doppler system, the third the color flow system, and the right-band column the B-mode system. Abbreviations are explained in the text.

Consequently CFI systems are limited to 6–32 samples per range gate, i.e. 6–32 Burst transmitted in each direction. This time limit puts severe constraint on all filters and estimators involved in the processing scheme. Hence, digital filters and early digitization are essential in CFI system to get sufficient fast and short responses.

In Figure 5.2, A block diagram of a basic CFI system is presented. The left most column represents a PW system while middle column is the color Doppler processor. Notice how the digitization takes place as early as possible.

Since strong stationary and quasi stationary echo are not filtered out before digitization a very powerful ADC is required. The right most columns depict B-mode circuitry.

In Doppler instrument only one parameter such as mean Doppler shift is extracted and shown. Hence, this method is less time consuming for estimating the mean velocity along the entire A line, without resorting to parallel processing must be devised. This is the last of CFI estimator.

Frequency estimation technique used in most CFI system is known as autocorrelation method. Here, the phase of autocorrelation function is calculated as a function of the interpulse duration time (i.e. 1/PRF). This is equivalent to comparing echo segment from consecutive A lines to one another and allows the phase change caused by Doppler shift of the RBCs to be estimated.

The mean Doppler shift and thus mean velocity can be calculated from the phase shift.

The autocorrelation can estimate the Doppler shift along an A line with as few as 3–4 samples. This requires all stationary echoes which are much stronger than blood flow signals to be removed efficiently. The calculations are performed in approximately one msec at PRF of 4 kHz.

An alternative estimation based on line domain correlation has been developed. In this method the velocity estimate is based on maximising the cross-correlation between small segments of two consecutive A lines.

Time domain flow imaging (under the name color velocity imaging) is not widely used by ultrasound equipment manufacturer. One major advantage of this technique is that it is much less susceptible to aliasing.

To get a real-time B-mode image as well as to visualize rapid flow changes, it is necessary to switch rapidly between imaging and Doppler acquisition.

Linear or phased array transducer with their electronic switching and beam steering capabilities are therefore the most common choice for CFI systems. Mechanical transducers have been employed in the past, but these are becoming increasingly rare on today's scanner.

Another problem is how to combine the pulse echo and Doppler data acquisition. In synchronous systems the received signal is split into two separate processing schemes, one for imaging and other one for Doppler. But requirement for optimal Doppler and optimal pulse echo are not similar. Therefore, even though very high frame rates are feasible, this is achieved at the expense of resolution and general image quality.

Alternatively, pulse echo and Doppler data can be acquired independently (an asynchronous system). This scheme allows the B-mode imaging and the Doppler pulses to be optimized separately. However, other compromises are required.

In every other pulse is used for imaging and alternatively Doppler, the available PRF is halved. This means a reduction in the maximum velocity measurable.

On the other hand, if many Doppler burst are employed interrupted by a single imaging pulse, the possible B-scan frame rate is reduced. Instead, a complete time sharing scheme is used. A whole image scan is performed and Doppler information is then collected over a time period which retains a reasonable frame rate (15 frames/sec).

Asynchronous data acquisition will mean missing the Doppler signal in periods during which B-mode image is being performed. Hence, it is necessary to generate a substitute signal. This is done by either repeating the last bit of Doppler acquisition or by synthesizing a Doppler filter signal. In CFI systems, the period of flow data acquisition can be minimized by reducing the overall number of Doppler scan times, the axial resolution and region of interest.

PROBLEMS IN COLOR FLOW IMAGING

As described, CFI system is based on the principles of PW Doppler scanner. Hence, aliasing is recurring problem especially since much lower PRF is used. Another problem arises because one simple characteristic, Doppler frequency representing the blood velocities in the sample volume over a one msec period is displayed, separated by long dead times.

A frame rate of 10 is not uncommon in CFI scanners which mean a rate of 10 interrogation and displays per sample volume per second.

Solid tissue motion is another CFI artifact. This is called flash artifacts is usually of very short duration, which makes it easy to recognise, although the artifact may obscure low flow particularly in the abdomen.

Since all color coding is performed relative to transducer, multiple flow beam angles may constitute a problem. Very tortuous vessel will be color coded in a wide range of lines, often with flow both towards and away from the transducer. This phenomenon is less noticeable in linear arrays where the angle of incidence is constant. In transducer with a sector shaped field of view even a straight vessel perpendicular to the transducer surface will be coded in multitude of hues. Due to very limited number of samples available for CFI estimator, these are more qualitative than their spectral counter parts (FFT) based processor as in CW, PW, and MG Doppler system consider a PW Doppler system. The sonogram provides a display of all Doppler frequency detected in a sample volume in each 10 msec period with 64-128 samples per Doppler waveform and display at a rate of 100 displays per second. Conversely in CFI system one Doppler shift is found for each 100 msec. More quantitative blood velocity information is then obtained from PW system.

CLINICAL ADVANTAGES OF COLOR FLOW IMAGING AND ITS LIMITATIONS

Technical Efficiency

Perhaps the greatest advantage of color flow imaging is technical efficiency. When moving blood is encountered, the vessel lights up even if the vessel is too small to be resolved on the gray scale image. Because vessels stand out in vivid color, they may be located and follow much more easily than with gray scale instruments. Further more basic judgment about blood flow can be made easy with color flow imaging (Figs. 5.3 and 5.4). One can quickly determine the presence or absence of flow, the direction of flow and the presence of local flow disturbances and therefore sonographer can quickly examine long vascular segments such as vascular bypass graft, with relative ease.

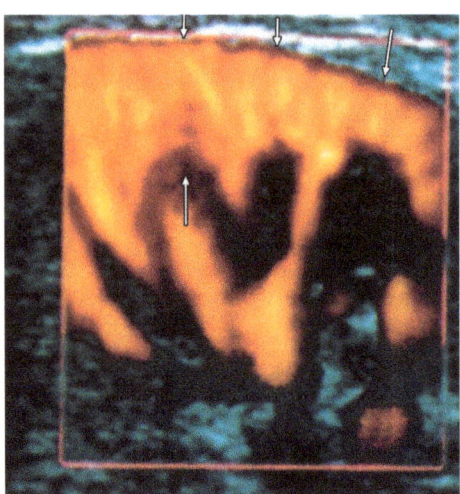

Fig. 5.3: Color amplitude image of a kidney. Conventional color flow image shows the presence of a range of frequency shifts in the cortical region of the kidney and noise in the tissue.

KEY POINTS

Advantages of CFI
- Its greatest advantage is that when US encounters with moving blood even very small vessel are displayed by providing color.
- Presence or absence of flow can be easily recognized.
- CFI simplifies differentiation between vascular and non-vascular structure.
- Flow assessment in entire lumen.

Disadvantages of CFI
- Reduced flow rate.
- Display mean velocity
- Aliasing occur such as the PW Doppler system.

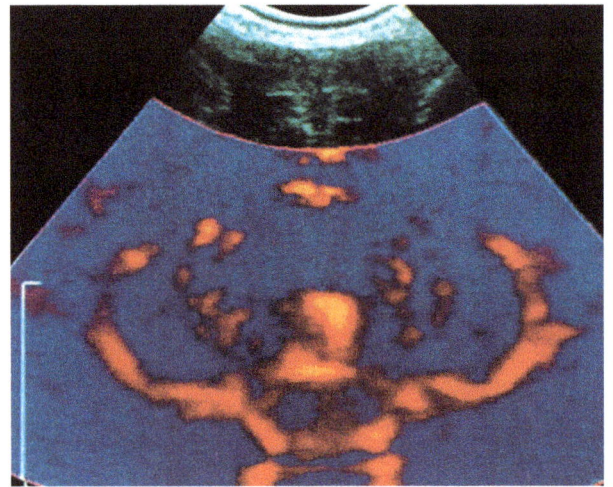

Fig. 5.4: This power Doppler image of the cranial vasculature uses a blue background which enhances flow detection because noise is converted to a uniform blue color.

Furthermore, color flow imaging facilitates the examination of vessels such as calf veins and renal arteries.

Assistance in Sorting Out Abdominal Anatomy

Another advantage of color flow imaging simplifies differentiation between vascular and non-vascular structure, which is particularly useful in the abdomen. One of the most obvious applications is sorting out porta hepatis anatomy. The bile ducts, which do not exhibit flow, may be differentiated visually from the hepatic artery and portal vein, in which flow is seen.

Flow assessment in entire lumen, a major advantage of color flow imaging is the depiction of blood flow throughout a large segment of a vessel, rather than solely at the Doppler sample volume. Because flow features are visible over a large area, localized flow abnormalities are readily apparent and are less likely to be overlooked than with gray scale Duplex methods.

The sonographer is immediately made aware of the location of any flow abnormalities which speeds up the examination and permit rapid assessment of long segment of vessels for obstruction and other pathology.

Visual Measurement of Stenosis

As compared with gray scale ultrasound, color flow imaging makes it easier to define the residual lumen in stenotic vessels permitting more precise visual measurement of arterial stenosis. Direct, visual stenosis measurement remains problem prone however, due to vessel tortuosity and acoustic shadows from calcified plaque.

Differentiation of Severe Stenosis and Occlusion

The ability of color flow imaging to detect low velocity flow in a tiny residual lumen may facilitate the differentiation between occlusion of an artery and near occlusion with a trickle of residual flow.

Limitations of Color Flow Imaging

Flow information is qualitative because:

1. Flow image is based on the average Doppler shift within the vessel, rather than the Peak Doppler shift. Average Doppler shift is not helpful for actually putting a number on a stenosis. Furthermore, average Doppler shift is lowered by flow disturbances.

2. It is not corrected for Doppler angle.
3. Only a few frequency levels are shown.

Because color flow images are qualitative, Doppler spectrum analysis must be used to derive quantitative flow data.

Low Pulse Repetition Frequency (PRF) and Frame Rate (FR)

A very large number of data must be processed by the color flow instrument to give each pixel and each television frame. Because of long processing time it may lead to serious effect on the gray scale and color. Doppler images are therefore acquired with reduced PRF and reduced frame rate. Reduced PRF may have the following effect:

- The B-mode image may be degraded because fewer data are available to build up the image.
- Doppler aliasing may occur due to Nyquist limits.
- Low PRF and low FR may limit the visualization of rapidly moving cardiac or vascular event. For example, cardiac valve motion may be less clearly seen with color flow scanning than with the gray scale scanning.
- Low frame rates may produce image flicker. If the frame rate is reduced below 15 frames/sec in the lumen, eye no larger blurs the ultrasound images into a moving picture.
- *Flow detection is angle dependent:* Blood flow is not detected with color flow device in vessel that are perpendicular to the ultrasound beam. A false positive diagnosis of vascular occlusion may occur if a vessel is approximately perpendicular to the ultrasound beam. This is particularly severe problem when curved array scanners are used for color Doppler imaging.
- *Flow direction is arbitrary:* Color of vessel on the CFI is not an absolute indication of flow direction. The color is assigned relative to the transducer. The operator may reverse the color scheme (arteries blue and vein red) simply by reversing the orientation of transducer or by pushing a button on the instrument. To determine the true direction of flow, the operator must closely observe the orientation of the vessel relative to the transducer or refer to a vessel in which the flow direction is known such as aorta.
- *Color flash:* With CFI, anything within the FOV that moves to the transducer is shown in color.
  In the abdomen peristaltic motion, cardiac motion or transmitted pulsation from great vessels may generate blotches of color on the ultrasound image called color flash which can obscure structure of interest.
  The color flash problem is particularly apparent in the upper abdomen because of the heart motion.
- *Visible bruit:* It is a peculiar, but useful flow phenomenon that can be seen with color flow imaging. A mark of color is seen within the soft tissue adjacent to the blood vessel; this color effect is caused by vibration of the vessel. This vibration in-turn is caused by a severe flow disturbance within the vessel; a visible bruit suggests severe arterial stenosis but caution is advised in interpreting, this finding because several flow disturbances may sometime occur in the absence of a significant stenosis.

Optimizing Color Flow Image Quality

The CFI is derived from weak scattered US waveform RBCs. Hence, flow detection is particularly susceptible to ultrasound instrument settings. The following set of rule may help sonographer to obtain adequate flow information when it is difficult.

Doppler Angle

Since this angle affect the CFI so when flow is absent in vessel one can move the color flow box or transducer to improve the Doppler angle.

Velocity Range

If the instrument is set to detect arterial velocities, it is not sensitive to venous velocities or vice versa. Hence, use proper PRF to take care of velocity range to level appropriate for the vessel of interest.

Field of View

If depth of field is shown on image, always use optimal depth.

Color Box Size

It is best to use a small color box especially when examining vessels deep within the body.

Power and Gain

If gray scale image is prioritized the color flow image suffer and vice versa. If any trouble in detecting flow, shift the image processing priority towards color.

Thump Control

It refers to electronic filtering that removes color artifacts generated by the heart or vascular pulsations. Thump control is not needed in smaller peripheral vessels and should be set as low as is practical.

Wall Filtering

If wall filter is set too high, low frequency signals generated by low velocity flow are eliminated. The wall filter is designed to eliminate low frequency noise but if it is set too high, it also eliminates flow information. It may be a major problem for detection of venous flow or evaluating small intrarenal arteries.

Very Slow Flow

Power Doppler may be more sensitive to the presence of slow flow than standard color Doppler imaging and it may be useful to switch to this modality when vessel appears occluded.

POWER DOPPLER FLOW IMAGING

As the name implies, this is a Doppler method, but differs from standard Doppler methods in that power or intensity of Doppler signal is measured and mapped and thus ignores the velocity of Doppler signal detected from each location.

In power Doppler system the density of red blood cells is depicted as opposed to their velocity (Fig. 5.3).

The amplitude and this intensity or a power of back scattered signal depends on the number of RBCs present within the sample volume, the size of vessel and the attenuation of intervening tissue. Since the Doppler frequency shift information is not utilized, power Doppler images is non-directional and does not suffer from aliasing.

The advantages of this modality over color flow imaging are therefore:

1. Power Doppler imaging is said to be more sensitive in detecting blood flow. 10–15 dB of improved sensitivity have been reported. Hence, smaller vessels and vessels with flow slow can be imaged. The reason, why smaller vessels are visualized in power Doppler is that the display dynamic range has been increased by sacrificing part of the available information (velocity and direction) and by increasing the persistence of the display flow signals. This allows the color priorities to be increased then producing the apparent increase in sensitivity.

   Since more dynamic range can be used because of noise that would overwhelm the standard color flow imaging can be arising a uniform background color, e.g. light blue. Hence, anything that represents noise is blue (Fig. 5.4) and anything that represents flow is another color (usually gold).

2. As described earlier power Doppler imaging is not affected by aliasing. Even the aliased portion of signal has the power and can be displayed as flow (Fig. 5.5).
3. Power Doppler is significantly less angle dependent (unless the angle becomes so close to perpendicular that the Doppler signal are below the flow detectable threshold of color processor) so, angle effects are usually ignored.
4. Power Doppler display improves in functional lumen definition. The difference between Doppler frequency shift from a sample volume close to the vessel wall and from one partially overlapping the wall will be very small. However, the number of red blood cells insonated within the two sample volumes will be quite different and therefore, so will the amplitude of the back scattered signals.

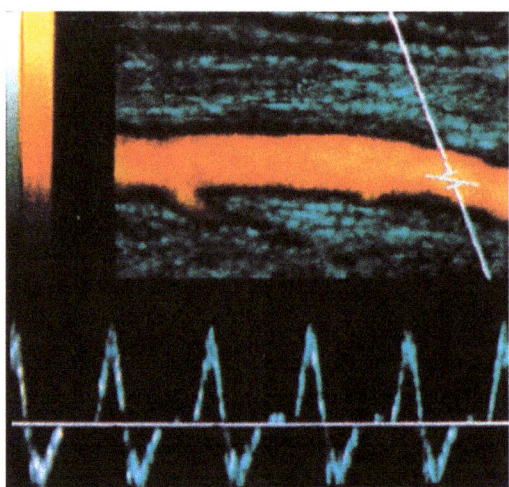

Fig. 5.5: Quantitative spectral information can be obtained in power Doppler mode.

5. Power Doppler imaging has one final advantage that has been appreciated since the advent of ultrasound contrast agents. Power Doppler imaging is less subject to blooming than the standard color Doppler imaging. Blooming is the spread of color outside of the blood vessel that occurs when amplification of Doppler signal is too great.

Blooming is particular problem when contrast agent is used to improve the detection of blood flow. Intravenous injection of the echo-enhancing agent greatly increases the Doppler signal intensity, causing over amplification and severe blooming. With power Doppler blooming does not occur.

In spite of its potential advantages over color Doppler, power Doppler imaging has two major limitations.

1. Frame rate is slow, which render this imaging method useless for rapidly moving vessels, rapidly moving patients (especially children) and areas subject to respiratory or cardiac motion.

   To compensate motion induced artifacts power Doppler significantly increase weighted temporal averaging (high frame to frame averaging). This technique reduces motion artifacts but increases the display response time (i.e. color map seems to lag behind the gray scale image).

2. Power Doppler imaging does not provide flow direction information and therefore cannot assess effects such as pulsatility and flow reversal.

The power Doppler depicts the density of red blood cells in vessel and should be used as an adjunct to conventional mean frequency velocity based color flow imaging.

HARMONIC IMAGING

Harmonic imaging relies on inherent property of microbubbles to resonate at specific frequency once they have encountered the ultrasound beam. Each compound has a specific resonant frequency and various subharmonic frequencies. The resonant frequency is largely dependent upon the particle size. Extensive studies on animal suggest that this may be a method to further enhance the effect of contrast agents.

Harmonic imaging requires an ultrasound machine which can transmit the sound beam at a specific frequency and receive at the resonant frequency. The resonant frequency is twice that of the transmitting frequency. The signal to noise ratio is improved because in theory only the echoes arriving back to the transducer from the object are displayed. That means that images are displayed from contrast fill objects other are removed from the display.

This is important particularly useful when conventional US imaging is limited by motion artifacts examples include imaging of heart and vessels seen in renal artery, located deep in the abdomen adjacent to the pulsating aorta.

Chapter 6

Contrast Agents in Ultrasound

INTRODUCTION

The major motivation and need for the current rapid rate of development of contrast agents for ultrasound lies in the nature of the current performance limits of ultrasound and color Doppler. At present most Duplex and color Doppler imaging systems are capable of detecting flow from vessels whose lumina lies below the resolution of the image. The detection of such unresolved flow using Doppler systems can be demonstrated simply by using a Duplex scanner to create a power Doppler image of the kidney in which vessels not visible on gray scale image become visible using Doppler mode. These vessels are the arcuate and the interlobar branches of the renal arteries. Their diameter is known to be less than 100 µm and therefore below the resolution limits of the image. However, as we progress distally, the blood flows more slowly as the rate of bifurcation increases giving lower Doppler shift frequencies and the quantity of blood in a given volume of tissue also decreases, weakening the back scattered echo. Eventually a point is reached at which the vessel cannot be visualized and the Doppler signals cannot be detected.

Two factors determine where that point will lie—Doppler shift frequency and echo strength.

First the velocity of blood must be sufficient to produce a Doppler shift frequency that is distinguishable from that produced by the normal motion of tissue and second the received intensity of the backscattered ultrasound must provide adequate signal strength for detection by the transducer above the acoustic and electric noise of the system. Using a higher frequency ultrasound helps in both aspects. The Doppler shift frequency corresponding to a given flow velocity increased in proportion to the transmitted sounds frequency and the backscattered intensity increases with the fourth power of transmitted frequency as predicted by the Rayleigh relationship.[1] In practice the penetration of sound through tissue places an upper limit on the ultrasound frequency that can be used.

For deeper vessels of the abdomen ultrasound frequencies above 5 MHz produce blood echoes whose amplitude at the skin surface is too small for detection by most current systems. In this and many other applications involving small vessels, it is the strength of the backscattered echo rather than Doppler shift frequency that defers the smallest vessel from which Doppler signals can be detected. It also defines the scale of vasculature. It is possible to detect in a neovascularized mass or a collateral vessel to a vascular occlusion. For larger vessels the effect of increasing the echo from blood is to enhance the signal to noise ratio which again determines detectability in such vessels as the renal artery or the middle cerebral artery when approached transcranially. There is then clear clinical potential for contrast agents capable of enhancing the echo of moving blood especially in systemic arterial system.

The principal requirements for an ultrasound contrast agent are that it should be easily introducible into the vascular system, be stable for the duration of the diagnostic examination, have low toxicity and modify one or more acoustic properties of tissues that determine the ultrasound imaging process.

The essential mechanisms whereby microbubbles act as echoenhancers are same as pertain to scattered echoes elsewhere, the echo intensity is proportional to change in acoustic impedance as the sound beam crosses from blood to the gas in bubbles. The impedance mismatch at such an interface is very high and essentially all the incident sound is reflected though all will not travel back to the transducer. However, though the reflection is near complete by itself.

This would not produce a very effective enhancing agent because microbubbles are very small and present in only small numbers. The reflectivity is proportional to the sixth power of the particles diameter and directly to their concentration.

Rather the intense echogenicity of microbubbles results from the fact that they resonate when insolated and this makes them behave as though much larger and thus more echogenic than a rigid bubble of the same diameter (10^{14} × or larger). Maximizing this resonance is a critical aspect of this design. Obviously the microbubbles must be made small enough to cross the capillaries (<7 μ) and like any other mechanical resonance system, the critical frequency depends on their diameter. It is a most fortunate coincidence that microbubbles in this size range happen to have their resonance frequencies in the 2–15 MHz. This most fortunate coincidence makes microbubbles such extremely effective reflectors that even in the low concentration after they have been dispersed throughout the systemic circulation, they produce some 20 dB of enhancement in echo strength-an increase of some 100 folds. Range of ultrasound frequencies that are used for clinical diagnosis microbubbles at (1-7 μ diameter) do not diffuse across the endothelium. So, there is no interstitial phase of enhancement. Thus, they are essentially markers for the blood pool (or for any other body space into which they have been placed) and their distribution is similar to those of tagged red cells. Typically the effective duration of vascular enhancement is a few minutes after which the microbubbles dissipate although, this model is complicated by evidence that some microbubbles are taken up by the phagocytic cell systems and these have liver/spleen specific effects.

The techniques for making microbubbles have been devised both to control their size and to make them sufficiently stable to provide a clinically useful enhancement time of at least a few minutes.

Levovist

It consists of galactose ground into tiny crystals whose irregular surfaces act as nidation sites on which air pockets form when it is suspended in water. A trace of palmitic acid is added as a surfactant to stabilize the resultant microbubbles which therefore are in effect tiny soap bubbles.

Optison

It represents another class of microbubbles with a shell formed by sonicating a solution of human serum albumin. The resulting capsules are filled with a perfluorocarbon gas (perfluoropropane) whose high molecular weight shows dissolution and thereby prolongs the enhancement for several minutes.

Sonovue

It is a family of microbubbles whose membrane consists of phospholipids. In this case, the gas is sulphur hexafluoride[5,6] which diffuses slowly like perfluoro compounds.

Extensive preclinical and clinical trials have demonstrated an excellent safety profile for intravenous injection of microbubbles. The total amount used is minute (less than 200/mL in the case of a dose of levovist and their small size makes embolization most unlikely.

The main unwanted effect is a mild and transient local discomfort at the injection site which results from the high osmolality of this agent.

THE IMPACT OF CONTRAST ENHANCEMENT

The arrival of the contrast agent some seconds after peripheral venous injection in the portion of the systemic vasculature is marked by a dramatic increase in signal strength. In spectral Doppler, this is seen as intensifying of the gray scale of the spectrum for spectral Doppler examinations that fail because of lack of signal strength, the effect of the contrast agent is to rescue the examination.

In color Doppler, the parameter mapped to color is the estimated Doppler shift frequency, which corresponds to the relative blood flow velocity. Color should therefore remain unaltered by contrast enhancement, what does change is the range of locations from which color signals are detected. The effect of contrast agent is to raise the signals from small vessels above that threshold to that point at which they are effectively detectable on a color image. Thus, more vessels appear in a contrast enhanced ultrasound image.

KEY POINTS

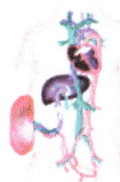

- Arcuate and interlobar branches of renal arteries and arteries less than 100 μ) has low resolution to make image.
- Hence, shift frequency and echo strength determines the visualization of small vessels.
- Contrast agents increases both above and hence act as echo enhancer.
- Echo enhancers are microbubles—levovist, optisan, and sonovue.
- Non-vascular use—tubal patency in infertility, ureteric reflux in children with urinary tract infections.
- Vascular use—cardiac, transcranial, carotid, and renal.

Studies have demonstrated the capacity of contrast agents to increase the technical success rate of Doppler ultrasound, for example—in clinical transcranial Doppler studies of middle cerebral artery administration of 10 mL of levovist in concentration of 200, 300, 400 mg/mL resulted in dose dependent increases in both surgical intensity and duration of enhancement. At a concentration of 400 mg/mL levovist increased the Doppler signal by approximately 25 dB. The time to peak enhancement was between 30 and 60 seconds and duration of enhancement was reported to be sufficiently long to be clinically useful.[2]

If the target vessel is larger than the flow detectable, the impact of the agent may be to shorten the examination time. In one study, levovist halved the examination time for the Duplex investigation of renal artery stenosis.[3] Yet another study[4] suggested improved accuracy in measuring peripheral vascular velocity when contrast is used.

In a satisfactory color Doppler study of the abdomen one use of the agent might simply be to enable a higher ultrasound frequency to be used, exploiting the agent to counter the higher tissue attenuation. In such a case, contrast enhancement translates into higher spatial solution.

Alternatively the color system may be set to use fewer pulses per scan line (that is a lower ensemble length) while still achieving the same sensitivity to blood flow by means of contrast enhancement. The agent will then provide the user with a higher frame rate.

An important general concept in the practical use of microbubble enhancing agents is their fragility, so that, they are readily destroyed by the insolating beam. In some situation strategies to preserve them improve their visualization significantly. The most important example is in echocardiography where the entire microbubble population generally passes through the ultrasound beam. A major increase in both the amount and duration of enhancement can be achieved by scanning intermittently (triggered by ECG) rather than continuously such approaches allow gray scale visualization of myocardial perfusion.

If the bubbles in a tissue slice are deliberately destroyed, then their reappearance is related to the rate of inflow of fresh bubbles which depends on the tissue flow rate. This destruction-reperfusion approach has been used for the myocardium and can be expected to be useful also in kidney and other abdominal organs.

As microbubbles resonate in the ultrasound beam they behave like a musical instrument and emit harmonic signals at double their resonance frequency. If a scanner is modified to detect these harmonic signals and use those to form the image or Doppler trace, the confusing clutter signal from tissue stationary or moving are suppressed and a cleaner image or trace is produced.

In harmonic mode, echoes from the contrast agent are received preferentially by means of a bandpass filter whose center frequency is at the second harmonic. Echoes from the solid tissues as well as from red blood cells themselves are suppressed.

The particular potential application of this entirely new diagnostic method is the detection of blood flow in small vessels surrounded by tissue that is moving in the branches of coronary arteries or in the myocardium[5] itself as well in the parenchyma of abdominal organs.[6]

Another way to improve the signal/clutter ratio[8] is to use a pair of pulses to form each B-mode line, the second of each pair being inverted in phase. The final image line is formed by summing the two resultant echo trains. Since the echoes from linear reflectors such as tissue, are inverted they cancel out but the non-linear response of the microbubbles means that their echoes are not exactly symmetrical in the compression and expansion phase and so they do not cancel out. This phase inversion scan mode has similar effect in reducing clutter as the harmonic mode but with the important advantage of retaining the full spatial resolution of B mode which is compromised in the latter because a narrow band pulse must be used.

CLINICAL APPLICATIONS

Non-vascular Use

Contrast agents have been used to evaluate tubal patency in infertility and ureteric reflux in children with renal tract infections.

Echovist is installed into the uterine cavity via a small Foleys catheter and using transvaginal sonography tracking of the echogenic contrast along the tubes and into the adnexal peritoneum is observed to establish tubal patency (Figs. 6.1 to 6.3). Some false negative results may be obtained due to tubal spasm and it does not offer the same anatomical detail as HSG when tubal surgery is an option. However, it a simple OPD procedure and is radiation free.

For vesicoureteric reflux, levovist is instilled into the bladder as for conventional MCU. The lower ureters and renal pelvis are examined transabdominally as the bladder is filled to stimulate micturition. Sensitivity seems to be higher than for X-ray MCU, perhaps because there are no time constraints on imaging and the level of reflux can be assessed using the same criteria. Avoidance of radiation is an obvious advantage though the posterior urethra is not well seen. So, it may not be possible to replace the initial investigation in boys. For girls and for all follow-up studies, the US MCU has become standard in many pediatric departments.

Contrast Agents in Ultrasound | **39**

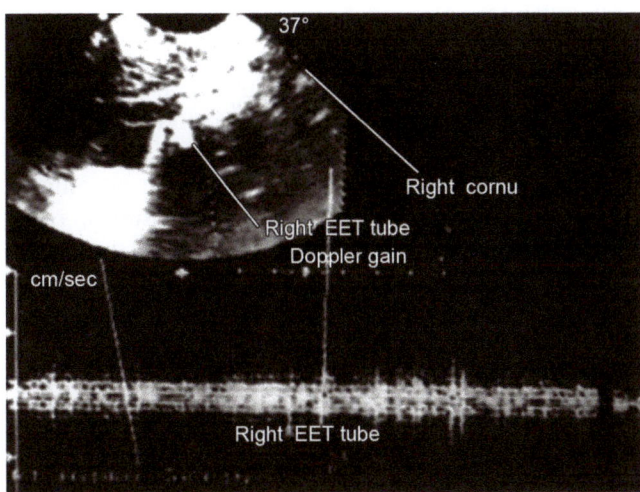

Fig. 6.1: Hydrosalpinx-contrast agent (Agitated Hemocele) with Duplex mode.

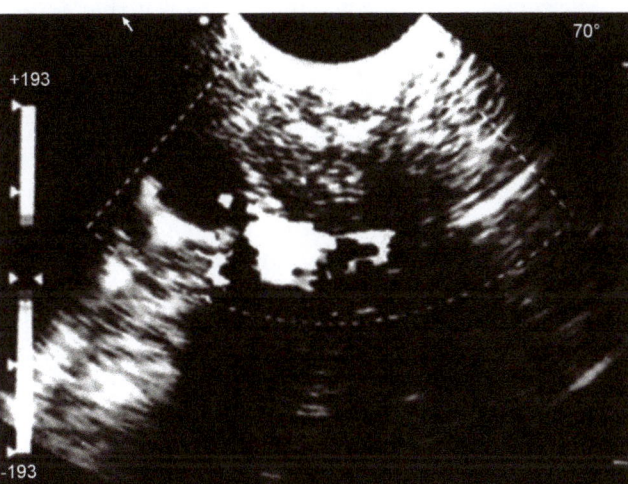

Fig. 6.2: Color mode—Patent tube.

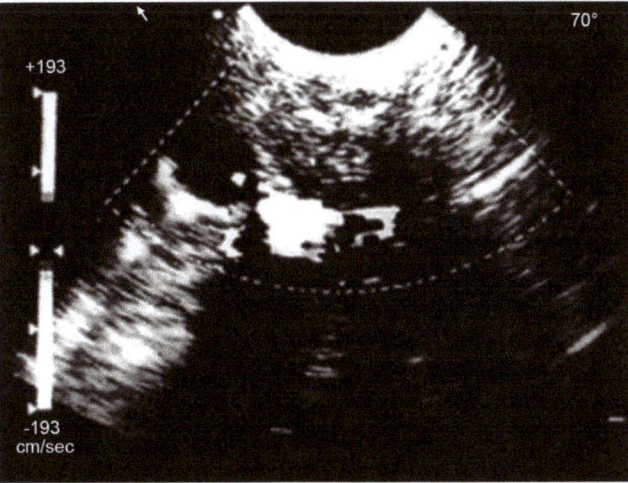

Fig. 6.3: Distal turbulence demonstrated by contrast agent (Agitated Hemocele).

KEY POINTS

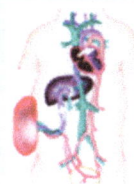

- Transcranial, carotid, renal, portal vein, peripheral, arterial, IVC, and venous.
- Functional uses of contrast Doppler.
- Mature scar—no vascularity while tumour recurrence shows marked vascularity.
- Hepatocellular carcinoma—fill in arterial phase while regenerating nodule and adenocarcinoma fill slowly.

Vascular Uses

Cardiac

The use of contrast media is to opacify the cardiac chamber. This improves delineation of the left ventricular endocardial border and allows better estimates of left ventricular function and measurement of ejection fraction. In many cardiology units, microbubble enhanced echocardiography has replaced isotope studies (particularly the MUGA scan) for left ventricular function. It is cheaper, quicker and avoids ionizing radiation.

The development of means to detect microbubbles in the myocardial capillaries is making myocardial perfusion estimates possible and ultrasound contrast stress echo studies are becoming more widely used. The possibility of studying the coronary arteries directly is also becoming an option.

TRANSCRANIAL DOPPLER

Transcranial Doppler (TCD) is a typical field where Doppler signals are routinely difficult to obtain because of the attenuation by the skull. Microbubbles improve signal intensity overcoming this technical difficulty. It allows a more complete depiction of the cerebral arterial system and basal veins. It is especially useful in depicting lesion with low blood flow velocities and low flow volume.

Cavernoma appears as echogenic areas with slow flow on Doppler. Flow within cavernoma themselves is undetectable but after Levovist enhancement, mean peak systolic flow velocities of 10–15 cm/sec are seen. Contrast enhanced TCD may therefore be especially useful in the intensive care unit as well as intra operatively and during postoperative follow-up.

As long as, there is good ultrasonic window through the temporal bone arteriovenous malformations can be detected without the need for enhancement because of their high velocity flows which is often bi- or multidirectional. Microbubbles may enhance delineation of the entire malformation and reveal even occult AVM.

Aneurysms, characteristically identified as sharp systolic bidirectional Doppler signal with a machine like noise may be detected on unenhanced TCD but can be diagnosed with higher accuracy and at a smaller size with contrast enhanced TCD. Enhanced Doppler can be expected to assist in the management of subarachnoid hemorrhage in detecting possible sources of hemorrhage and in monitoring arterial spasm.

The diagnosis of cerebral vascular stenosis is based on demonstrating aliasing on color Doppler supported by characteristic changes in the Doppler frequency spectrum especially high velocities. In patients with poor signal transmission through the temporal bone, microbubble enhancement reduces the failure rate and may be especially helpful in distinguishing high grade stenosis from occlusion. Low volume flow at high grade stenosis may be missed on transcranial ultrasound because the signals are weak, exactly as with the extracranial carotid arteries.

The increased signal intensity after microbubble enhancement allows a complete three-dimensional reconstruction of the circle of Willis and improves the delineation of tumor feeding vessels and the identification and localization of highly vascularized areas within the tumor. Additionally 3D display may rescue the examiner dependence of vascular ultrasound by allowing off line analysis. It may also help overcome some of the limitation of access to cerebral vessel by allowing display of reformatted sections in planes that cannot be obtained directly.

To date harmonic imaging has been disappointing in transcranial Doppler because the stimulation of microbubbles to resonate in a non-linear mode depends upon achieving a higher acoustic intensity than for simple resonance and this is difficult to achieve through the attenuating skull bone. The recently described technique of wideband harmonic imaging seems to be less dependent on sound pressure suggesting a potential for transcranial imaging.

CAROTID DOPPLER

Echo enhancement by contrast allows carotid Doppler to be performed by less skilled operators and with inexpensive scanners so the technique could become more widely used. Enhancement may also lead to better delineation of plaque ulcers. The ability to improve demonstration of trickle flow in very light stenosis is of undoubted clinical value because these patients benefit from endarterectomy whereas surgery is of no benefit once the internal carotid artery has occluded.

RENAL DOPPLER

Preliminary studies have shown that Levovist improves the diagnosis of significant renal artery stenosis by substantially reducing the failure rate for both the main renal arteries and for changes in intrarenal waveforms. This resulted in fewer false negative and false positive results when compared to digital subtraction angiography. This could increase the value of ultrasound screening for renovascular hypertension to the extent that microbubble enhancement becomes a routine part of investigation. Ultrasonic diagnosis of renal vein thrombosis is difficult because access to the renal veins may be limited and also because the process commonly starts in small veins at lobar level and then propagates to the main renal vein. By this stage collaterals open up both at the capsule and in the renal hilum thus the demonstration of venous signal at renal hilum does not completely exclude renal vein thrombosis. Better delineation of the venous anatomy following enhancement may prove to be an important application of microbubbles though there are no reports on this use.

Microbubble enhancement provides valuable added confidence in the diagnosis of acute transplant occlusion affecting the surgical anastomosis.

PORTAL VEIN DOPPLER

Echo enhanced Doppler provides useful information in a failed Doppler study. Enhancement allows a decision between a technical failure and true absence of flow. This situation is common is cirrhosis because of the highly attenuating liver and because the portal vein flow velocity may be very low. A confident diagnosis of portal vein patency can be achieved more often so that DSA can be avoided in some cases.

PERIPHERAL ARTERIAL DOPPLER

Signal strength is improved by microbubble enhancement and this is likely to prove helpful in improving signals from segments where shadowing from calcific plaques attenuates the signals and from very light stenosis where the flow velocity drops (trickle flow). In addition contrast speeds up to procedure. Levovist has been shown to improve the signals from leg arteries in a clinical trial but the diagnostic advantage has not been evaluated systematically.

INFERIOR VENA CAVA

Inferior vena cava (IVC) thrombosis is occasionally difficult to diagnosis especially in the infrarenal portion which is often obscured by intestinal gas. A microbubble enhancing agent might be very useful here and for the same reason, in the iliac veins in the pelvis. Echovist injected into a vein in the foot improves visualization of the cava and of the flow disturbances around caval filters. Whether a microbubble injected into a distant (antecubital) vein would also be useful has not been studied systematically.

PERIPHERAL VENOUS DOPPLER

Unenhanced Doppler may fail in the diagnosis of deep vein thrombosis especially where the leg is swollen or obese and in diagnosis of below knee deep vein thrombosis. As with other vascular beds these problems amount to between a few and 10%.

A problem with microbubbles is the dilution of contrast agent because of the large volume of these capacitance vessels as reflected in the partial success reported for Echovist injections directly into veins of foot when compared to limited value of Levovist injected into an antecubital vein. Since this is such an important clinical problem, active research continues and it may be that infusion techniques will improve the clinical usefulness of microbubble agents for DVT.

FUNCTIONAL USES OF CONTRAST DOPPLER

The clinical applications can be divided into those that interrogate the entire hemodynamics of an organ and those that study only one region, for example, a tumor. There have been two main whole organ studies looking at the liver and the transplanted kidney.

For the liver either the inflow or the outflow can be chosen and in both the principle is to separate the venous from the arterial signals because the normal balance whereby some 25% of hepatic flow is arterial is shifted towards much higher proportions in diseases where there is arteriovenous shunting especially cirrhosis and malignancy.[7]

The inflow measurements were originally made by estimating the flow in the hepatic artery and portal vein using conventional spectral Doppler to obtain the mean flow velocity and multiplying this by the vessels area to obtain the Doppler perfusion index: unfortunately the excellent results initially reported have proved to be difficult to reproduce but a microbubble enhanced DPI promises to be more easily reproduced. In this method a bolus of contrast is tracked using a power Doppler gate that covers both artery and vein and the relative slopes of the two arrival curves are used to derive the two values. In the outflow method a spectral Doppler gate is placed over a hepatic vein and the relative slopes of the two arrival curves is used to derive the two values. In the outflow method a spectral Doppler gate is placed over a hepatic vein and the arrival time of an IV bolus is measured. In both cirrhosis and metastatic disease the arrival time is much earlier than in patients with chronic hepatitis or controls and this may allow early detection and avoid the need for biopsies. For the transplant kidney a spectral doppler gate that covers the artery and the vein and is used to track the arrival time of the bolus and from these the true arteriovenous transit can be calculated.[8] It seems to be longer in rejection than in acute tubular necrosis and so unnecessary biopsies might be avoided.

The regional approach has been used for malignancies seeking to improve differential diagnosis by revealing features of neo-vascularization for example in the liver.[9]

Many studies in the breast show that the arrival time in cancers is earlier than in benign masses though some cases of benign breast change have been confusing especially those that have an inflammatory component.[10]

The lack of vascularity in mature scars in comparison to the marked vascularity of tumor recurrence has emerged as a proven clinical tool for this problem. In liver a variety of temporal patterns have been described that are generally similar to those seen in triple phase CT. Malignancies especially hepatocellular carcinomas fill during the arterial phase a few seconds after injection while regenerating nodules and hemangioma fill slowly, the latter typically from the periphery and usually in complete (Figs. 6.4A to D). Focal nodular hyperplasia shows similar temporal features to malignancies though their liver specific phase discriminates them well (Figs. 6.5A to C).

An interesting way to make use of the fragility of microbubbles is to set up an infusion for steady blood level, apply a destructive pulse to a region of interest and then with non-destructive interrogating pulse watch for reperfusion as the slice fill with microbubbles. This reperfusion kinetic method has been applied to the myocardium where it shows great promise as a way to detect regional perfusion defects caused by anastomotic failures or by rejection.

The liver specific phase of microbubbles seen after the agent has cleared from larger vessel is an example of tissue targeting. It occurs with agents that are phagocytosed by the res such as (sonovist and sonazied) but also with levovist. Clinically this phase is significant because many lesions particularly malignancies do not take up the agents and so are highlighted as microbubble poor spaces.[11]

In this phase, the microbubbles are not moving so conventional doppler does not detect them and they are not obvious on gray scale. Non-linear modes such as color doppler stimulated acoustic emission (SAE) or the phase inversion mode (PIM) imaging are needed for their depiction. The effect is transient especially with a fragile agent such as levovist because it depends on bubble destruction and so special scanning approaches have to be used taking care to minimize inadvertent exposure to

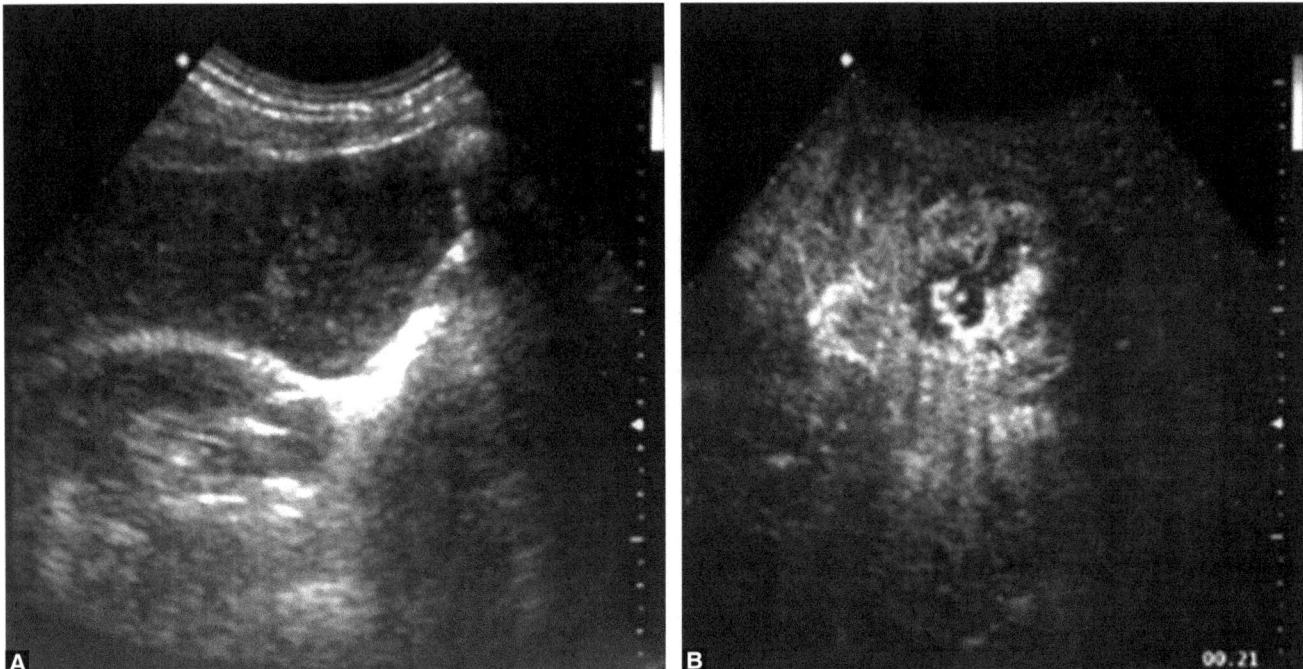

Figs. 6.4A and B: Hepatocellular carcinoma (A) Gray scale image shows a well-defined mixed echogenicity mass lesion in the liver; (B) Early arterial phase image of the lesion after contrast administration shows peripheral enhancement.

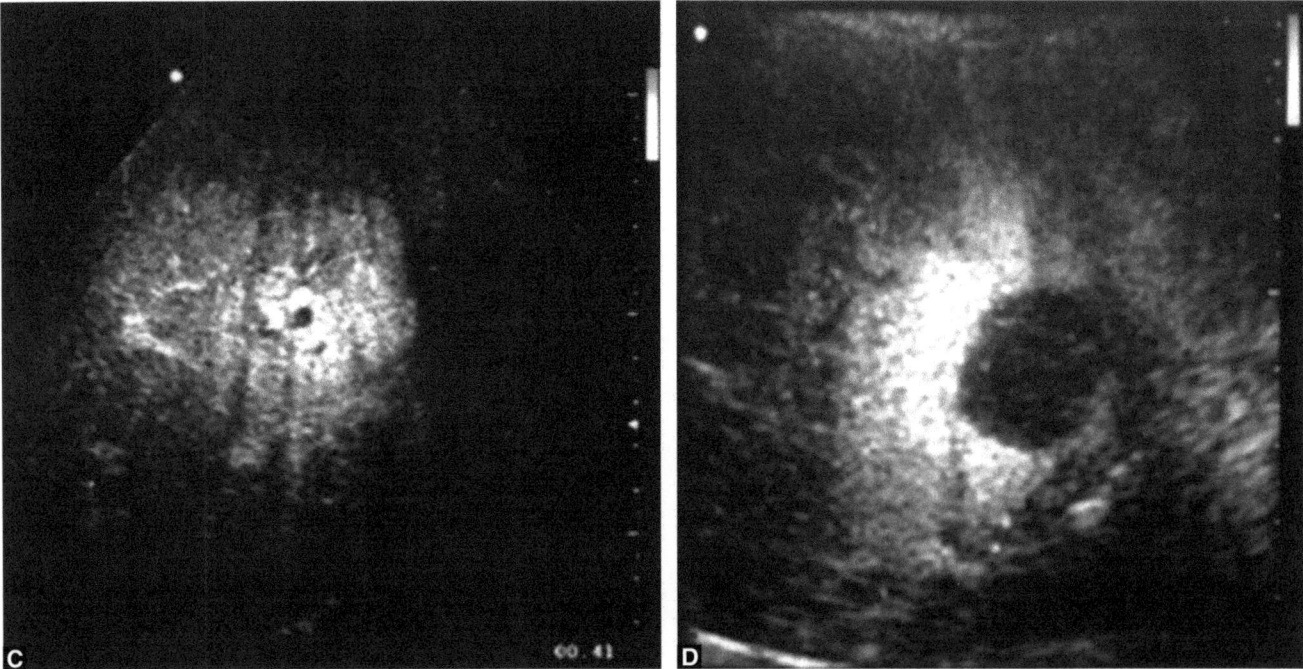

Figs. 6.4C and D: Hepatocellular carcinoma (C) Progressive centripetal enhancement in the lesion is evident in late arterial phase; (D) In the late phase, surrounding liver enhances more than the lesion from which contrast has been washed out, leading to increased lesional conspicuity.

the ultrasound. Allowing the vascular phase to clear (3 min with levovist) then scanning with slow sweeps through the region of interest and then reviewing the images in the cine loop is one practical approach. The scanner needs to be set for maximum output power using a low frequency and with the transmit few at the region of interest maximizing the SAE effect but it may also be possible to employ phase inversion techniques in a non-destruction mode. The effects can be produced in all subjects but are weaker when sound attenuation is high and with levovist fade over 30 min: the best effect is achieved 5-15 min after injection.

The SAE reveals most types of focal lesion as color defects and the increase in conspicuity is striking (Figs. 6.6A and B). In a specific study where two blinded

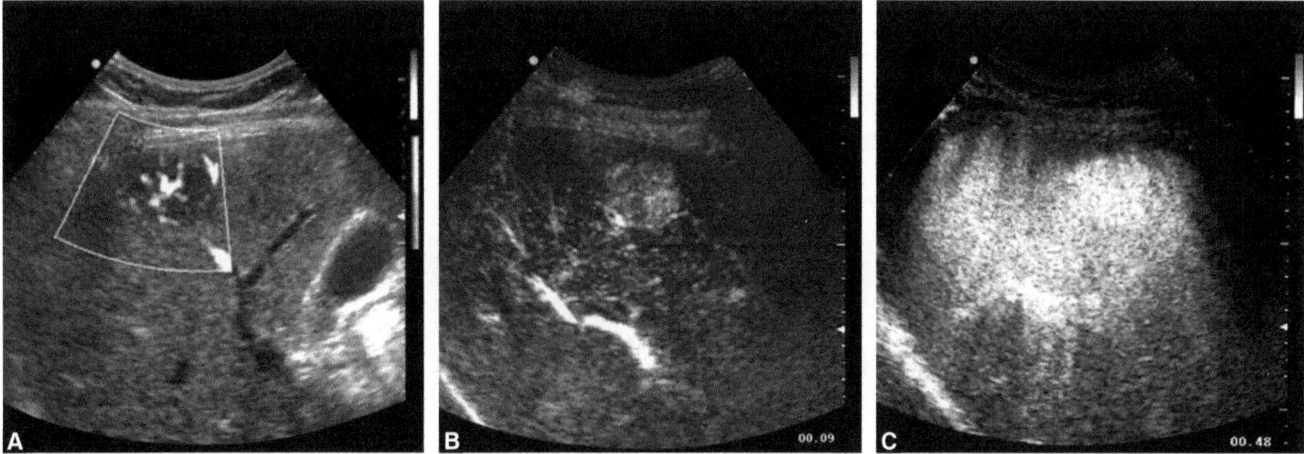

Figs. 6.5A to C: Focal nodular hyperplasia (A) Increased vascularity is evident on power Doppler imaging; (B) Increased vascularity is also seen in early arterial phase, after contrast administration. A branch of right hepatic artery is also well visualized; (C) Late arterial phase image shows progressive contrast enhancement.

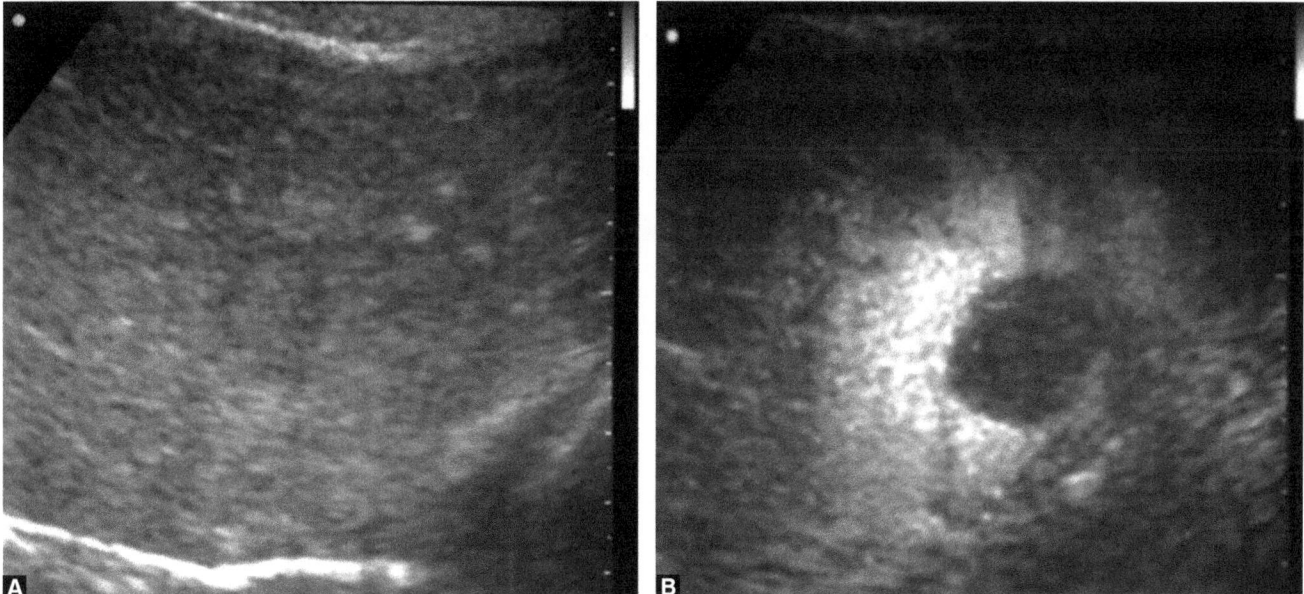

Figs. 6.6A and B: (A) A baseline sonogram shows an ill-defined hypoechoic lesion in the liver; (B) After contrast administration, lesion appears as a color defect and becomes more conspicuous.

observers scored the SAE signal intensity. Both scored all 15 metastases as low SAE with significantly more signal in 4 hemangiomas and in other benign lesions. One observer was able to distinguish hemangiomas from metastases completely, while the other scored an overlap in only one case (a metastasis with moderately high SAE). Scores similar to the surrounding liver were seen in two cirrhotic nodules, two focal fatty change and four focal nodular hyperplasia. High SAE activity seemed to correlate with a benign etiology and scanning in sae mode improved specificity. Initial evaluation of suspected cases of fnh in sae mode might replace sulphur colloid radionuclide scanning.

Pim provides better spatial resolution so that new lesions smaller than 1 cm in diameter can be seen.[12] It exploits the non-linearity of microbubble behavior based on the fact that bubbles are easily expanded by a negative pressure but progressively resist compression by increased pressure. Thus they respond differently to the compression and rarefaction phases of the ultrasound wave and this information can be extracted by summing the echoes from each scan line from two pulses of inverted phase. Tissue returns opposite signals which cancel out but microbubbles give different signals and do not cancel completely. The system has a reduced frame rate but selects for the location of the microbubbles and retains the spatial resolution of gray scale imaging. In a preliminary study of 12 patients being screened for liver metastases strong gray scale signals filling the liver parenchyma were elicited while metastasis appeared as defects even if they were isoechoic on conventional ultrasound.

A multicenter study including 128 patients suspected of having liver metastases confirmed these results with greatly improved sensitivity especially for small (subcentimeter) lesions, fewer false positives and detection of some lesions that were too small to be detected on CT but were seen on gadolinium enhanced MRI.

Although, focal diseases in the liver is the most important application, these agents also collect in normal spleen and this has proved to be useful in distinguishing splenunculus from lymphadenopathy and in detecting small intrasplenic masses such as in lymphoma.

Limitations of both these methods include their transient effect fall off in the far field and artefacts such as shadowing. A difficulty with liver specific phase imaging using levovist is obtaining proof of the nature of the defects seen because the transient effect makes biopsy almost impossible.

This may be resolved with the more persistent agents undergoing clinical trials.

Stimulated acoustic emission (SAE) has relatively poor spatial resolution but has the advantage of intrinsic segmentation since it uses the color doppler circuitry the color signals can easily be separated from the gray scale component so that the exact corres-pondence between the bubble signature and the lesion or tissue seen on gray scale is apparent. PIM has the same spatial resolution as gray scale but the bubble and tissue components are inextricably enlarged and so the two signals cannot be separated.

A recently introduced mode, agent detection imaging (ADI) offers a combination of both features. A development of SAE but using power doppler it depicts the bubble destruction signature as a color overlay with the same spatial resolution as the underlying gray scale scan. It offers the combination of excellent spatial resolution and the ability to view the background and the bubble signals together or separately so that the precise location of the microbubbles can be determined.

The therapeutic potential of microbubbles is a topic of active research.[13,14] They may be used in two ways, to enhance the effects of high intensity focused ultrasound (HIFU) by increasing the amount of energy deposited or by acting as vehicles for therapeutic agents. In this mode, the loaded microbubbles are ruptured at the desired site by applying sufficiently intense sound to achieve a local high concentration of agent, thrombolytic agent or an anticancer drug.

REFERENCES

1. Burns PN. Interpreting and analyzing the Doppler examination. In: Taylor KJW, Burns PN, Wells PNT (Eds). Clinical Applications of Doppler Ultrasound. New York: Raven Press: 1995.pp.55-99.
2. Bauer A, Becker G, Krone A, Frohlich T. Transcranial Duplex sonography using ultrasound contrast enhancers. Clin Radiol. 1996;51:19-23.
3. Missouris CG, Allen CM, Balen FG. Noninvasive screening for renal artery stenosis with ultrasound contrast enhancement. J Hyperten. 1996;14:519-24.
4. Tschammler A, Viesr G, Schindler R. Ultrasound contrast media in vitro studies. J Ultrasound Med. 1993;12:S33.
5. Porter TR, Xie F, Kriesfeld D. Improved myocardial contrast with second harmonic transient ultrasound response imaging in humans using intravenous perfluorocarbon exposed sonicated dextrose albumin. J Am Cell Cardiol. 1996;27:1479-501.
6. Kono Y, Moriyasu F, Yawada K. Conventional and harmonic gray scale enhancement of the liver with sonication activation of a US contrast agent. Radiology. 1996:201.
7. Albrecht T, Blomley MJ, Casgron DO. Non invasion diagnosis of hepatic cirrhosis by transit time analysis of ultrasound contrast agent. Lancet. 1999;353:1579-83.
8. Blomley M, Albrecht T, Eckersley R. Renal arteriovenous transit time measured noninvasively using bolus injections of microbubble contrast. Radiology. 1998;209:461.

9. Wilson SR, Burns PN, Muradati D. Harmonic hepatic US with microbubble contrast agent: initial experience showing improved characteri-sation of haemangioma, hepatocellular carcinoma and metastasis. Radiology. 2000;215:153-61.
10. Albrecht T, Patel N, Cosgrove DO. Enhancement of bower Doppler signals from breast lesions with the ultrasound contrast agent Echogen emulsion: subjective and quantitative assessment. Acad Radiol. 1998;5(Suppl):S195-8, discussion S199.
11. Albrecht T, Blomley M, Wilsons. Improved detection of metastatic liver lesions using pulse inversion harmonic imaging with Levovist a multicenter study. Radiology. 2000; 1685.
12. Harvey C, Blomely M, Eckersley R. Improved detection of hepatic malignancies using pulse inversion mode in the late phase of enhancement with the ultrasound contrast agent Levovist (SHU 508A): Early experiences Radiology (Submitted) 1999.
13. Ho SY, Barbarese E, D'Arrigo JS. Evaluation of lipid coated microbubbles as a delivery vehicle for Taxol in brain tumor therapy. Neurosurg. 1997;40:1260-6, discussion1566-8. Porter TR, Leveen RF, Fox R. Thrombolytic enhancement with perfluorocarbon exposed sonicated dextrose albumen microbubbles. American Heart Journal. 1996;132:964-8.

Cerebrovascular Doppler Sonography

Doppler ultrasound is the principal investigation for patients with possible carotid disease. Indications for Doppler ultrasound of neck arteries are:
- Transient ischemia (TIAs) <24 hours
- Reversible ischemic neurological deficit (rind)
- Preoperative-in high risk groups
- Mild stroke in younger patients, in resolution
- Non-focal symptoms possibly vascular (atypical cases)
- Pulsatile masses
- Following endarterectomy
- Suspected trauma or dissection, including the trauma to vertebral vessels
- As screening measure
- Subclavian steal syndrome
- Posterior fossa ischemia.

A completed stroke does not warrant a carotid Doppler examination as endarterectomy is not likely to be offered, whereas definite benefit is shown for patients with severe stenosis with symptomatic ischemia who undergo endarterectomy in terms of risk for subsequent stroke trials. For asymptomatic bruits value of surgery is less clear.

To know the degree of significant stenosis in relation to need for carotid surgery, studies were conducted in North America and Europe. These two trials differed somewhat in methodology and also in the results. Whereas, North American trial demonstrated some improvement by surgery for the patients with stenosis >50% and definite improvement for stenosis >70%, the European trial put the percentage at 60%, above which the surgery reduced the risk of stroke. Also because of different methods of measuring stenosis the 70% stenosis in the European trial corresponded to 50% reduction in North American trial. Whereas, North American trial compared diameter of stenosed vessel with the normal vessel more distally whereas in European trial, stenosed vessel diameter was compared with the expected normal vessel diameter at the same level. Both trials compared the results with angiography of stenosis which remains the gold standard despite being interobserver assessment, invasive and with interobserver variability.

Patients who are to undergo surgery for peripheral or coronary artery disease, aneurysms or other vascular disease are also at risk and hence, candidates for carotid Doppler sonography.

Following endarterectomy, reocclusion may develop over next 24–40 hours, neointimal hyperplasia between 1–2 years or restenosis over seven years. Therefore, follow-up with carotid ultrasound is mandatory.

TECHNIQUE

For carotid arteries, the patient lies supine with pillow under shoulders and neck turned to opposite side to open the anterior triangle of the neck. Generally, 7-10 MHz frequency transducer is used and transverse scanning from sternoclavicular region up in the neck is first done, followed by longitudinal scanning to outline both carotid arteries (Fig. 7.1). Particular scan plane can be recommended and variety of planes might be used to define the anatomy optimally. In the region of carotid bulb reverse flow may be seen, helping the identification and minimizing the time required. Spectral Doppler is required to assess and quantify the abnormal flow. In the color mode, the position of maximum Doppler shift is sought and cursor is placed accordingly. The angle of insonation and gate range is optimized. The velocity setting and wall filters are adjusted and maximum shift is located by obtaining waveforms.

Cerebrovascular Doppler Sonography | 47

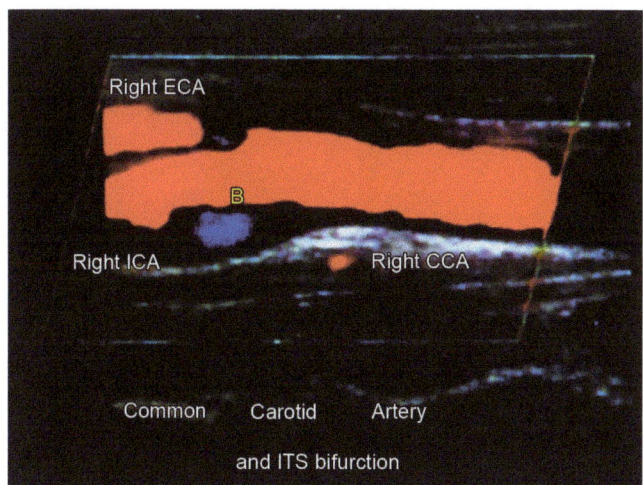

Fig. 7.1: Normal longitudinal color Doppler flow image of the common carotid artery (CCA) and its bifurcation with flow reversal (blue area) appearing at early systole or peak systole.

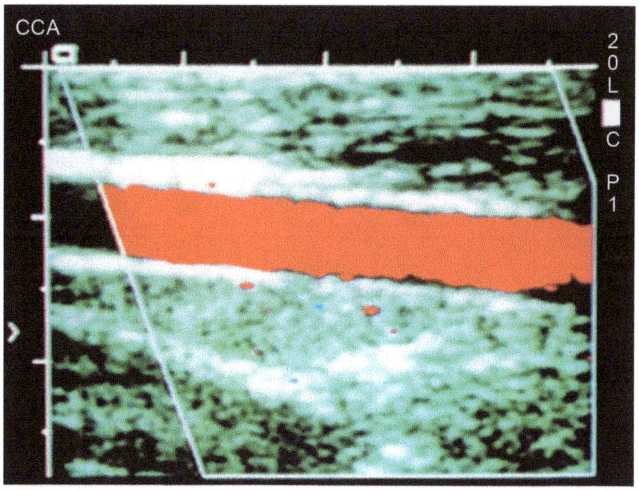

Fig. 7.2: Color Doppler image of common carotid artery (CCA) showing uniform filling of lumen, suggesting presence of laminar flow.

It is important to identify external carotid artery separate from the internal carotid artery, more importantly in the presence of disease, where the distinction may be even more difficult as the significant disease alters the waveform characteristics, blurring the distinction between external carotid and internal carotid flow. In such situations, tapping the superficial temporal artery over zygoma induces the fluctuations in blood flow only in the external carotid artery. Scanning the orbit for the reversal of flow in the ophthalmic artery confirms the significant carotid artery occlusion.

Common carotid and internal carotid artery (ICA) show laminar flow on color image (Fig. 7.2).

The external carotid artery (ECA) may normally be identified by appearance of cervical branches low in the neck, location and particular waveform characteristics such as more pulsatile flow with little flow in diastole (Fig. 7.3) (high resistance pattern) and the prominent dicrotic notch. In contrast to this internal carotid artery shows less pulsatile flow with relatively high diastolic flow and localized widening of bulb at the origin (Fig. 7.4). Waveform of CCA resembles that of ICA (Fig. 7.5).

The intimal thickness is best measured when the carotid artery is in longitudinal section with the ultrasound beam orthogonal to it, and is taken on the far wall, in the magnified image. The cursors are placed between luminal margin of the inner line and the inner margin of the outer line. The normal values are taken to be less than 0.8 mm. (Fig. 7.6).

For the vertebral arteries during the longitudinal scanning in carotid plane the scan plane is rotated laterally till it comes to overlie the lateral masses of cervical vertebrae, the vertebral artery being visible in between the gaps. The artery can also be sought for, low in the neck between the

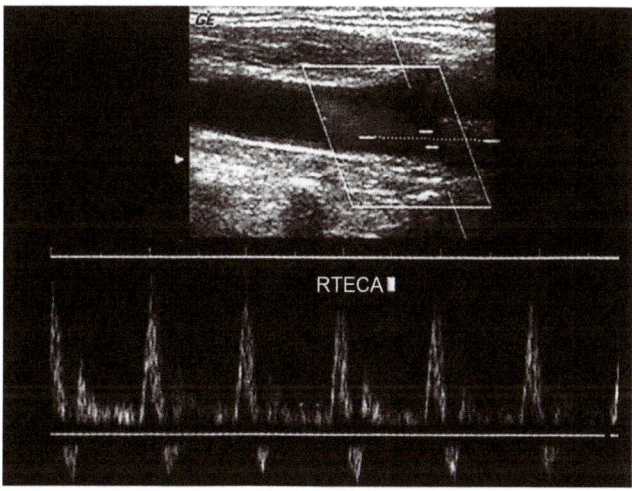

Fig. 7.3: Waveform of normal external carotid artery (ECA) showing triphasic waveform characteristic of arteries supplying muscular bed.

vertebral column and subclavian artery or high in posterior neck when it passes around the lateral mass of atlas. It is also important to evaluate both vertebral arteries at least at two different locations, one lowest and another highest in neck to avoid misinterpretations and missing abnormality in the course of vertebral artery.

The direction of flow in the vertebral arteries should be noted to identify the phenomenon of the subclavian steal. The color flow in the vertebral arteries should be similar to that of the common and internal carotid arteries. This phenomenon can be unmasked in the latent cases by asking patient to do some muscular work by arm or inducing the reactive hyperemia in the arm muscles or by occluding

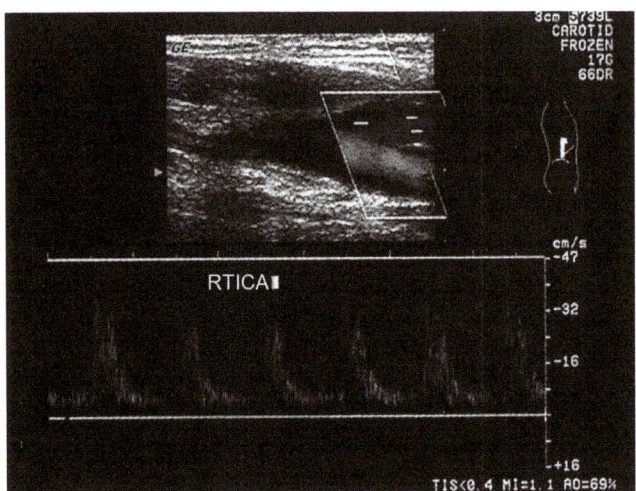

Fig. 7.4: Normal waveform of right internal carotid artery (RTICA) persistent flow is seen during diastole. Spectral window can also be appreciated.

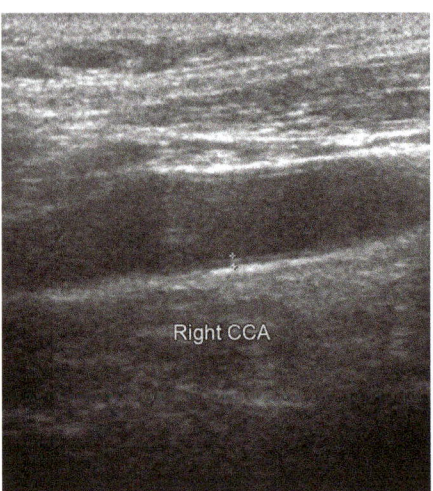

Fig. 7.6: Gray scale image showing how to measure the intimal media thickness in carotid artery.

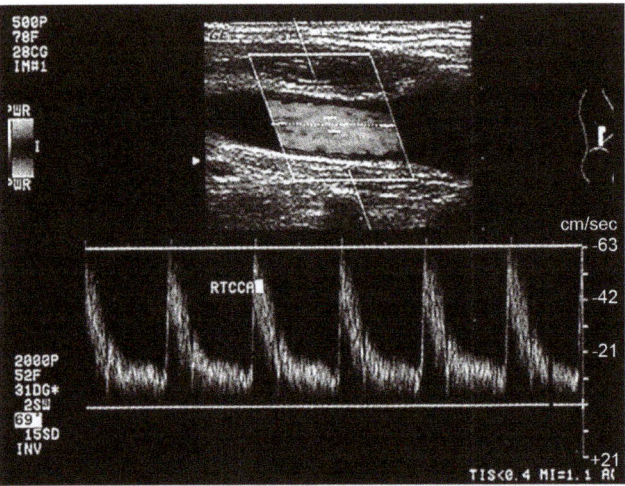

Fig. 7.5: Pulse Doppler of normal carotid artery shows sharp systolic peak with antegrade flow during diastole.

brachial artery with a pressure cuff for 2-3 minutes and then releasing the cuff.

The spectral flow pattern in the vertebral arteries is similar to that of internal carotid arteries with relatively higher diastolic flow except for the PSV which is relatively lower in vertebral arteries.

ABNORMAL FINDINGS

The normal and abnormal flows can be quickly distinguished. The color Doppler is helpful. Though color variations may be seen with cardiac cycle, no areas of persistent color change are seen normally, the presence of which indicates abnormal or turbulent velocity implying the disease in the vessels. The severity of disease or stenosis in the arteries can be quantified either by velocity measurements in the area of narrowing or by direct visualization and measurement of the stenosis.

DOPPLER CRITERIA

In the normal vessels, the peak velocity measurements are taken from common carotid artery about 2-3 cm below the bifurcation, from the internal carotid arteries about 2-3 cm above the bulb and from the external carotid artery about 1-2 cm above the bifurcation.

In the diseased arteries the waveforms are obtained from the areas of maximum velocity. The final position of the sample volume is determined by sound of Doppler shift as well as by the imaging on the screen. When color Doppler is not available it becomes necessary to reduce the size of sample volume and move it slowly around area of stenosis till maximum shift is seen as well as heard, on the speakers.

The internal carotid artery supplies the low resistance capillaries of cerebrum and therefore shows flow throughout the cardiac cycle with appreciable flow even during diastole. The external carotid artery on the other hand supplies the tissues of neck and scalp which have higher resistance and only minimal flow if at all is seen in diastole. Besides, dicrotic notch following peak systole is a rather prominent feature of the waveform.

Of the various indices used for measurements of blood flow, the most important are the peak systolic velocity, end diastolic velocity and the ratio of peak systolic velocities of the internal and the common carotid arteries. The exact normal values and those belonging to different degrees of the stenosis have been quoted differently by various authors because they vary from center-to-center and one equipment to another and on the techniques used. Every center should optimize values for itself, it needs to be pointed out.

The physiological variations due to heart rate (tachycardia), cardiac output, contralateral stenosis or occlusion may affect velocities potentially misdiagnosing the mistakenly pathological velocities. In such cases velocity ratios rather thin single peak velocity should be referred to as a general increase in velocity affect flow in both internal and external carotid arteries, as against the local flow in the internal carotid artery. Otherwise peak systolic and diastolic values refer to just the internal carotid arteries and not to the external carotid and the common carotid arteries.

Very severe degree of stenosis (>90%) with very narrow lumen, results in weak signals and low velocities because of small blood flow through the residual lumen. Hence, it is important to change the settings of the equipment to those geared to detect very low intensity, low velocity signals unless the false diagnosis of occlusion instead of stenosis is made, and the patient gets denied the benefit of surgery. In fact ignoring the subtotally occluded vessel and allowing it to occlude may lead to permanent risk of stenosis of 5% per year.

At the point of maximal narrowing in the carotid vessel the velocity of the moving blood typically increases because of the restriction of the arterial lumen. The compensatory flow develops in collaterals from ipsilateral external carotid artery, vertebral artery or contralateral vessels. This decreases the amount of blood being delivered to diseased artery as a function of increasing stenosis. The positive association is maintained until the stenosis is somewhere near 90-95%.

At the point of maximal narrowing and for about 2 cm distally, despite increased blood velocities cohesive flow is maintained which tends to get dissipated further downwards, because of jet phenomenon. For a distance 1-2 cm therefore, it is possible to get a relatively accurate Doppler tracing in terms of velocity increase caused by stenosis. The point of maximal stenosis however is sometimes masked by calcification. Further a zone of turbulence is established 1-2 cm distal to the area of stenosis. The color Doppler offers a good estimate of the direction of the blood flow. This is achieved by taking multiple longitudinal projections until one projection allow a velocity jet of sufficient magnitude to be measured. It is important to ensure that correct angle correction is applied for the measurement. A deficient algorithm for angle correction especially for linear array transducers leads to the over estimation of stenosis.

The waveforms obtained also depend upon conditions remote from the site of measurement of the disease at a site proximal such as aortic valve abnormalities or stenosis at carotid origin, tend to affect the waveform. The significant distal disease in carotid siphon also increases the pulsatility at proximal sites. Occlusion or severe stenosis in the contralateral carotid artery results in the increased flow velocity in the remaining carotid.

Suggested diagnostic criteria for Doppler diagnosis of various degrees of stenosis are given in Table 7.1.

Criteria for assessing the severity of carotid artery stenosis are shown in Figures 7.7A and B.

Some observers feel that taking only one velocity whether systolic or diastolic for estimating stenosis does not take into account other considerations such as cardiac output change, etc. They propose instead-Internal carotid artery to common carotid artery (at a point 2-4 cm distal to bifurcation) peak systolic velocity ratio to allow for corrections due to change in cardiac output or arrhythmias. But this suffers from the limitation induced by compounding of error in the individual measurement of each velocity. The other velocity ratios proposed are end diastolic velocity in the internal carotid artery divided by and diastolic velocity in the common carotid artery (ii) peak systolic velocity in the internal carotid artery divided by end-diastolic velocity in the common carotid artery.

However, few facts are to be kept note of. Common carotid artery velocities are higher by as much as 10-20 cm near the origin and decrease near the bifurcation. Also, blood flow tends to be more consistent approximately 3 cm from the bifurcation.

DIRECT STENOTIC MEASUREMENTS

This can be either by the diameter reduction or area reduction method. The diameter measurement is quicker

TABLE 7.1: Suggested diagnostic criteria for Doppler diagnosis of various degrees of stenosis.

Diameter reduction	PSV (cm/sec)	PDV (cm/sec)	Systolic VICA/VCCA	Diastolic VICA/VCCA	% Spectral broadening
0	<110	<40	<1.8	<2.6	<30
1–39	<110	<40	<1.8	<2.6	<40
40–59	<130	<40	<1.8	<2.6	<40
60–79	>130	>40	>1.8	>2.6	>40
80–99	>250	>100	>3.7	>5.5	>80

(PSV: peak systolic velocity; PDV: peak diastolic velocity; VICA: velocity in the internal carotid artery; VCCA: velocity in the common carotid artery)

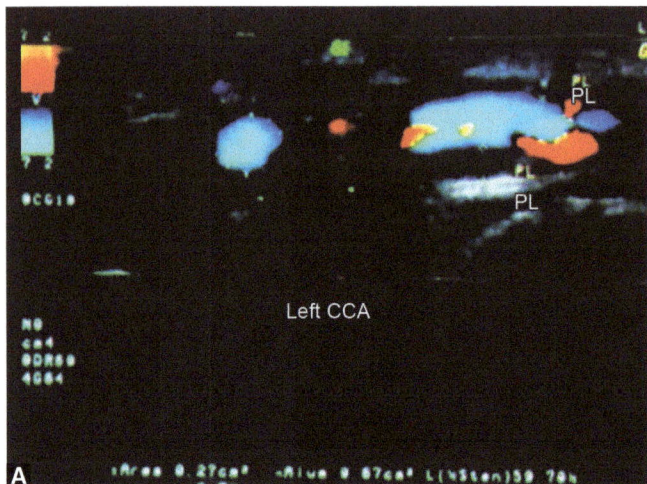
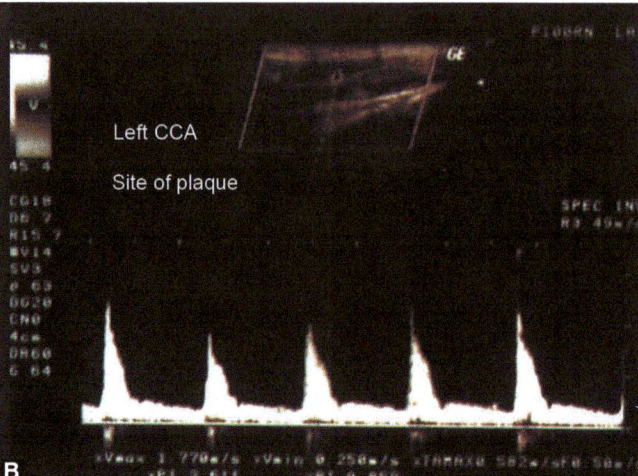

Figs. 7.7A and B: (A) CDFI of the common carotid artery shows approximately 60% area stenosis; (B) Duplex scanning through the area of stenosis demonstrates increased peak systolic velocity, consistent with >60% luminal narrowing (STENOSIS).

but area reduction measured in the transverse section does take into account the effect of asymmetrical plaques. A reduction of diameter by 50% will correspond to the area reduction of approximately 70% and these two are not just interchangeable as such. For the purpose of measurement in the transverse image color and power Doppler are helpful but it needs to be ensured that Doppler gain settings are set optimally so that not only better assessment of boundaries of residual lumen be made but also the distinction between peripheral poorly reflective plaque and inadequate color filling because of suboptimal gain settings be made.

The distinction between complete occlusion and severe stenosis which is important from treatment point of view can be achieved with color Doppler. The accuracy of Doppler ultrasound as described in the literature is quite high. As per one report Doppler had an overall sensitivity of 96%, specificity as high as 86% and negative predictive value of 94%, positive predictive value of 89% for the significant stenosis (diameter <50%).

PLAQUE CHARACTERISTICS

It has been known that softer, more delicate lipid-rich plaques are more likely to fracture and dislodge than firm, more fibrotic, coherent plaques. Based on the plaque characteristics it has been suggested that symptoms relating to carotid artery disease are more common with echopoor type 1 and 2 than echo-reflective type 3 and 4.

Classification (Steffen) of Plaque Morphology

Type 1 : Predominantly echo poor with thin reflective cap (Fig. 7.8)

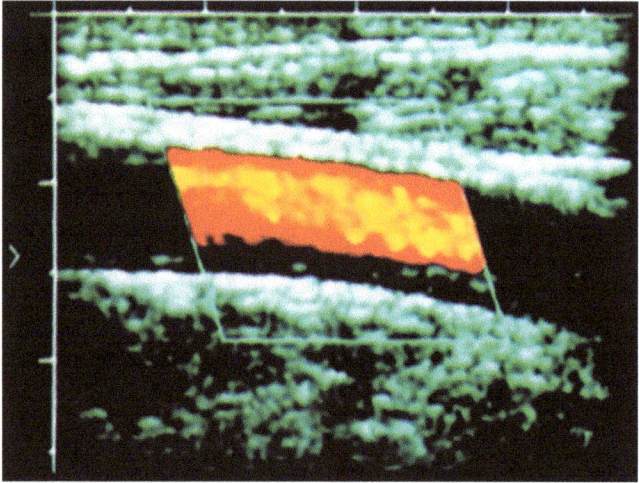

Fig. 7.8: Power Doppler image of common carotid artery showing smooth, thin, homogeneous plaque in the posterior wall.

Type 2 : Substantially echo poor with small areas of increased reflectivity (Fig. 7.9)

Type 3 : Predominantly reflective lesions with areas of low reflectivity accounting for less than 25%

Type 4 : Uniformly reflective types.

There can be various complications which the plaques might undergo. They may undergo hemorrhage which may suddenly increase in size. The surface disruption may lead to release of plaque content in the bloodstream. The thrombus may form on the ulcerated surface and may break off with distal embolization. The results of correlating the risk of stroke with attempted ultrasound visualization of ulcerated plaques and intra-plaque hemorrhage have not been very successful. There are a few limitations of ultrasound interpretations of surface characteristics

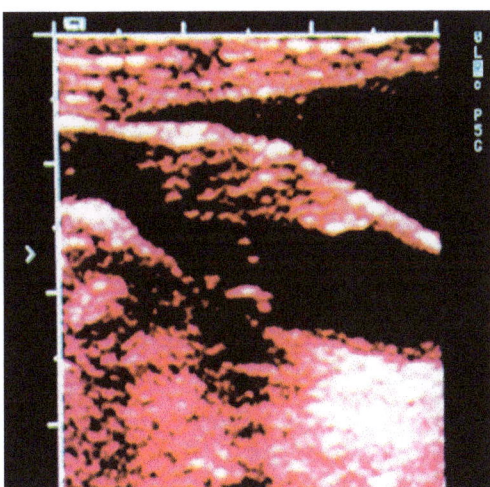

Fig. 7.9: B-mode image of distal common carotid artery showing a homogeneous plaque causing significant narrowing of lumen.

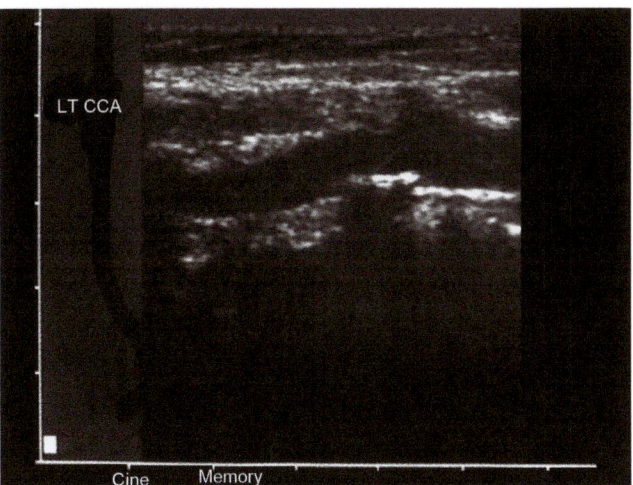

Fig. 7.10: B-mode image of common carotid artery shows a densely calcified plaque in the posterior wall with posterior acoustic shadowing.

as well. The echopoor areas in the plaque may be due to hemorrhage or due to an aggregation of lipids. The apparent ulceration on sonography may be due to a breach on the plaque surface or because of an irregular but intact surface. Further, some plaques might be visualized clearly while others may not show a clear outline. However, overall a homogenous, smoothly outlined, predominantly reflective plaque is less likely to have symptoms while a heterogeneous, irregular, echo-poor lesion is more likely to have symptoms or complications.

Based on signals or echogenicity the plaques can be characterized as higher intensity, hyperechoic or isoechoic. The high intensity and hyperechoic signals are comparable to the fascial layers or, adventitial layer of the artery while isoechoic signals are compared to those returning from muscle of neck. Both of these represent fibrous constituents of plaque. It is helpful to differentiate them from hypoechoic signals within the plaque which by definition have echogenicity similar to blood and represent lipid, hemorrhage or smooth muscle proliferation.

The newer advances in ultrasound technology allow rendering of 3D reconstruction of acquired images and help improve conspicuity and better define the extent of pathology. This can be used to advantage for showing complex tortuousity of carotid arteries and their branches.

Contrast enhanced imaging of carotid arteries can be done by injecting US contrast agents or by altering the sensitivity of ultrasound machine to detect signals emitted by moving blood. This can be helpful for evaluating patients with difficult anatomy. Further, contrast agents improved conspicuity of luminal interface and improve visualization and characterization of plaque and analyse residual lumen. Further improvement is achieved by the digital encoding scheme that increases ultrasound delivery and also increase signal intensity or reflected signals of returning echoes from moving blood cell. This has the potential for mapping more accurately plaque characteristic such as ulceration.

An almost totally hypoechoic plaque or the one which is centrally hypoechoic with a rim of increased echogenicity is classified as homogeneously hypoechoic. On the other hand a plaque which is homogeneously echogenic is classified as homogenously hyperdense plaque. Of heterogeneous plaques, the one with >5% plaque elements hyperechoic are labeled as heterogeneously hyperechoic while those with more than 50% hypoechoic are calcified plaques may also be seen (Fig. 7.10) classified as heterogeneous hypoechoic.

Surface characters of plaque too may have some impact in patients with acute neurological symptoms because of extent of surface irregularity and its relation to transient ischemic attack like symptoms. By definition an ulcer is an inter-plaque defect or excavation greater than 2 × 2 mm. Unfortunately, neither gray scale ultrasound nor angiogram is very sensitive or specific in this regard. Color Doppler may help by showing areas of flow reversal within the matrix of plaque.

A classification has been prescribed incorporating the plaque characteristics, surface outline and degree of stenosis into one. This classification (Thiele) is as given below:

1. Hemodynamic
   H_1 0–20% diameter reduction : Normal to mild
   H_2 20–60% diameter reduction : Moderate
   H_3 60–80% diameter reduction : Severe
   H_4 80–90% diameter reduction : Critical
   H_5 occluded (Fig. 7.11)
2. Morphological components
   P_1 homogeneous
   P_2 heterogeneous

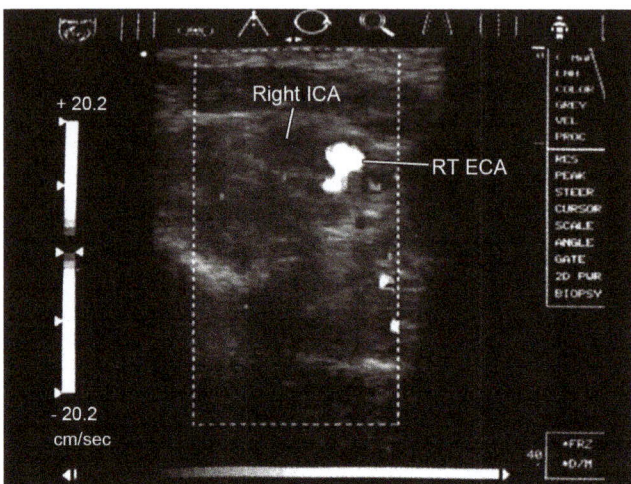

Fig. 7.11: Transverse color flow image just above the carotid bifurcation shows complete lack of color filling of internal carotid artery suggesting thrombosis. External carotid artery shows normal flow.

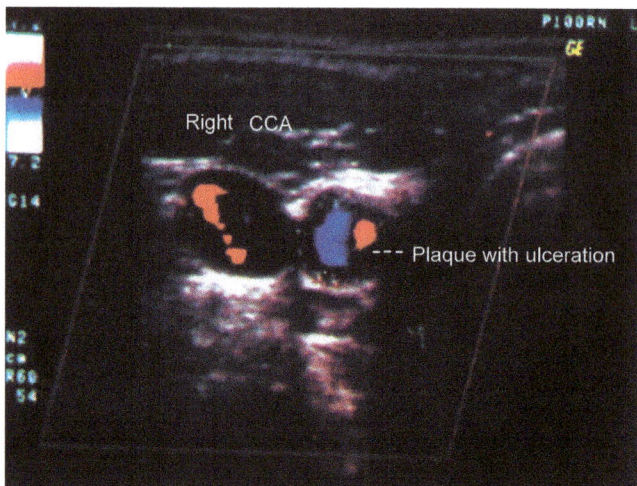

Fig. 7.12: Transverse color Doppler image of common carotid artery shows a hypoechoic plaque with area of reversed low velocity flow suggesting presence of plaque ulceration.

3. Surface characteristics
   S_1 smooth
   S_2 irregular (defect <2 mm)
   S_3 ulcerated (defect >2 mm) (Fig. 7.12).

A lesion classified $H_4 S_2 P_2$ as above will correspond to the 80% diameter reduction. The degree of narrowing can also be quantified in terms of area stenosis (Figs. 7.13A to C).

Carotid Occlusion

While carotid stenosis, even the critical one may be salvageable by surgery but carotid occlusion is not. Hence, distinction is of clinical importance and should be made by color Doppler, power Doppler or by the use of echo-enhancer agents. A number of pitfalls need to be avoided as small external carotid artery branches close to the occluded internal carotid artery. Another pitfall is when internal carotid artery occludes while external and common carotid arteries are patent. The waveform in common carotid artery might reflect external carotid artery circulation with reduced or absent diastolic flow. On the other hand, in case of significant diversion of flow to internal carotid circulation via ophthalmic and meningeal arteries the waveform is more like internal carotid artery with substantial diastolic flow, called the internalization of external carotid artery. Still another situation may arise because occlusion of the common carotid artery may not always result in the occlusion of internal carotid artery. While the patency might be maintained by the retrograde collateral flow down the external carotid artery, these patients still remain at the risk of significant brain ischemia in the distribution of the internal carotid artery.

KEY POINTS

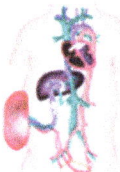

Carotid Doppler
- For stenosis–PSV, PDV, systolic and diastolic pressure and % of spectral broadening should be taken into consideration.
- In plaque—symptoms related to carotid artery are more common with echopoor type 1 and 2 than echo reflector type 3 and 4.
- Contrast enhanced imaging—improve visualization and characteristics of plaque.

Carotid Dissection

The causes can be as variable as spontaneous, because of atheroma, extension of the aortic dissection up the carotids, following hyper-extension neck injury or iatrogenic during angiography. The appearances on ultrasound too may vary. There may be complete occlusion of vessels or a smoothly tapered stenosis with or without hematoma or thrombosis of false lumen might be recognizable. Alternatively, on Doppler ultrasound double lumen with variable flow pattern in two channel may be seen. Recanalization of occluded lumen may be seen in as high as 60% of the cases.

Pulsatile Neck Masses

Pulsatile neck masses can be due to prominent carotid bulb, ectatic neck arteries, enlarged lymph nodes adjacent to carotid sheath, carotid artery aneurysm or carotid body tumors. Prominent and ectatic arteries can be easily made by Doppler ultrasound. Enlarged nodes too can be easily

Cerebrovascular Doppler Sonography

made out. Fixity or invasion to carotid sheath is made out by scanning while patient swallows.

Carotid Aneurysms

May arise because of mural degeneration, atheroma or following trauma. While aneurysm itself may be visible on ultrasound, patent lumen above carotid aneurysm may not be clearly seen. The evidence of flow in the ophthalmic artery on the same side may not indicate patency, as it may come from opposite side via circle of Willis.

Carotid Body Tumors

Characteristically spread and separate the two arteries, the internal and external carotids. Poorly reflective and highly vascular mass is seen on ultrasound at bifurcation. The external carotid artery may show low resistance pattern.

VERTEBRAL ARTERIES

The clinical significance of the disease in the vertebral arteries as compared with the carotid arteries is far less clear, because basilar artery and posterior circulation is supplied by two vertebral arteries and connected to circle of Willis allowing compensatory flow unless both vertebral arteries are narrowed. Failure to visualize vertebral arteries in the locations suggested (as above) might be due to congenital absence or hypoplasia. The altered waveform may be seen because of localized disease in the form of color and spectral evidence in the segment being examined. Alternatively, damped waveforms may be due to involvement of proximal vertebral artery or subclavian disease.

In case of proximal subclavian stenosis, phenomenon of subclavian steal may occur. Blood reaches affected arm down (instead of up) the ipsilateral vertebral artery from posterior circulation which itself gets supplied from opposite side. Thus posterior circulation get stolen. The direction of flow can be made out on Doppler.

Transcranial Doppler Ultrasound

In the neonates the assessment of midline intracranial structures dates back to the days of A scan. The high quality images and Doppler studies could be obtained recently through fontanelles and thin calvarial bones recently. In 1982 Aaslid first described pulsed transcranial Doppler for adults. Since then techniques of pulsed transcranial Doppler have been further refined. More recently improvement in technology has allowed realtime color transcranial Doppler, providing useful physiological,

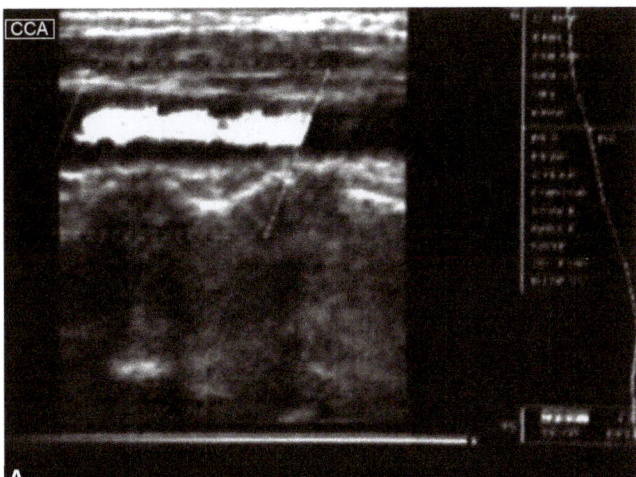
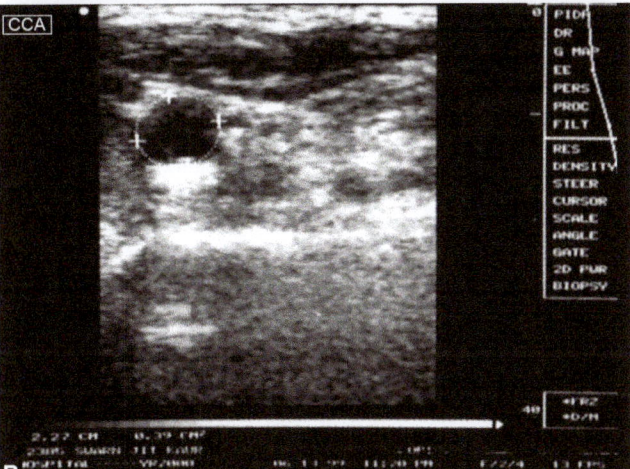
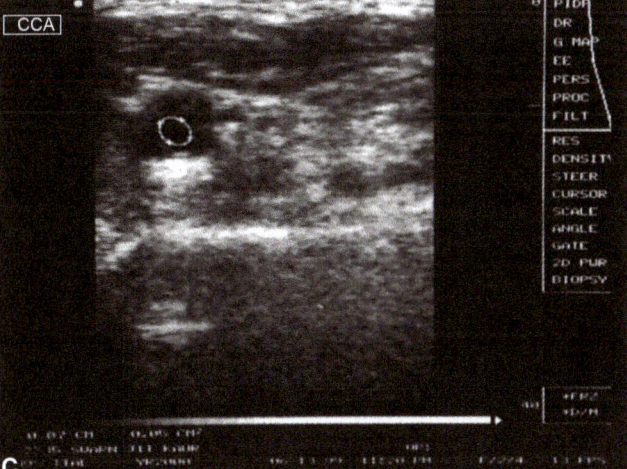

Figs. 7.13A to C: (A) Color Doppler image of common carotid artery shows narrowing of lumen due to circumferential wall thickening; (B) Transverse section showing circumferential wall thickening; (C) Measurement of area of vessel and residual lumen by electronic calipers shows 87% area stenosis.

pathological and pharmacological information and also including intraoperative and postoperative monitoring of endarterectomy patients.

The main problem in the transcranial Doppler is attenuation and scattering of ultrasound beam by vault not only at soft tissue/bone interface but also at multiple interfaces in the skull vault. The attenuation is greater in older patients, females and the black subjects.

Anatomy

The internal carotid artery as it exits up the cavernous sinus at the base of brain in the region of basal cisterns divides into three branches. The anterior cerebral artery turns forwards, up and medially to run around corpus callosum. The middle cerebral artery passes laterally into the sylvian fissure and then posteriorly and superiorly in the fissure towards the parietal region. The two vertebral arteries enter the skull through foramen magnum and form the basilar artery at the base of the brain at the lower border of pons. The basilar artery runs anterior to pons to divide at its upper border into two posterior cerebral arteries. The posterior cerebral arteries pass around cerebral peduncles supply the occipital lobe.

The complete, classic circle of Willis is seen only in 50-60% of cases, the most common variation is absence or hypoplasia of anterior cerebral artery (20%), the supply being maintained by the opposite anterior cerebral artery through anterior communicating artery. Similarly proximal posterior cerebral artery may be absent, the supply coming from the ipsilateral internal carotid artery via posterior communicating artery (30%).

Examinations Technique

The three main access portals are transtemporal, suboccipital and transorbital window.

The transtemporal window renders visualization of circle of Willis and all it's major branches. The transorbital window provides alternative access for internal carotid arteries, anterior cerebral artery, and ophthalmic artery. The low frequency (2 MHz) is used with maximum possible sensitivity settings and maximum possible power for adult except in transorbital window to avoid excessive insonation and damage to lens. For neonates, lowest possible power output is to be maintained regardless of the window to be used.

Transtemporal Window

The side of this window is quite big and search is to be made for the thinner segment. The generous application of gel is required to avoid air-pockets trapped between hairs of patient. The transducer is to be placed above and in front of external auditory meatus and a transverse (axial) section is taken. Failure to visualize the cerebral peduncle, third ventricles and perisellar region constitutes inadequate visualization. Good visualisation of brain ensures proper and successful Doppler scan of blood vessels unless pathological. In 10 percent of cases (elderly) completely impenetrable temporal bone is present precluding visualization. Ipsilateral middle cerebral artery (MCA) can be traced back to the region of the circle of Willis and to subsequent branches with some cranial caudad angling of the probe. It may not be possible to get full circle of Willis on one scan and the communicating arteries may not be seen at all because of their small size or congenital absence. The direction of flow is to be noted particularly in the proximal anterior cerebral arteries (ACAs), as they are the major source of collateral pathways. Spectral Doppler gives this information rather than power Doppler which is more sensitive for locating the flow. The use of echo enhancer agents improves visualization considerably above either of these. The proximal and distal segments of PCA are visible around the peduncles to the inferior aspect of occipital lobe. The termination of basilar artery is seen in 56% of cases more often with power Doppler.

The internal carotid artery (ICA) is examined by angling probe interiorly lying as it is in the region of the foramen lacerum and then angling it progressively more superiorly. The ICA termination is also visualized by turning transducer through 90% and scanning medial side of middle cranial fossa, requiring several planes because of the curves of carotid siphon.

Suboccipital Window

The location is midline posteriorly at the level of hairline and directing probe upwards towards the foramen magnum. The visualization is improved by scanning just to the side of midline to avoid dense midline ligaments. The third part of vertebral artery is seen running upwards towards foramen magnum. The junction of vertebral arteries to from basilar artery may be seen if it lies low enough.

Transorbital Window

The beam is directed upwards and medially towards the apex of orbit. The structures visualized are ophthalmic artery, carotid siphon and the contralateral ACA. With power output reduced to minimum, transducer is put over closed eyelid using sterile aqueous gel instead of ultrasound gel. The color transducers being heavy and bulky find limitation with this approach but need to do so is reduced as ACAs are well-visualized by transtemporal approach.

The flow in the ophthalmic artery should be assessed close to the orbit rather than just behind the eye as the flow in the retinal artery is towards the eye. There is collateral circulation in the mid and posterior orbit between orbital branches of external carotid artery and ophthalmic artery to supply circle of Willis in case of ipsilateral ICA blockade.

Transcranial Pulsed Doppler

The ordinary transcranial Doppler has a role to play when color Doppler equipment is not available or cannot be used example in theaters where the space at the side of patient head is insufficient.

Using the transtemporal window the bifurcation can usually be detected at a depth of 65 mm and the flow in MCA is towards the probe while that in the ACA is away from it. Both arteries are then followed by adjusting the greater and lesser depth. The MCA is located at a shallow depth of 35 mm while ACA is located between 65-75 mm and angulating more anteriorly. The patency of ACA can be confirmed by the flow reversal in response to compression of ipsilateral carotid in the neck, but is to be avoided.

The PCA is located by angulating the probe posteriorly, at a depth of 55 mm as it curves round brainstem. The signal direction is towards that of probe normally. Further down as PCA is tracked medially to termination of BA at a depth of >5 mm signal is biphasic. Small changes in probe angle are required to trace the path of the arteries.

The carotid siphon is identified at 55-70 mm through transorbital approach. The direction of flow obviously varies as per anatomy, i.e. towards the probe in lower part and away from the probe in the upper part). The vertebral arteries are located through suboccipital approach at 40-70 mm. The origin of basilar artery is 15 mm deeper at 70-80 mm and passes anterior to brainstem still deeper at 100 mm.

The highest velocities are seen in the MCA followed by ACA, PCA, BA, and the ICA in the last. All velocities decline with age. The peak or mean MCA velocities should not vary by more than 20%.

	Peak velocities (Age 40–60 years)		Mean velocities	
	Mean	Range	Mean	Range
MCA	91	57–125	58	35–81
ACA	86	46–127	53	32–74
PCA	60	19–101	37	17–56

Applications

Applications of color and pulsed TCD are:
- Identification of occluded/stenosed arteries and collateral pathways
- Investigation in the setting of vasospasm complicating SAH
- Investigation of brain death
- Assessing the venous system
- During carotid surgery and neuro-intensive care
- Emboli detection
- Estimating the cerebral perfusion reserve
- Detection of intracranial aneurysms and identifying large feeders to AVMs.

Indications vary from institution to institution and also depend upon the logistic involved. Color Doppler systems are more bulky. Hence, for ICU, theater or immobile ward patient, smaller pulsed system is used though color Doppler gives better waveform and velocity information. Pulsed Doppler system is better for monitoring cerebral perfusion reserve and emboli counting.

Cerebral Perfusion Reserve

Prior to carotid endarterectomy the ability of cerebral vessels to dilate in response to breath-holding, CO_2 rebreathing or acetazolamide challenge is noted. Some vascular surgeons do not find this useful. They think adequacy of patency of anterior and posterior communicating arteries (collateral pathways) is enough.

Emboli Counting

It is done by identifying characteristic embolic noise correctly. It requires sensitive equipment, time (minimum 20 minutes recording, optimally 60 minutes), quality control and rigorous training. Emboli are more frequent with tight stenosis, before starting aspirin therapy. They might also be present with heart valves, though that remains unproven. A related application of embolus detection is identifying patent foramen ovale.

Patient Monitoring

By pulsed, TCD is done when prolonged monitoring is required, e.g. neurointensive care, during neurosurgical operations or carotid arterial operations. The MCA is insolated with probe fixed to temporal region with a head band. A fall in diastolic velocity and increase in pulsatility give indirect measure of cerebral flow and rising ICP.

The TCD is used by some surgeons during carotid endarterectomy for monitoring. The effect of clamping carotid is monitored to assess the need for shunting. Also, during shunt insertion and removal tiny air embolisms is a part of procedure though showers of multiple and recurrent embolism is a cause for concern. Particulate emboli produce coarser sound. Postoperatively, cerebral blood flow is to be monitored.

Ischemic Stroke

Color TCD is better for this purpose. It is useful for monitoring the revascularization therapy or to detect intracranial stenosis which might be the cause for TIAs in patients in whom no disease in the neck is present.

Subarachnoid Hemorrhage

To diagnose ischemic neurological deficit. The intracranial velocities always rise following SAH and if severe enough can result in neurological defect or deterioration of consciousness. The diagnosis includes excluding other causes of neurological deterioration and by finding markedly elevated velocities (e.g. >150 cm/sec) in MCA. The velocities may be elevated in all or one artery. It may not be consistently predicted which patient will develop vasospasm, based on velocity measurements.

Aneurysms and AV Malformations

Though initial results have shown promise it is early to say whether ruptured or unruptured aneurysms can be reliably shown.

Cerebral Venous Thrombosis

The TCD can be used to assess the intracranial veins and venous sinuses. In superior sagittal sinus blockage venous flow is increased in veins running parallel to MCA to the cavernous sinus thus bypassing blocked sagittal sinus. A variety of abnormal drainage patterns may be identified though reliability of this is being questioned.

Transcranial Doppler Sonography

INTRODUCTION

Transcranial Doppler (TCD) sonography is an emerging technique in which a hand held transducer is used to measure velocities within the circle of Willis and vertebrobasilar system through regions of calvarial thinning, orbits or foramen magnum. This technique is very useful in certain clinical conditions to assess the intracranial vasculature, because it is a noninvasive, nonionizing and a portable technique that is safe for serial or prolonged studies. However, variations in arteries and lack of a good temporal window can be source of error or incomplete studies. Therefore, for proper use of TCD, understanding of its limitations, knowledge of cerebral hemodynamics and vascular anatomy as well as correlation with clinical situation is necessary.

BASIC INSTRUMENTATION

For TCD, excellent signal-to-noise ratio is necessary. Therefore, the available TCD machines have a lower bandwidth and secondarily a larger and less well-defined sample volume than most other pulse Doppler instruments. TCD is performed using low frequency transducer (2-3 MHz), sensitive to Doppler frequencies up to 10 kHz without aliasing and adjustable levels of transmitted sound energy ranging from 10 mW/cm^2 to the currently recommended maximal level of 100 mW/cm^2. Commercially available TCD scanners with color capability have recently been introduced (Fig. 8.1). Transcranial color Duplex sonography technique allows correction of angle of insonation resulting in more accurate estimation of flow velocities. It is also more reproducible and shortens the examination time.[1]

Recently, TCD machines with dual monitoring capability have become available in which two transducers are used

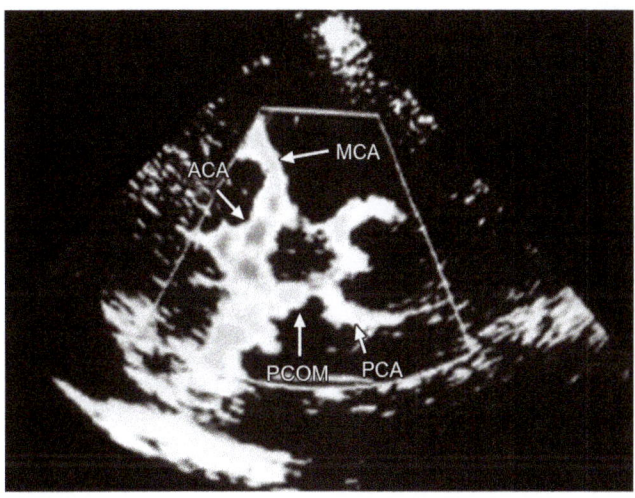

Fig. 8.1: Color Duplex TCD image (transtemporal window) shows circle of Willis including middle cerebral artery (MCA), anterior cerebral artery (ACA), posterior cerebral artery (PCA) and posterior communicating artery (PCOM)

to monitor two arteries simultaneously. These probes are synchronized to insonate during the silent period of the other probe. This dual monitoring capability gives better assessment in monitoring during carotid or cardiac surgery. They are also useful to distinguish carotid or cardiac source of emboli and shorten the examination time in emboli detection techniques. Special high frequency transducers (20 MHz) are also available to directly assess the intracranial arteries during surgery.[1]

TECHNIQUE AND NORMAL PARAMETERS

Before starting the intracranial vascular examination, the examiner should ascertain the status of extracranial arteries, because changes in the extracranial system will reflect on intracranial vessels.

The preferred position for the examiner is at the head end of the bed. The patient's head should face forward or, to the side during the insonation. The patient should be resting comfortably to avoid major fluctuations of PCO_2 (alteration in arterial PCO_2 will alter intracranial flow) and movement artifacts.

Ultrasonic Windows

The transmission of ultrasound through the cranium is a significant problem. Experiments have shown that loss of ultrasound energy depends upon the thickness of the skull. Therefore, loss of transmission varies greatly in different parts of the skull in the same patient, and from patient to patient. The temporal window is an attractive area for ultrasound evaluation because of absence of bony specula and is generally the most useful site of the examination.[2] The other useful TCD approaches are transorbital, suboccipital, and submandibular approaches.[1,2]

Another important concept to understand is regarding the vessel identification. Most of the TCD machines used worldwide do not have the color imaging capability. Therefore, instead of direct visual identification, other criteria are described for vessel identification as listed in Table 8.1.[1]

KEY POINTS

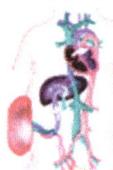

TCD: Technique and windows
- **Technique:**
  - Examiner should be at the head end of the bed
  - Patient head forward or to the side during insonation
- **Ultrasonic windows:**
  - Transtemporal
  - Transorbital
  - Suboccipital
  - Submandibular

TABLE 8.1: Criteria for vessel identification.

Cranial window used
Depth of sample volume
Direction of blood flow
Distance over which the vessel can be traced (traceability)
Relationship to TICA-MCA-ACA junction
Angle of transducer
Relative blood velocity (MCA > ACA > PCA = BA = VA)
Response to compression maneuvers

(ACA: anterior cerebral artery; BA: basilar artery; MCA: middle cerebral artery; PCA: posterior cerebral artery; TICA: terminal internal carotid artery; VA, vertebral artery)

Transtemporal Window

The gel-coated transducer is placed just anterior to the external auditory canal. At the depth of approximately 65 mm, flow can be detected towards the transducer, which is due to middle cerebral artery (Fig. 8.2). By decreasing the depth in approximately 5 mm increments, the artery can be traced, confirming that it is middle cerebral artery. After this the bifurcation of the terminal internal carotid artery is identified at depth of 60–65 mm by its bidirectional flow (Fig. 8.3). Terminal internal carotid artery shows bidirectional flow because sample volume generally includes origin of both middle and anterior cerebral arteries. Anterior cerebral artery can be insonated at depth of 75 mm by tilting the transducer anterosuperiorly (Fig. 8.4). It shows the flow away from the transducer. After returning to the bifurcation of terminal internal carotid artery and tilting the transducer inferiorly, the examiner can obtain a tracing of the terminal portion of the internal carotid artery. It characteristically exhibits the lowest velocity of the anterior vessels because of the large angle of insonation necessary for localization.

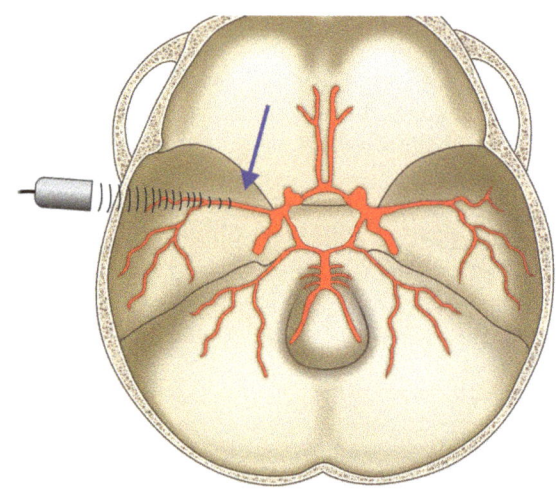

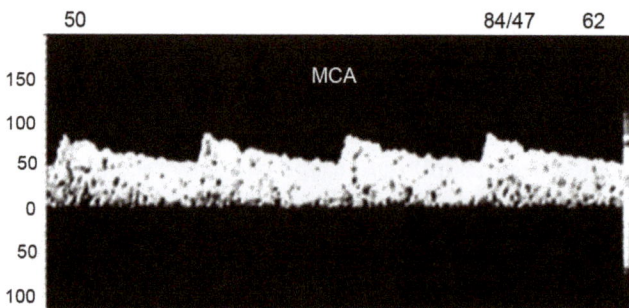

Fig. 8.2: Middle cerebral artery: Picture depicting middle cerebral artery insonation through transtemporal approach and spectral waveform from the artery showing low resistance waveform with flow towards the transducer.

Transcranial Doppler Sonography

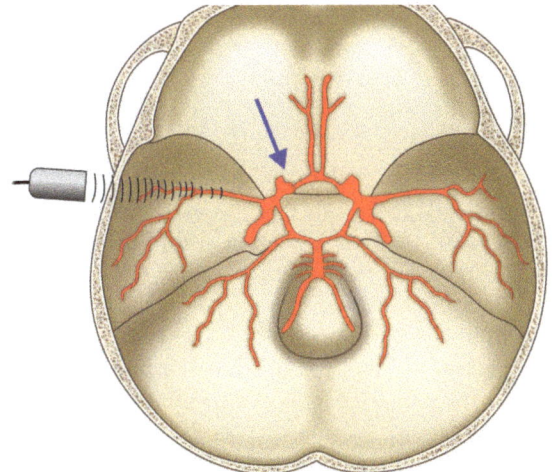

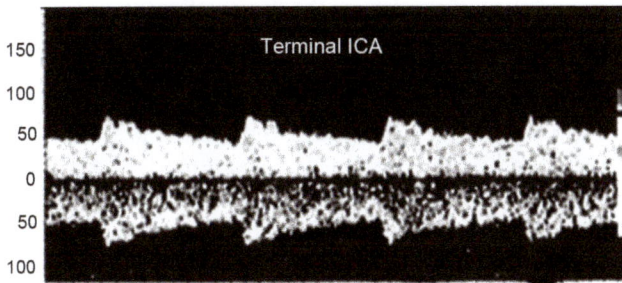

Fig. 8.3: Internal carotid artery (terminal portion): Picture depicting terminal carotid artery insonation through transtemporal approach and spectral waveform from the artery showing typical bidirectional flow.

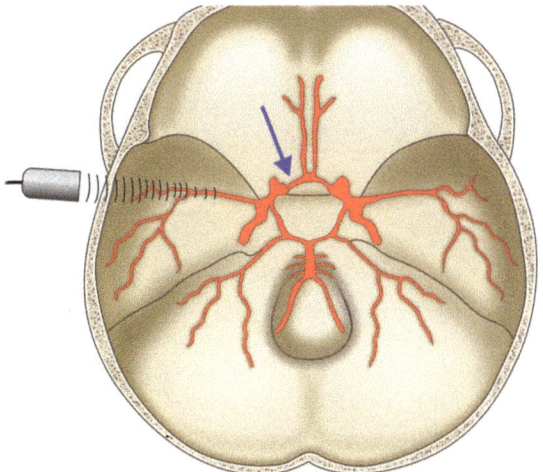

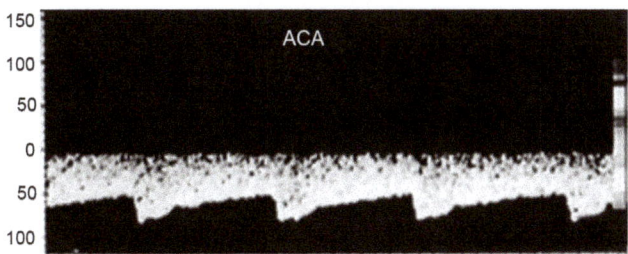

Fig. 8.4: Anterior cerebral artery: Picture depicting anterior cerebral artery insonation through transtemporal approach and spectral waveform from the artery showing low resistance waveform with flow away from the transducer.

Finally, the posterior cerebral artery (PCA) can be insonated at depth of 60–75 mm by tilting the transducer posteroinferiorly. The posterior cerebral artery can than be tracked to the basilar artery (BA) at approximately 75 mm depth and from there to the contralateral posterior cerebral artery (80–85 mm). The display of bilateral blood flow at the junction with the BA and the change in flow direction within the contralateral posterior cerebral artery can be useful features to identify the posterior cerebral artery.

Transorbital Window

Gel-coated transducer is gently applied on the closed eyelid and lowest acoustic intensity (10 mW/cm^2) is used to minimize the risk of eye damage.[3] Ophthalmic artery is usually insonated at depth of 45–60 mm by scanning in the axial plane with slight medial angulation. By tilting the transducer slightly superiorly and inferiorly, the carotid artery is insonated at depth of 60–75 mm. Ophthalmic artery shows pulsatile (triphasic) flow, while internal carotid artery shows less pulsatile (biphasic) flow. Parasellar portion of the internal carotid artery shows flow towards the transducer, whereas flow in the genu portion is bidirectional and away from the transducer in the supraclinoid portion.[1]

Transforaminal (Suboccipital) Window

The transforaminal window is optimally accessed with patient seated and head flexed slightly forwards. The transducer is placed between the posterior margin of the foramen magnum and the posterior arch of the first cervical vertebra. This approach is useful to insonate the vertebral and the basilar arteries. By aiming the transducer at the nasal angle with slight lateral angulation, vertebral arteries can be localized at depth of 65–85 mm with the blood flow away from the transducer. If the transducer is angulated relatively inferiorly and the depth is decreased, the extracranial portion of the vertebral arteries can be localized. Basilar artery can be scanned at depth of 90–120 mm by scanning directly in the midline and can be tracked from the vertebral artery junction onwards.[1,2]

Submandibular Approach

By this approach the retromandibular and more distal extradural portion of the internal carotid artery can be evaluated. Transducer is placed in submandibular portion and angled superiorly and posteriorly near the angle of mandible and internal carotid artery can be tracked up to the depth of 80-85 mm where it bends to form the carotid siphon.[4]

The typical insonation depths and flow velocities are shown in Table 8.2.

In many individuals compression tests may be necessary to identify certain arterial segments unequivocally. These maneuvers are particularly valuable in assessing the collateral pathways. Compression tests during TCD examinations can be performed on the carotid arteries, low in the neck with two fingers, or on the vertebral arteries at the mastoid slope.[2] There is a slight risk of causing an embolism from plaques during the compression tests. Therefore, they should be performed by experienced investigators after performing a B-mode examination of the carotid arteries. The possible effects of compression maneuvers on intracranial flow are listed in Table 8.3.

Subarachnoid Hemorrhage and Vasospasm

Most common cause of subarachnoid hemorrhage is the rupture of intracranial aneurysm into the subarachnoid space. It can also occur due to vascular malformations, vasculitis or trauma. In a significant percentage of patients, no definite cause is found. After the hemorrhage, focal or diffuse spasm of intracranial vessels can occur. This spasm peaks between 11 and 17 days after the bleed and then gradually subsides.[5-7] In a significant percentage of patients, ischemic deficits occur due to the vasospasm and it remains a significant clinical problem. TCD has been used to detect vasospasm based on increased flow velocities in these arteries due to decreased cross sectional area of the vessel (Fig. 8.5). Bedside TCD monitoring can accurately document the development and resolution of vasospasm, aiding in assessment of risk of ischemic neurological complications. It is also useful to time the surgery or to take decisions regarding therapies such as induced hypervolemia and hypertension, calcium channel blockers, transluminal angioplasty or intra-arterial papaverine treatment.[1]

The TCD is most accurate in detecting vasospasm in the middle cerebral artery as compared to other intracranial arteries. The relatively superficial and predictable location of middle cerebral artery, compared to other arteries of the circle of Willis, allows easier localization. Also, unlike the anterior cerebral arteries and other arteries, middle cerebral artery rarely acts as a route for collateral circulation.[1,5-7]

TABLE 8.2: Summary of vessels identification criteria.

Artery	Window	Depth (mm)	Direction of flow (relative to transducer)	Relation to TICA-MCA-ACA Junction	Velocity (cm/sec)	Response to carotid Compression
MCA (M1)	Transtemporal	45–65	Towards	At	46–86	↓, 0
MCA-ACA bifurcation	Transtemporal	60–65	Bidirectional	At	—	↓, 0
ACA	Transtemporal	60–75	Away	Anterosuperior	41–76	↓, 0, r
PCA (P1)	Transtemporal	60–75	Toward	Posteroinferior	33–64	0, ↓ (fetal origin: ↓, 0)
PCA (P2)	Transtemporal	60–75	Away	Posteroinferior	33–64	0, (fetal origin: ↓, 0)
TICA	Transtemporal	60–65	Toward	Inferior	30–48	0, r
Ophthalmic artery	Transorbital	45–60	Toward	—	21–49	0
CS, Supraclinoid	Transorbital	60–75	Away	—	50–60	0, r
CS, Genu	Transorbital	60–75	Bidirectional	—	—	0, r
CS, Parasellar	Transorbital	60–75	Toward	—	50–60	0, r
Vertebral artery	Transtemporal	65–85	Away	—	27–55	—
Basilar artery	Transtemporal	90–120	Away	—	30–57	—

Note: Anterior and posterior communicating arteries are detectable only with transcranial Doppler sonography if they act as collateral routes of circulation (i.e. exhibiting increased blood flow).

(ACA: anterior cerebral artery; CS: carotid siphon; MCA: middle cerebral artery; PCA: posterior cerebral artery; r: reversal of flow; TICA: terminal internal carotid artery; ↓: decreased flow)

TABLE 8.3: Effect of compression tests of the common carotid arteries on various vessels segments and their diagnostic meanings.

Insonated vessels segment	Findings at rest	Effect of ipsilateral CCA compression test	Effect of contralateral CCA compression test	Functional meaning of compression test
MCA (M1/M2)	Normal flow velocity, flow toward probe	↓ or ↓↓ or [STOP]	0 or [↓]	Confirmation of vessel identity
ACA (A1)	Normal flow velocity flow away from probe	[↓↓] or [STOP] or with D	[0] or ↑ or ↑↑ with or without D	Confirmation of vessel identity, presence or absence of potential anterior collateral pathway
ACoA	No signal available	[↑↑ with D and flow toward probe]	↑↑ With D and flow away from the probe	Confirmation of existence of ACoA
	Indistinguishable from contralateral ACA	O or ↑ or ↑↑	[↓↓] or [STOP] or with D	See ACA
	Contralateral ACA ipsilateral ACA	See ACA	0 or ↑ or ↑↑	See ACA
PCA (P1)	Normal flow signal, flow toward probe	0 or ↑ or ↑↑	O or ↑	Confirmation of vessel identity and presence or absence of potential collateral pathway
PCA (P2)	Normal flow signal	0 or ↑, or ↓↓ or [STOP] if ICA supplied	O or [↓]	Confirmation of vessel identity and type of PCA supply differentiation of basilar and/or supply
ICA blood				
PCoA (transtemporal or transorbital)	No signal available Indistinguishable from PCA or AMCA branches without compression maneuvers Alternating flow	n nonembryonal type: With D or ↑↑ With D With flow toward probe in vicinity of PCA With flow toward probe during transorbital insonation. In embryonal type" ↓ or ↓↓ or *↓ or #↓	No reaction thus far	Confirmation of existence of PCoA differentiation of posterior and anterior collateral pathway, differentiation of basilar or ICA blood supply
DVA	Normal flow signal away from probe	0 or ↑	0 or ↑	Confirmation of existence of vessel
BA conclusive insonation	Normal flow signal away from probe	0 or ↑ or [↑↑]	0 or ↑ or [↑↑]	Confirmation of existence of posterior collateral pathway differentiation from carotid vascular tree within large depth
ICA, C2-C4 segments of collateral siphon, (transorbital approach)	Normal flow toward probe away from probe, or bidirectional	[STOP] or ↓↓ and/or [with D]*	0 or ↑	Exclusion of silent ICA occlusion, analysis of potential pathways
ICA-C1, (transtemporal approach)	Low-frequency flow toward probe Indistinguishable from MCA (M1)	[STOP] or ↓↓	0 or ↑	Analysis of potential collateral pathways differentiation from MCA often possible

(CCA: common carotid artery; MCA: middle cerebral artery; ↓: slight decrease of flow velocity; ↓↓: strong decrease of flow velocity; [ ]: very rare event; 0: no effect; ACA: anterior cerebral artery; #↓: reversal of flow towards or away from transducer; D: local distortion of blood flow due to relative stenosis; ↑: slight increase of flow velocity; ↑↑: strong increase of flow velocity; ACoA: anterior communicating artery; PCA: posterior cerebral artery; P1: precommunicating part of PCA; P2: postcommunicating part of PCA; ICA: internal carotid artery; *↓: alternating flow; DVA: distal vertebral artery; BA: basilar artery.) This list reflects our present experience but may not be complete. It refers to findings in normal subjects.

*Due to jet of PCoA collateral channel, overlap of ↓↓ and ↑↑ signals is possible.

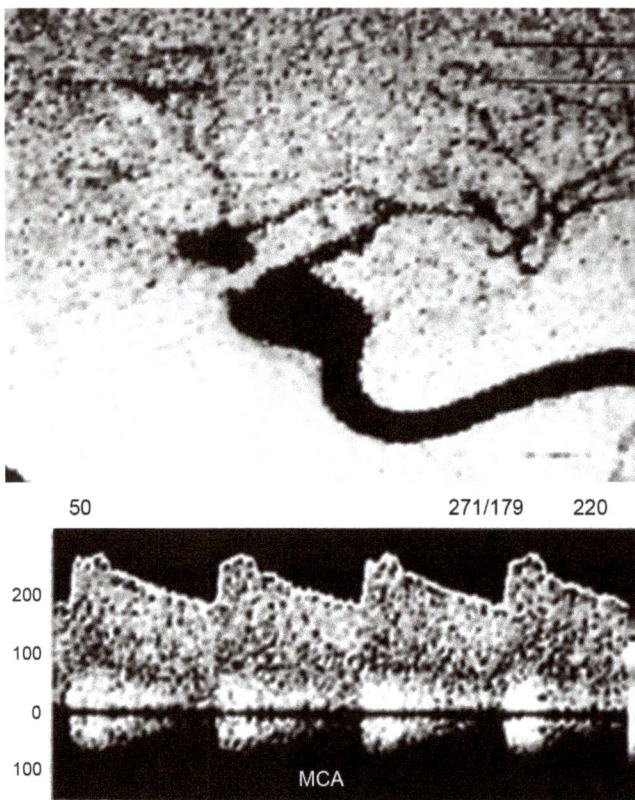

Fig. 8.5: Subarachnoid hemorrhage-vasospasm: IADSA image in a case with subarachnoid hemorrhage showing aneurysm arising from anterior communicating artery with marked spasm of internal carotid, middle cerebral and anterior cerebral arteries. Spectral waveform from middle cerebral artery shows increased velocities (220 cm/s) and spectral broadening, diagnostic of spasm.

Therefore, accelerated blood flow in the middle cerebral artery is typically due to vasoconstriction rather than increased blood flow. TCD sensitivity and specificity to detect vasospasm have been reported in range of 84-94% and 89-90%, respectively, in two large studies.[8,9] Statistically significant correlation between flow velocities and stenosis has also been demonstrated for terminal internal carotid artery, posterior cerebral artery, vertebral artery and basilar artery.[10, 11] The relative lack of accuracy in anterior cerebral artery can be due to anatomic variations (atretic A1 segments), or aberrant course (with suboptimal angle of insonation) or because anterior cerebral artery may frequently act as collateral route of blood supply.[10]

In general, mean middle cerebral artery flow velocities up to 120 cm/s correlate with mild angiographic vasospasm. Mean middle cerebral artery flow velocities between 120 cm/s and 200 cm/s correlate with moderate angiographic vasospasm (25-50% diameter narrowing), whereas flow velocities more than 200 cm/s imply severe angiographic vasospasm (greater than 50% narrowing).[12]

In addition, the rate of rise of velocities can predict the site of vasospasm induced ischemia. A rise of more than 25% over previous day and greater than 200 cm/s often occur 2 days before onset of clinical vasospasm and infarction in the middle cerebral artery territory[13] (Fig. 8.6). To exclude the possibility that increased flow velocity in middle cerebral artery relates to vasospasm rather than increased flow, the middle cerebral artery to internal carotid artery velocity ratio can be determined. Normally, the ratio is 1.7 ± 0.4; a ratio above 3 indicates middle cerebral artery vasospasm that would be visible angiographically, whereas ratio over 6 suggests severe vasospasm with attendant risk of infarction.[5]

However, it is important to be aware that some studies have demonstrated lack of correlation between flow velocities, clinical grade, change in blood flow and neurological deficit.[10] Errors may arise because of arterial variations or different resting diameters in different population groups. Coexisting proximal hemodynamically significant lesion (due to pre-existing extra or intracranial disease or due to vasospasm of proximal intracranial internal carotid artery) may also result in false negative studies. Increased intracranial pressure in cases with subarachnoid hemorrhage may also change cerebral perfusion pressure and result in change in flow velocities. Change in blood pressure, volume status or PCO_2 variations may also give rise to change in flow velocities with resultant difficulty in interpretation. Therapeutic interventions may also result in change in flow velocity and the sonographers should be aware of any of these factors before making a diagnosis. The sonographer and clinician must carefully consider the patient's clinical findings, the flow velocities from all vessels in their likelihood of reflecting vasospasm, the limitations of TCD technique, and, in some cases correlation with CBF and neuroimaging data.[10] Analysis of all available data may then permit optimal interpretation and use of TCD results.

ARTERIAL STENOSIS AND OCCLUSION

Although, middle cerebral artery or carotid siphon stenosis are responsible in only a small percentage of ischemic strokes, a timely diagnosis may be crucial in preventing a major ischemic event. This is important because in Asian populations, intracranial vascular diseases are two or three times more common than European populations.[14] Previously, these clinical conditions went undiagnosed because angiography which was used to study intracranial arteries, is an invasive investigation with potential complications. Noninvasive means to investigate intracranial stenosis such as TCD have radically changed the situation. If intracranial stenosis is detected,

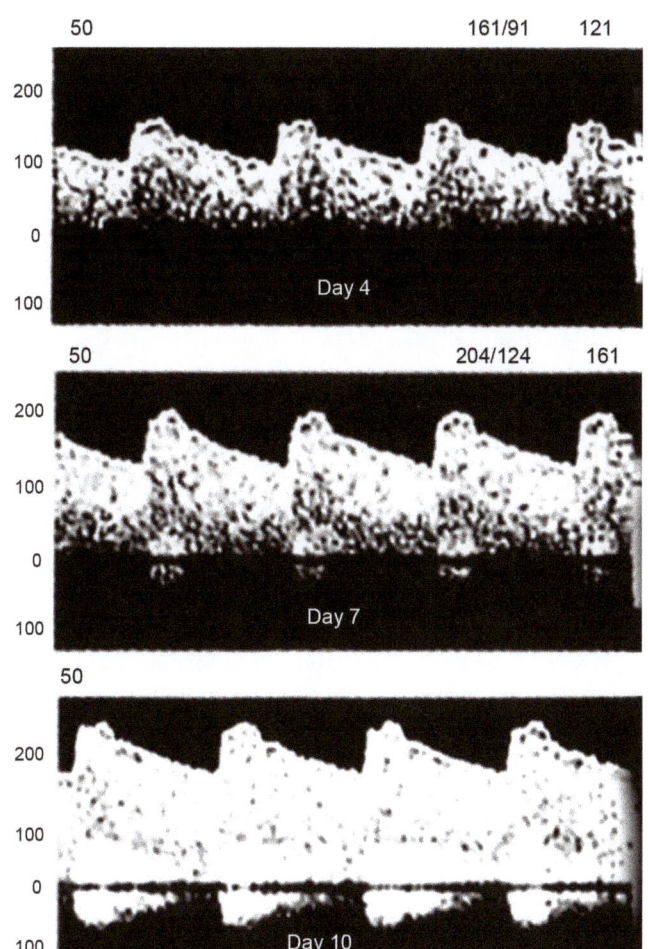

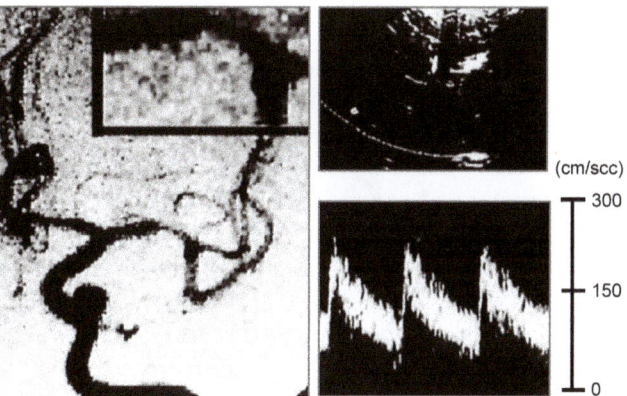

Fig. 8.7: Middle cerebral artery stenosis: IADSA image in a patient with transient ischemic attacks in left middle cerebral artery shows significant stenosis of middle cerebral artery. Special waveform (shown on the left side) had shown significantly increased velocities (200 cm/s) in this artery.

Fig. 8.6: Subarachnoid hemorrhage with vasospasm- serial studies: Spectral waveforms from left middle cerebral artery in a case with subarachnoid hemorrhage shows mildly increased velocity (121 cm/s) at day 4 (A). Progressive increase in velocity (161 cm/s) seen at day 7 (B) and day 10 (220 cm/s). This patient developed ipsilateral middle cerebral artery infarct. Therefore, evolution of vasospasm can be observed by TCD and rapid rise in flow velocities can be a warning signal for significant vasospasm and subsequent infarction.

appropriate medical therapy can be started or in selected cases intracranial angioplasty can be done.

MIDDLE CEREBRAL ARTERY STENOSIS/OCCLUSION

Middle cerebral artery is a common site for intracranial stenosis. TCD can diagnose middle cerebral artery stenosis with high reliability with reported sensitivity for stenosis/occlusion 94.1/85.7% and specificity for stenosis/occlusion 96.7/100%.[15] Most important finding to diagnose middle cerebral artery stenosis is a "focal" segment with increased velocities (Fig. 8.7), other various features are also described as listed in the Table 8.4.[15]

Velocities exceeding the corresponding site of the contralateral artery by 30 cm/s and unassociated with turbulence or low-frequency noise indicate a moderate stenosis with a diameter narrowing of approximately 40–50%. High-grade stenosis (more than 50% diameter narrowing) produces all the abnormalities listed in Table 8.4. Very high-grade stenosis (90% or more) result in velocities of 200 cm/s or more.

Acute middle cerebral artery occlusion may not produce any signal. To exclude technical factors for lack of insonation, ipsilateral anterior cerebral artery and posterior cerebral artery should at least be insonated. Increased velocities in anterior cerebral artery and posterior cerebral artery may indicate collateral flow through leptomeningeal anastomosis and further supports the diagnosis of middle cerebral artery occlusion.[16,17] Limitations of middle cerebral artery stenosis diagnosis on TCD include inability to distinguish it from very distal carotid siphon stenosis and difficulty in diagnosing stenosis beyond M1 segment.

CAROTID SIPHON STENOSIS

The ultrasonic features of carotid siphon stenosis are similar to those of middle cerebral artery stenosis. Typical findings in a case of siphon occlusion include markedly reduced flow velocities in proximal ICA and the common carotid artery. The flow signal is characterized by reverberating systolic low flow within the blind stump and by absence of any flow during the diastole. In patients with intact circle of Willis with carotid occlusion reversal of flow in the ipsilateral A1 segment of anterior cerebral artery may also be demonstrated.

TABLE 8.4: Criteria for diagnosis of stenosis in the main stem of the middle cerebral artery.

Acceleration of flow
Flow velocity change must be "circumscribed"
Flow velocity becomes damped distal to the stenosis
Side-to-side difference of mean flow velocity of at least 30 cm/s
Circumscribed, disturbed flow
Spectral broadening
Increased low-frequency components (during systole in low grade stenosis, during the entire cycle in high grade stenosis)
Arterial wall calibrations
Non harmonic low frequency noise
Musical murmurs

Unpredictable topography of carotid siphon and the osseous openings within the orbits may cause difficulty in evaluation of carotid siphon stenosis. In addition, ipsilateral posterior communicating artery, when it functions as a collateral channel may have increased flow velocities and it may be misdiagnosed as carotid stenosis due to its proximity to the carotid artery.

Moya-moya disease is a progressive cerebrovascular disorder with bilateral occlusion of the basal circulation and development of collateral blood supply. This disease may be diagnosed by TCD (Figs. 8.8A to H).[18,19] Intracranial internal carotid and middle cerebral arteries may show high or low velocities depending upon the stage of disease. Increased flow velocities are seen in the earlier stage while decreased flow velocities in these arteries are seen in the later stage. Increased flow velocities may also be seen in posterior cerebral and ophthalmic arteries because of the collateral flow.

Posterior Circulation

The distal vertebral artery can be a site for atherosclerotic disease or dissection. Significant stenosis of vertebral or basilar artery may be diagnosed by occipital approach. However, TCD evaluation of these vessels is difficult and requires considerable expertise. Ultrasonic features of stenosis or occlusion are similar to describe above. Dolicoectasia of all or portion of the vertebrobasilar system may be suggested by TCD when a significantly lower than normal flow velocities are demonstrated, particularly on patients with clinical evidence of brainstem ischemia or cranial nerve deficits.[20] TCD has also been used to prove that decrease in blood flow due to neck rotation or hyperextension and concomitant vertebral artery narrowing is the cause of symptoms in positional vertebrobasilar ischemia[21] and the adolescent stretch syndrome.[22]

ASSESSMENT OF EFFECTS OF EXTRACRANIAL OCCLUSIVE DISEASE

Carotid Stenosis or Occlusion

Extracranial carotid Duplex sonography is a sensitive and specific investigation to detect stenosis of proximal internal carotid artery due to atherosclerotic disease or dissection. TCD is a useful adjunct to this investigation because it can be used to evaluate the effect of such lesions on cerebral hemodynamics by measuring intracranial flow velocities (Figs. 8.9A to C), demonstrating the presence or absence of collateral routes of circulation, and testing autoregulation.[23-26] It can also be used to demonstrate embolic phenomenon and to depict "tandem" lesions.[23-26]

When a high-grade stenosis or occlusion of the internal carotid artery is present, TCD may demonstrate a decrease in mean blood flow velocity, with diminished pulsatility because of vasodilatation in the distal arterial circulation. Increased velocities in contralateral anterior cerebral artery, ipsilateral posterior cerebral artery, anterior communicating and posterior communicating arteries[23-26] may demonstrate presence of collateral circulation. The presence of functioning anterior communicating artery is indicated by increased velocity in contralateral anterior cerebral artery and reversal of flow in the ipsilateral anterior cerebral artery. Similar findings are shown in posterior communicating artery collateral flow from posterior cerebral artery to internal carotid artery. TCD can be used to demonstrate the presence or lack of improved intracranial blood flow after extracranial-intracranial arterial bypass surgery.[27]

Subclavian Steal Syndrome

The subclavian steal can occur when a high-grade stenosis or occlusion of a subclavian artery occurs proximal to the vertebral artery origin. Flow in basilar artery is usually not affected unless there is a high-grade stenosis in the vertebral artery supplying the steal.[28,29] Duplex examination of vertebral artery is the primary method used to diagnose this disease. TCD can be used as adjunct and both methods can be used to suggest whether lesion is incomplete or complete. Incomplete steal effects cause a decrease in systolic blood flow velocity and, when more severe, alternating blood flow direction in the vertebral artery on the side of the subclavian lesion. When the complete reversal of blood flow is demonstrated, it is called as complete steal.[28,29] Basilar artery blood flow is resistant to any critical changes resulting from the steal mechanism. In fact, it has been reported that even in symptomatic patients most vertebrobasilar symptoms are caused by cerebral microangiopathy rather than a large artery flow disturbance.[2,30]

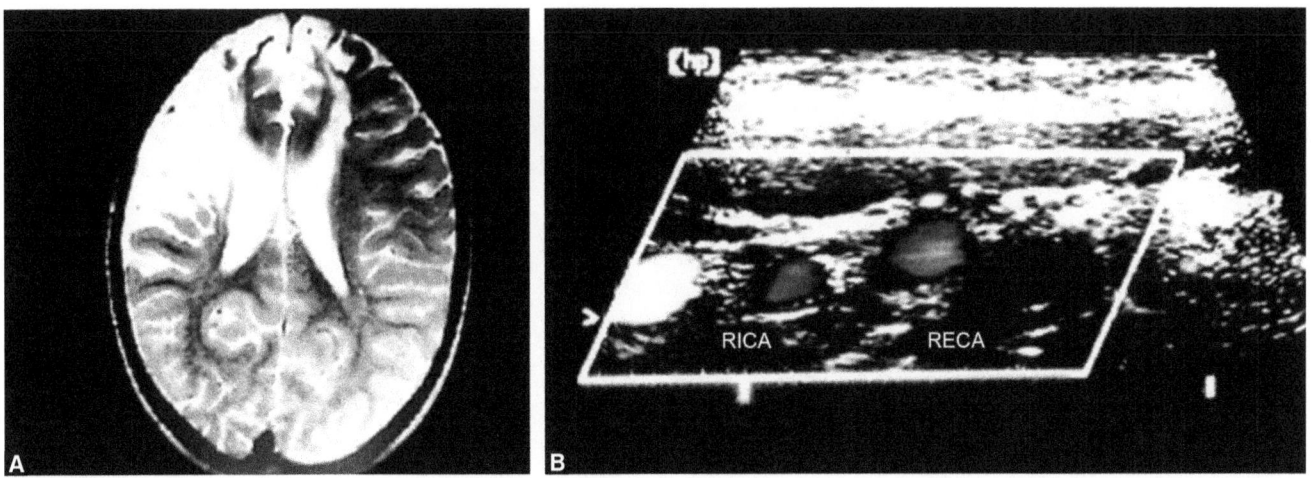

Figs. 8.8A and B: Moya-moya disease: Axial T2-weighted image (A) in a child with repeated strokes shows multiple infarcts. Color Doppler image (B) in neck region shows internal carotid artery is smaller than external carotid artery.

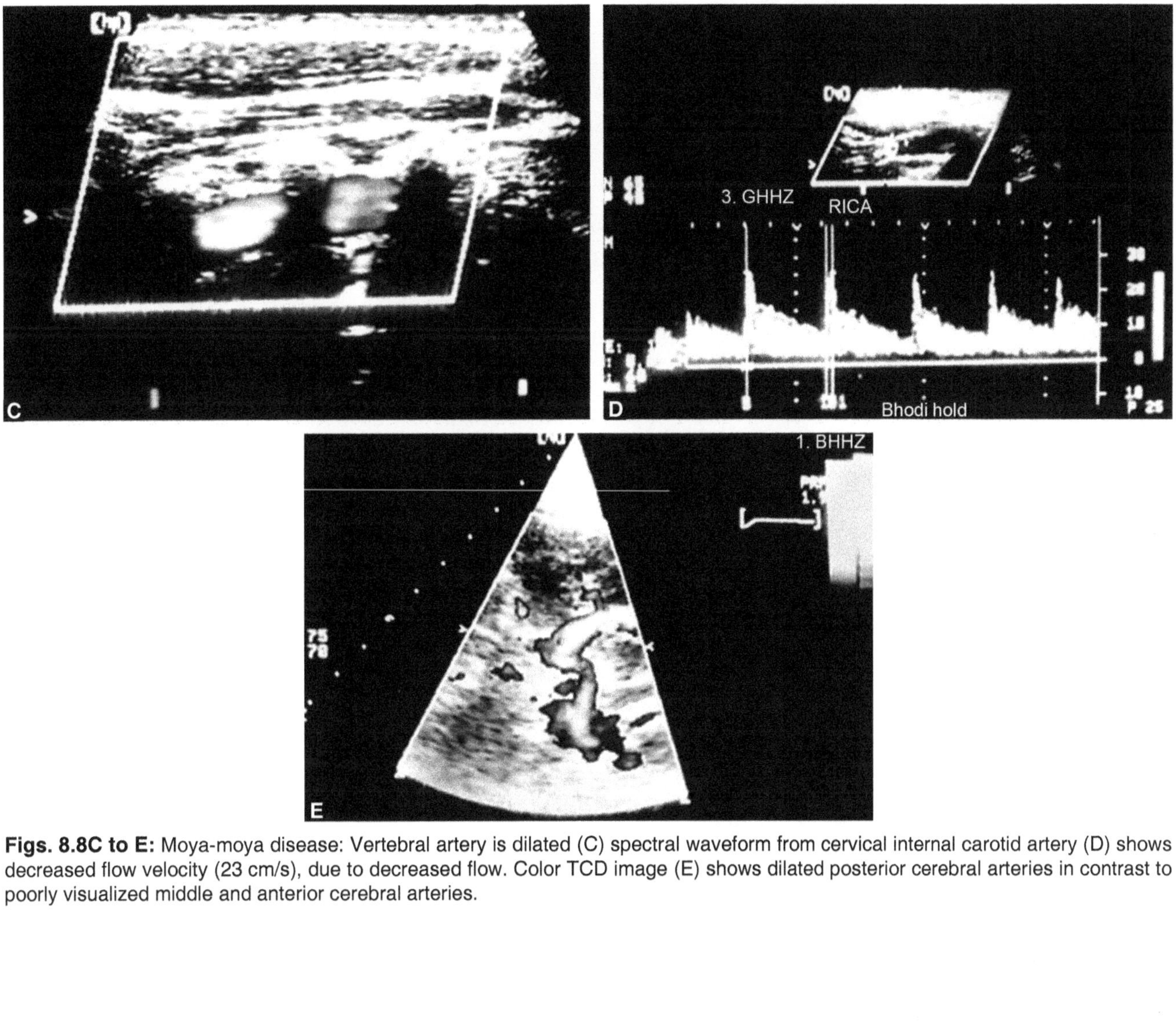

Figs. 8.8C to E: Moya-moya disease: Vertebral artery is dilated (C) spectral waveform from cervical internal carotid artery (D) shows decreased flow velocity (23 cm/s), due to decreased flow. Color TCD image (E) shows dilated posterior cerebral arteries in contrast to poorly visualized middle and anterior cerebral arteries.

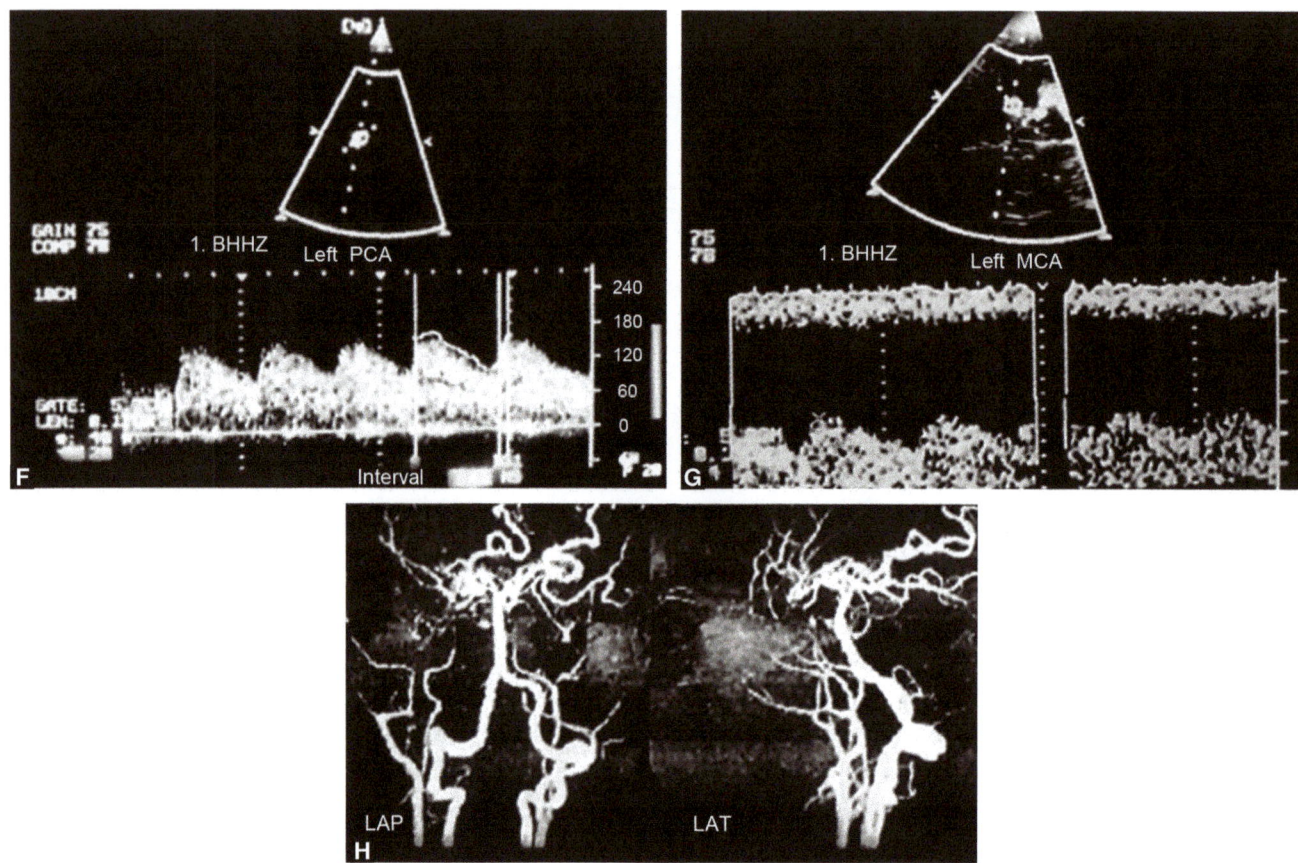

Figs. 8.8F to H: Moya-moya disease: Spectral waveform from posterior cerebral artery (F) shows increase flow velocities (160 cm/s) because it is providing collateral flow while middle cerebral artery (G) shows decreased flow velocity (28 cm/s) because of the proximal obstruction. These findings considered together are consistent with B/L intracranial internal carotid artery stenosis/occlusion (Moya-moya pattern). MRA (H) confirms the diagnosis. This case illustrates the need to evaluate the extracranial arteries for proper interpretation of TCD findings.

EMBOLI DETECTION

The TCD can be used to detect microemboli in the intracranial arteries. Both solid (atheromatous material) and gaseous emboli can be detected. Microemboli can be detected because they are much larger than the red blood cells and much more sound is reflected from them, which produce a pathognomonic high amplitude "spike" (Fig. 8.10). Doppler instrumentation used for emboli detection should have a high dynamic range (in excess of 50 dB) and the receiver should enable measurement of the signal power increase caused by emboli, which may be more than 40 dB.[31,32] Gain or automatic control may further extend the dynamic range, and this is mandatory for gaseous embolus detection because these usually overload the Doppler instrumentation.

Although use of emboli detection in day-to-day clinical work is still not very well-defined, potential uses of embolic signal monitoring are listed in Table 8.5.[32]

Artifacts, too, may cause power increase in the Doppler spectrum and may be mistaken as emboli. They are usually due to electrical interference, fast movements of the probe, or bumping of the probe. These artifacts can be distinguished from microemboli because the signal arising due to them is bidirectional, low frequency, and coincident with transducer impacts, motion, or electrical switching transients.[31,32]

INTRAOPERATIVE AND PROCEDURAL MONITORING

Carotid Endarterectomy

Intraoperative complications of carotid endarterectomy are mainly due to ischemia during cross-clamping, hyperemic phenomenon, or embolization of atheromatous or gaseous materials. TCD has been used to assess ischemia after cross-clamping in these patients, by monitoring the middle cerebral artery flow and status of collateral routes.[32-36] If ischemia is

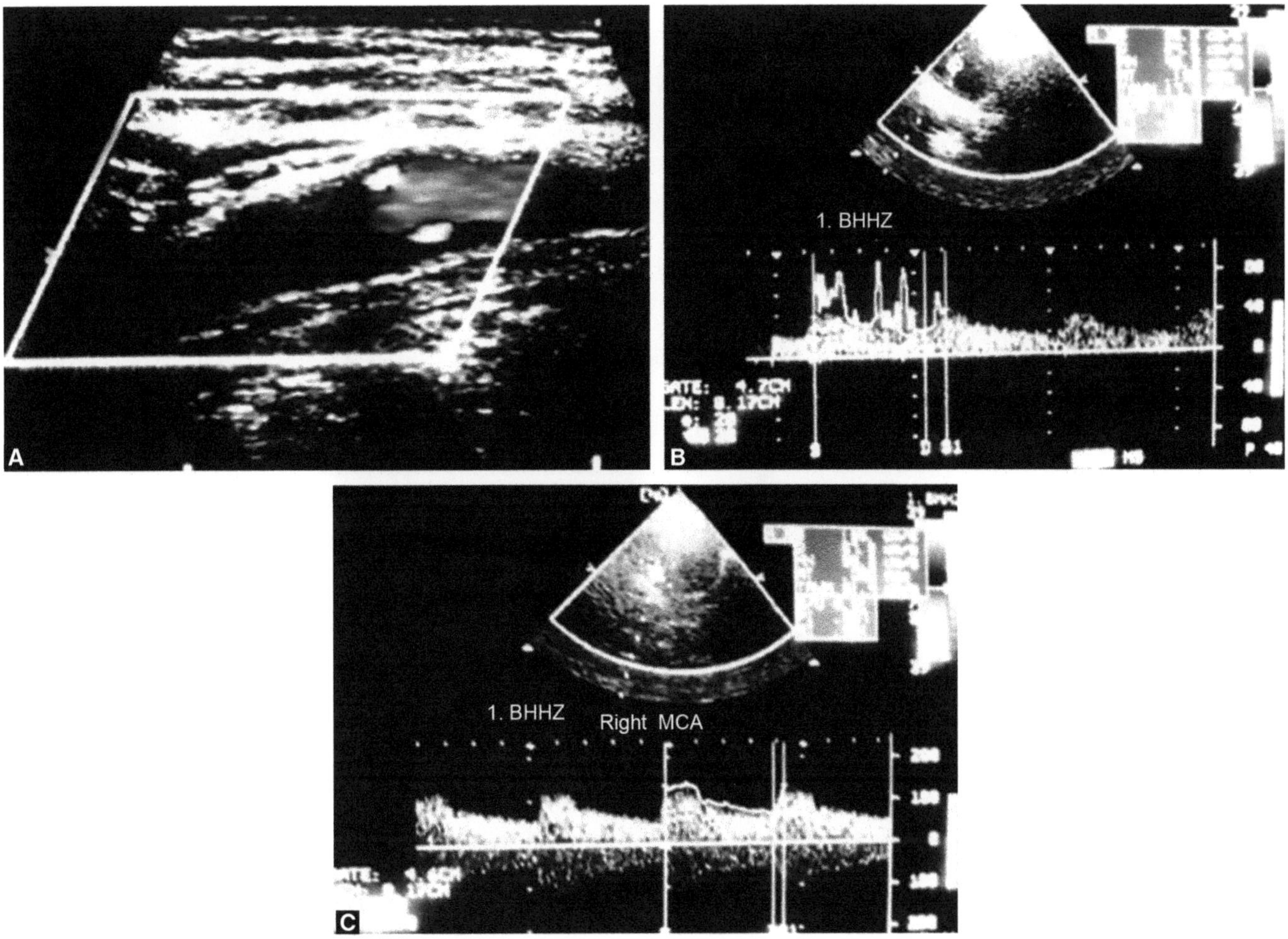

Figs. 8.9A to C: Cervical internal carotid artery block: intracranial hemodynamic effect: Color Doppler images (A) of left cervical internal carotid artery showing block in its proximal portion. TCD examination shows decreased velocity (39 cm/s) and therefore reduced flow in left middle cerebral artery (B) as compared to the contralateral (C) middle cerebral artery (102 cm/s).

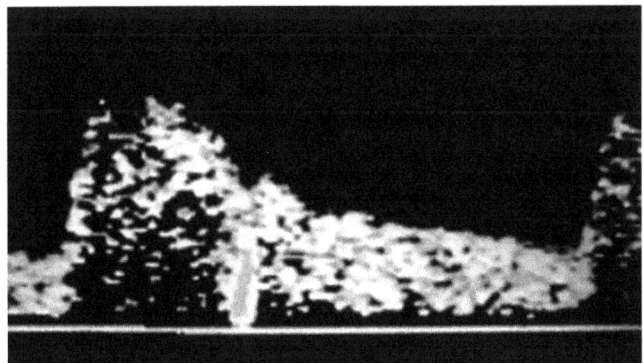

Fig. 8.10: Microemboli: Detection of middle cerebral artery embolus (bright- signal) in a patient with internal carotid artery plaque.

TABLE 8.5: Potential uses of emboli detection.

1. Localization of embolic source
2. Identification of at risk patients
    a. Carotid stenosis
    b. Cardiac embolism
    Prosthetic cardiac valves
    Native valve disease
    Atrial fibrillation
    Postmyocardial infarction
    Other cardiac embolic disease
3. Monitoring during procedures
    a. Cardiopulmonary bypass
    b. Carotid endarterectomy
    c. Coronary angiography
    d. Carotid angioplasty
4. Monitoring effectiveness of treatment
    Anticoagulation or antiplatelet therapy

suspected by this technique, a surgeon may take adequate precautions such as temporary shunt placement. Hyperemic phenomenon can occur after the surgery. It occurs because of sudden normalization of blood flow in part of brain in which autoregulation is impaired due to chronic ischemia. This may result in cerebral edema or hemorrhage and can be detected by TCD by demonstration of sudden and prolonged increase in flow velocities in the middle cerebral artery.[36,37] As stated before, microemboli detection during surgery by TCD is useful because it can warn the surgeon to modify the surgical technique.[32] It has been shown that significant deterioration in postoperative cognitive function may occur in patients in whom TCD detected 10 or more particulate microemboli during initial carotid detection.[38] Postoperatively, Doppler can be used to monitor the operative site in the neck and if indicated, the middle cerebral artery flow.[33-35]

Direct Intraoperative Doppler Sonography

Doppler probe may be placed directly on the intracranial vessels to evaluate them during neurosurgery. For this purpose, special transducers (up to 20 MHz) are needed which are capable of insonating the blood vessel by direct contact.[39] Velocity measurements using these systems may be inaccurate because of relatively large size of range-gated sample volume in relation to vessel size, but it is possible to determine vessel patency, direction of flow, presence of laminar or non-laminar flow, and change in flow velocity during the procedure.[39] Intraoperative Doppler sonographic technique has been used to monitor the graft during extracranial-intracranial bypass surgery.[39] It has also been used in aneurysm surgery to assess patency of the parent vessel after clip placement or to evaluate the anastomosis and distal cerebral flow during vascular bypass of unresectable aneurysms.[39]

Neuroradiologic Procedures

It has been demonstrated by TCD that large number of microemboli enters intracranial circulation during catheter angiography.[40] Most of these emboli are thought to be gaseous and occur most commonly during catheter flushing and injection of contrast medium. Although no case of transient or permanent ischemic deficits have occurred because of these emboli TCD can be used to improve angiographic techniques and to improve catheters, guide wires and flushing systems used during these procedures. TCD has also been used during the interventional procedures such as to monitor intracranial flow during balloon occlusion, so as to determine the efficacy of collateral flow.[41] It has also been used during angioplasty, thrombolysis and arteriovenous malformations treatment.[41,42]

Cardiopulmonary Bypass

The TCD enables a dynamic evaluation of cerebral blood flow during cardiopulmonary bypass as well as to detect emboli, which may occur during aortic cannulation or cardiac manipulation, or other surgical maneuvers.[32]

Brain Death

The accurate diagnosis of brain death is important, more so in view of issues that surround the transplantation of organs. TCD can be used to confirm cerebral circulatory arrest, although the diagnosis of brain death must be made by the physician on basis of clinical findings as well as result of diagnostic studies. Arrest of intracranial flow results in a characteristic pattern of to and fro blood flow which can be documented in the middle cerebral artery and other patent basal cerebral arteries.[43-45] This oscillating pattern is caused by systolic forward flow in the large basal arteries and diastolic reversal of flow produced by the microcirculatory obstruction and reflex contraction of the basal arteries.

Arteriovenous Malformations

In arteriovenous malformations, feeding arteries, nidus and draining veins display unusual hemodynamics related to increased blood flow velocity and vessel diameter, decreased arterial pressure, increased venous pressure and diminished or absent autoregulation. TCD shows increased flow velocities with reduced pulsatility in the feeder vessels.[46-48]

Maneuvers performed during TCD studies to document normal autoregulation produce no response in the vessels of arteriovenous malformations.[49] These abnormalities permit localization of arteriovenous malformation and assessment of the hemodynamic status. TCD has also been used to monitor the effects of surgical or endovascular interventions.[50] However, one should be aware that angiography remains the primary investigation for detection, assessment, and follow-up in cases of cerebral arteriovenous malformations.

Cerebral Trauma

The TCD has been used to demonstrate increased intracranial pressure after trauma.[1,51] In the early stage of increased intracranial pressure, increase in systolic velocity, a decrease in diastolic velocity, and increased pulsatility are demonstrated without an increase in the mean velocity (Figs. 8.11A and B). With further increase in intracranial pressure, diastolic velocity approaches zero as the intracranial tissue pressure equals diastolic pressure. Finally, reversal of diastolic flow demonstrable in the late stages of increased intracranial pressure heralds compromise of intracranial circulation.[1,51]

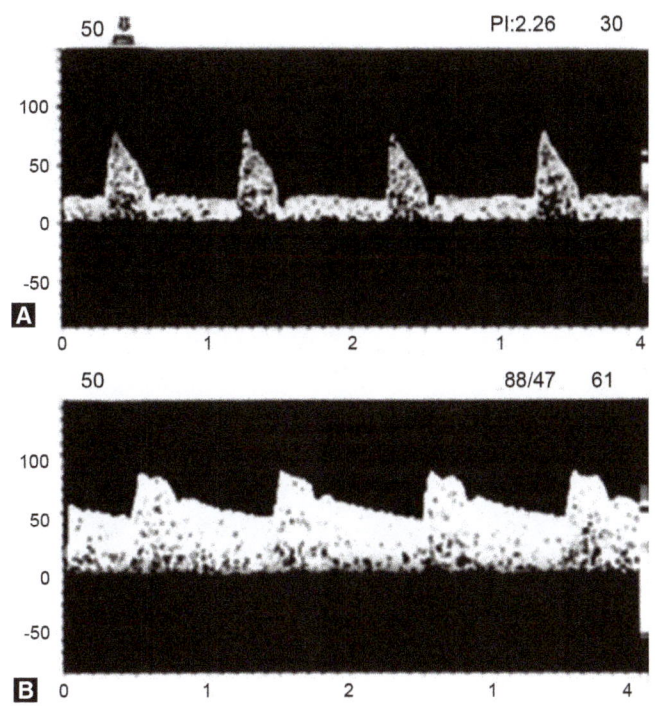

Figs. 8.11A and B: Trauma–raised intracranial pressure: Spectral waveform image of middle cerebral artery (A) in a case with significant head trauma shows decreased diastolic flow while the systolic velocities are well maintained (increased pulsatility). This finding indicates raised intracranial pressure in this clinical setting. Normal spectral waveform (B) is shown below for comparison.

After severe head injury, impairment of autoregulation may occur which will allow passive increase or decrease in cerebral blood flow secondary to changes in systemic pressure. Defects in autoregulation may be specifically suggested by TCD examination.[2]

After a head injury generalized decrease in cerebral blood flow velocities often occur and typically is followed by progressive increase in velocities beginning 2–3 days after the injury with peak velocities by day 5 or 7.[52,53] These velocity increases is thought to be due to vasospasm. In most cases permanent deficits due to this vasospasm are rare.

FUNCTIONAL RESERVE TESTING

The term cerebral autoregulation refers to the ability of cerebral arteries to maintain cerebral blood flow and therefore cerebral perfusion, at a relatively constant level despite fluctuation in cerebral perfusion pressure. If systemic pressure and consequently cerebral perfusion drops, dilatation of cerebral arteries occur which result in maintenance of cerebral blood flow.

Transeranial Doppler is an ideal test for detecting rapid changes in cerebral perfusion and cerebral autoregulation, because this technique allows observation of changes in flow velocities in real-time. Functional tests are aimed at evaluation of this reserve mechanism using various stimuli such as hypocapnia or hypercapnia, increased or decreased systemic arterial pressure.[2] A patient can be made to breathe room air followed by increasing concentrations of CO_2. Because of increased arterial PCO_2, peripheral vasodilatation, resulting in increased intracranial flow will occur. This will manifest as increased flow velocities in the cerebral arteries in TCD examination.[54] Therefore, autoregulatory response in a particular person can be assessed. Intactness of autoregulatory response implies that a drop in systemic arterial pressure can be counter balanced by vasodilatation of cerebral arteries to maintain adequate blood flow. The vasomotor response may become exhausted if the resistance vessels of brain are already maximally dilated as in cases with extracranial occlusive arterial disease.[2,55] This test can also be used in evaluating hemodynamic effects of various conditions in which reduced cerebral perfusion may occur, such as occlusive arterial diseases, migraine, hypoxia, high altitude exposure and, head trauma and in cases with arteriovenous malformation.[2]

OTHER USES

The TCD has also been used to assess hydrocephalus, pathophysiology of headaches, intracerebral aneurysms and cerebral veins. However, discussion of all these diseases is beyond the scope of this chapter. Readers are referred to several excellent texts covering these topics.[1]

CONCLUSION

Transeranial Doppler can be a tremendously useful investigation in many intracranial diseases such as vasospasm, stroke, and in monitoring during various operative and endovascular interventional procedures. It is also very useful to evaluate cerebral hemodynamics in various disease states for research purposes. It is an investigation, which is relatively inexpensive and free of risks. It can be repeated over the time and can be easily performed at the bedside or wherever a procedure or surgery is being performed (Table 8.6).

However, it also suffers from many inherent difficulties, few of which are common to Doppler examination elsewhere in the body, but some are particular to TCD evaluation as listed in Table 8.7.[4] It is operator dependent, and the examiner should be aware of anatomy and physiology of cerebral vascular system. To properly interpret the information, clinical correlation and as well as the status of extracranial arteries should be known and the examiner should be well aware of the limitations of this examination technique.

TABLE 8.6: Clinical applications of transcranial Doppler.

- Diagnosis of intracranial occlusive disease (individual and epidemiological aspects)
- Auxiliary test for extracranial occlusive disease in inconclusive extracranial test
- Evaluation of hemodynamic effects of extracranial occlusive disease of intracranial blood flow (e.g. internal carotid artery occlusion, subclavian steal)
- Detection and identification of feeders of arteriovenous malformations
- Preoperative compression tests for evaluation of collateralizing capacities of circle of Willis
- Detection of right to left shunts in the heart (e.g. patent foramen ovale) and paradoxical embolism
- Intermittent monitoring and follow-up of:
    - Vasospasm in subarachnoid hemorrhage and migraine
    - Spontaneous or therapeutically induced recanalization of occluded vessels
    - Establishment of collateral pathway after occluding interventions
    - Occlusive disease during anticoagulative or fibrinolytic therapy
- Continuous monitoring during:
    - Neuroradiologic interventions (e.g. balloon occlusion, embolization)
    - Short-term pharmacologic trials of vasoactive drugs and anesthetics
    - Carotid endarterectomy (shunt)
    - Cardiac surgery (ischemic encephalopathy, embolism)
    - Increasing intra-anterior cerebral artery pressure
    - Evolution of brain death
- Functional test:
    - Stimulation of cerebral vasomotor receptors with CO_2 or other vasoactive drugs (e.g. acetazolamide)
- Neuropsychologic tasks for hemispheric dominance (with simultaneous bilateral and TCD recording)

TABLE 8.7: Common sources of error and trouble spots.

- **Anatomic**
    - Variations and incomplete circle of Willis
    - Missing or hypertrophied anterior cerebral artery
    - Posterior cerebral artery stemming directly from the internal carotid artery
    - Atretic vertebral artery
- **Technical**
    - Absent temporal windows
    - Not identifying the best temporal window
    - Small temporal window
    - Too transparent a temporal window
- **Instrumentation**
    - Large sample volume
    - Exceeds Nyquist limits
    - Improper use and adjustment of gain control
    - Unknown Doppler angle
- **Interpretive errors**
    - Misinterpretation of hyperdynamic collateral channels as stenosis
    - Displacement of arteries caused by space-occupying lesions
    - Misdiagnosis of vasospasm as stenosis
    - Poor gold standard of angiography

REFERENCES

1. Lupetin AR, Beckman I, Asturi R, et al. Transcranial Doppler sonography. In: Orrison WW Jr (Ed). Neuroimaging. Philadelphia, WB Saunders. 1998.pp.411-43.
2. Otis SM, Ringelstein EB. Transcranial Doppler sonography. In: Zwiebel WJ (Ed). Introduction to Vascular Ultrasonography 4th edition. Philadelphia WB Saunders. 2000.pp.177-201.
3. Spencer MP, Whisler D. Transorbital Doppler diagnosis of intracranial artery stenosis. Stroke. 1986;17:916-21.
4. Otis SM, Ringelstein EB. The Transcranial Doppler examination: Principles and applications of transcranial Doppler sonography. In: Tegeler CH, Babikian VL, Gomez CR (Eds). Neurosonology. Mosby: St. Louis. 1996.pp.113-28.
5. Sieler RW, Newell DW. Subarachnoid hemorrhage and vasospasm. In: Newell DW, Aaslid R (Eds). Transcranial Doppler. New York: Raven. 1992.pp.101-7.
6. Aaslid R, Huber P, Nornes H. Evaluation of cerebrovascular spasm with transcranial Doppler ultrasound. J Neurosurg. 1984;60:37-41.
7. Harders AG, Gilsbach JM. Time course of blood velocity changes related to vasospasm in the circle of Willis measured by transcranial Doppler ultrasound. J Neurosurg. 1987;66:718-28.
8. Lindergaard KF, Nornes H, Bakke SJ, et al. Cerebral vasospasm diagnosis by means of angiography and blood velocity measurements. Acta Neurochir (Wien). 1989;100:12-24.
9. Creissard P, Proust F. Vasospasm diagnosis: Theoretical sensitivity of transcranial Doppler evaluated using 135 angiograms demonstrating vasospasm. Acta Neurochir (Wien). 1994;131:12-18.
10. Sloan MA. Transcranial Doppler monitoring of vasospasm after subarachnoid hemorrhage. In: Tegeler CH, Babikian VL, Gomez CR (Eds). Neurosonology. St. Louis: Mosby. 1996. pp.156-71.

11. Sloan MA, Burch CM, Wozniak MA, et al. Transcranial Doppler detection of vertebrobasilar vasospasm following subarachnoid haemorrhage. Stroke. 1994;25:2187-97.
12. Newell DW. Distribution of angiographic vasospasm after subarachnoid hemorrhage: implications for diagnosis by TCD. Neurosurgery. 1990;27:574-77.
13. Seiter RW, Grolimund P, Aaslid R, et al. Cerebral vasospasm evaluated by transcranial ultrasound correlated with clinical grade and CT-visualized subarachnoid hemorrhage. J Neurosurg. 1986;64:594-600.
14. Caplan LR, Gorelick PB, Hier DB. Race, sex and occlusive cerebrovascular disease. A review. Stroke. 1986;17:648-55.
15. Ley-pozo J, Ringlestein EB. Non-invasive detection of occlusive disease of the carotid siphon and middle cerebral artery. Ann Neurol. 1999;28:640-47.
16. Biass L, Duterte DL, Mohr JP. Anterior cerebral artery velocity changes in disease of the middle cerebral artery stem. Stroke. 1989;20:1737-40.
17. Zanette EM, Fieschi C, Bozzao L, et al. Comparison of cerebral angiography and transcranial Doppler sonography in acute stroke. Stroke. 1989;20:899-903.
18. Takase K, Kashihara M, Hashimoto T. Transcranial Doppler ultrasonography in patients with Moya-moya disease. Clin Neurol Neuro Surg. 1997;99(Suppl)2:S101-05.
19. Muttaqin Z, Ohba S, Arita K, et al. Cerebral circulation in Moya-moya disease: A clinical study using transcranial Doppler sonography. Surg Neurol. 1993;40(4):306-13.
20. Rautenberg W, Aulich A, Rotter J, et al. Stroke and dolichoectatic intracranial arteries. Neurol Res. 1993; 14(Suppl):201-03.
21. Weintraub MI, Khoury A. Transcranial Doppler assessment of positional vertelsrobasilar ischaemia [Letter]. Stroke. 1995;26:330-31.
22. Sturzenegger M, Newell DW, Douville CM, et al. Transcranial Doppler and angiographic findings in adolescent stretch syncope. J Neurol Neurosurg Psychiatry. 1995;58:367-70.
23. Schneider PA, Rossman ME, Torem S, et al. Transcranial Doppler in the management of extracranial cerebrovascular disease. Implication in diagnosis and monitoring. J Vasc Surg. 1988;7:223-31.
24. Cantelmo NL, Bakikian VL, Johnson WC, et al. Correlation of transcranial Doppler and non-invasive tests with angiography in the evaluation of extracranial carotid disease. J Vasc Surg. 1990;11:786-92.
25. Thiel A, Zickman B, Stutman WA, et al. Cerebrovascular carbon dioxide reactivity in carotid artery disease–Relation to intraoperative cerebral monitoring results in 100 carotid endarterectomies. Anesthesiology. 1995;82:655-61.
26. Silvestrini M, Troisi E, Cupini LM, et al. Transcranial Doppler assessment of the function effect of carotid stenosis. Neurology. 1994; 44:1910-14.
27. Cooperberg EB, Rudenev IN, Lavrentev AV, et al. Evaluation of hemodynamic effects of extracranial-intracranial arterial bypass in unilateral internal carotid artery occlusion. Cardiovasc Surg. 1993;1:704-08.
28. Von Reutern GM, Pourcelot L. Cardiac cycle-dependent alternating flow in vertebral arteries with subclavian artery stenosis. Stroke. 1978;9:229-36.
29. Klingelhofer J, Conrad B, Benicke R, et al. Transcranial Doppler ultrasonography of caroticobasilar collateral circulation in subclavian steal. Stroke. 1988;19:1036-42.
30. Ringlestein EB, Busker M, Buchner H. Evaluation of hemodynamic effects of subclavian steal mechanism as basilar artery blood flow with the help of transcranial Doppler sonography. Presented at the first International Conference on Doppler sonography. Rome, Italy, 1986.
31. Russell D, Brucher R. Embolus detection with Doppler sonography. Methods and Clinical Potential. In: Tegeler CH, Babikian VL, Gomez CR (Eds). Neurosonology. Mosby: St. Louis. 1996.pp.235-38.
32. Markus H, Russell D, Brucher R. Doppler embolus detection: Stroke treatment and prevention. In: Tegeler CH, Babikian VL, Gomez CR (Eds). Neurosonology. St. Louis, Mosby. 1996. pp.239-51.
33. Sundt TM, Sharbough FW, Anderson RE et al. Cerebral blood flow measurements and electroencephalographic changes during carotid endarterectomy. J Neurosurg. 1974;41:310-20.
34. Zuccarello M, Yeh H, Tew TM. Morbidity and mortality of carotid endarterectomy under local anesthesia. A retrospective study. Neurosurgery. 1988;23:445-50.
35. Ferguson GG. Intraoperative monitoring and internal shunts: Are they necessary in carotid endarterectomy? Arch Surg. 1987;122:305-07.
36. Magre TR, Davies AH, Baird RN, et al. Blood flow in the internal carotid artery and velocity in the middle cerebral artery during carotid endarterectomy. Cardiovasc Surg. 1994;2:37-40.
37. Jansen C, Springers AM, Moll FL, et al. Prediction of intracerebral hemorrhage after carotid endarterectomy by clinical criteria and intraoperative transcranial Doppler monitoring. Results of 233 operations. Eur J Vasc Surg. 1994;8:220-25.
38. Jansen C, Ramos LMP, van Heesewijk JPM, et al. Impact of microembolism and hemodynamic changes in the brain during carotid endarterectomy. Stroke. 1994;35:992-97.
39. Gilsbach JM. Intraoperative Doppler sonography in Neurosurgery New York: Springer-Verlag. 1983.pp.1-88.
40. Dagirmanjian A, Davis BA, Rothfus WE, et al. Silent cerebral microemboli occurring during carotid angiography: Frequency as determined with Doppler sonography AJR. 1993;161:1037-40.
41. Giller CA, Sterg P, Batjer HH, et al. Transcranial Doppler ultrasound as a guide to graded therapeutic occlusion of the carotid artery. Neurosurgery. 1990;20:307-11.
42. Giller CA, Purdy P, Giller A, et al. Elevated transcranial Doppler ultrasound velocities following therapeutic arterial dilatation. Stroke. 1995;26:123-27.
43. President's Commission. Guidelines for the determination of brain death. JAMA. 1981;246:2184-87.
44. Powers AD, Graeberg MC, Smith RR. Transcranial Doppler ultrasonography in the determination of brain death. Neurosurgery. 1989;24:884-89.

45. Petty GW, Mohr JP, Pedley TA, et al. The role of transcranial Doppler in confirming brain death. Sensitivity, specificity and suggestions for performance and interpretation. Neurology. 1990;41:300-03.
46. Lindegaard KF, Grolimund P, Aaslid R, et al. Evaluation of cerebral AVM's using transcranial Doppler ultrasound. J Neurosurg. 1987;65:335-44.
47. Hassler W, Steinmetz H. Cerebral hemodynamics in angioma patients: An intraoperative study. J Neurosurg. 1987;67:822-31.
48. Hassler W. Hemodynamic aspects of cerebral angiomas. Acta Neurochir. 1986;37(Suppl):1-136.
49. Hassler W, Burger R. Arteriovenous malformations. In: Newell DW, Aaslid R (Eds). Transcranial Doppler. New York: Raven. 1992.pp.123-35.
50. Petty GW, Massaro AR, Tatimichi TK, et al. Transcranial Doppler ultrasonographic changes after treatment for arteriovenous malformations. Stroke. 1990;21:260-66.
51. Hassler W, Steimetz H, Gawlowski J. Transcranial Doppler ultrasonography in raised intracranial pressure and in intracranial circulatory arrest. J Neurosurg. 1988;68:745-51.
52. Steiger HJ, Aaslid R, Stooss R, et al.: Trans-cranial Doppler monitoring of head injury. Relations between type of injury, flow velocities, vasoreactivity and outcome. Neurosurgery. 1994;34:79-85.
53. Compton JS, Teddy PJ. Cerebral artery vasospasm following severe head injury: A transcranial Doppler study. Br J Neurosurg. 1987;1:435-39.
54. Markwalder TM, Grolimund P, Seiler RW, et al. Dependancy of blood flow velocity in the middle cerebral artery on the end-tidal carbon dioxide partial pressure-a transcranial ultrasound Doppler study. J Cereb Blood Flow Metab. 1984;4:368.
55. Bullock R, Mandelow AD, Bone I, et al. Cerebral blood flow and CO_2 responsiveness as an indicator of collateral reserve capacity in patients with carotid arterial disease. Br J Surg. 1985;72:348.

Chapter 9

Doppler in Liver

LIVER

Sonography is considered to be the most effective primary investigation of choice is elucidation of liver pathology. Color Doppler sonography is a superb, noninvasive alternative to anteriography and phlebography.

The hepatic artery and portal veins are best interrogated by Doppler ultrasound of the porta hepatis using oblique intercostal scans.

TECHNIQUE

The abdominal vessels are insonated using established techniques. The Doppler sample volume is adjusted to encompass but not exceed the diameter of the vessel studied. The pulse-repetition frequency (PRF) is adjusted manually when aliasing occurs. Low PRF and lowest available filter of Doppler receiver are used. A low frequency (3 MHz) is chosen for examination of deep vessels and for detection of high velocities and a high frequency (5-7.5 MHz) transducer is used for the examination of superficial vessels, studies of children or detection of low blood flow velocities.

The portal vein is the most readily accessible vessel in the portal system. The entire length of the portal vein can be examined from an entire abdominal subcostal approach, using a right paramedian and slightly oblique plane.

The splenic vein is examined at the splenic hilum by angling the transducer to follow the long axis of the vessel.

The superior mesenteric vein is examined through a longitudinal right paramedian upper abdominal approach.

The hepatic veins usually are explored easily through an oblique, subcostal or intercostal approach, yielding excellent Doppler signals. The inferior vena cava is insonated along its visible length noting any localized increase in caliber and/or flow velocity.

The hepatic artery is insonated at its origin at the celiac axis and where it crosses the portal vein. Intrahepatic branches are examined adjacent to portal venous branches. The splenic artery was examined concomitantly with the vein, at the splenic hilum and within the spleen.[1]

NORMAL PATTERNS

Portal Veins

Approximately 25% of the flow into the liver is supplied by hepatic artery, the remainder by the portal vein. Normal portal venous flow is hepatopetal and is usually monophasic with some fluctuation due to respiration and cardiac activity (Figs. 9.1A and B). Thus when color flow is being used to assess the portal vein, flow into the liver will conventionally appeared.

Hepatic Artery

The hepatic artery can be identified in most patients at porta hepatis lying between the portal vein and common bile duct. In a small percentage of patients, this anatomy may be altered and the hepatic artery may lie anterior to the bile duct. Color flow imaging allows rapid differentiation of bile duct from hepatic artery. The hepatic artery waveform characteristically has a high diastolic phase due to the low resistance of the hepatic vascular bed.

Hepatic Veins

The hepatic veins characteristically have a triphasic waveform which reflects right atrial and inferior vena cava

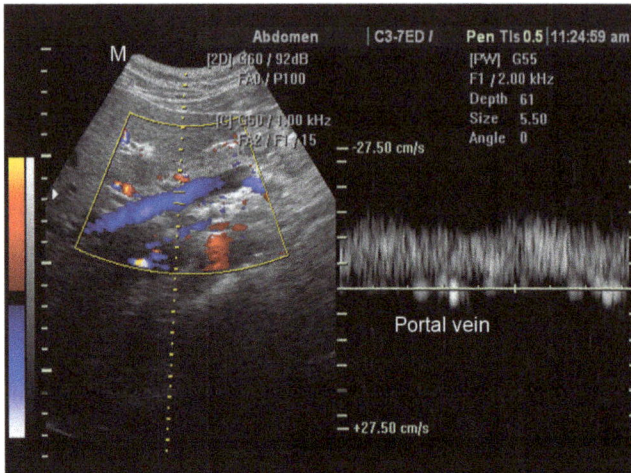

Fig 9.1A: Duplex Doppler showing normal portal venous waveform.

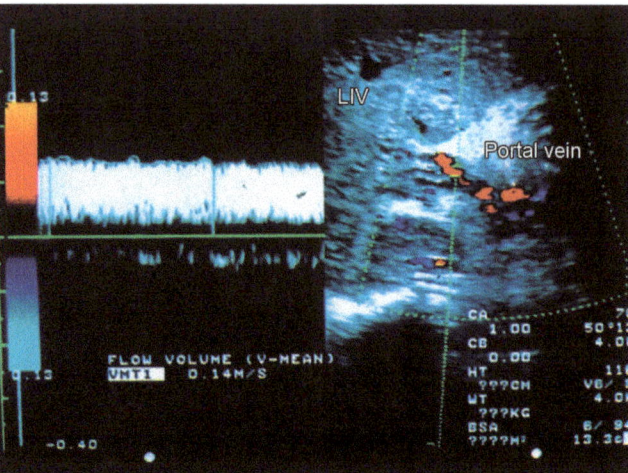

Fig. 9.1B: Duplex Doppler evaluation of portal vein showing portal venous flow pattern. Loss of phasic variation is noted.

pressures (Fig. 9.2). This result in flow in the hepatic veins being predominantly coded blue, i.e. away from the probe on the color Doppler.[2]

Physiological Variations

1. *Respiratory variations: Caliber* variations of vessels of the portal venous system during deep inspiration are easily observed with real-time equipment. A significant caliber increase is noted during inspiration in normal patients. This increase (50–100%) is particularly clear at the level of the splenic and superior mesenteric veins. During expiration, the caliber of the splenic and superior mesenteric veins always rapidly decreased. Caliber variations in the portal trunk were either very slight or completely absent.[3]
2. *Variations due to posture:* In normal patients, shift from supine to sitting position significantly decrease portal venous velocity, cross-sectional area of portal vein and portal venous flow. This effect of posture is attributed to absence of values in the splanchnic venous system.[4]
3. *Variations due to physical exercise:* During physical exercise, vasodilation in the muscular vessels takes blood away from the splanchnic system. Hence, immediately after exercise, the cross-sectional area of the portal vein and portal venous flow were significantly decreased. After ten minutes post-exercise, portal venous velocity, the cross-sectional area of the portal vein and portal venous flow seen to return to the basal pre-exercise values.[4]
4. *Postprandial variations:* Studies show that eating causes vasodilatation and flow increase in the splanchnic system. An increase in the diameter of portal vein and

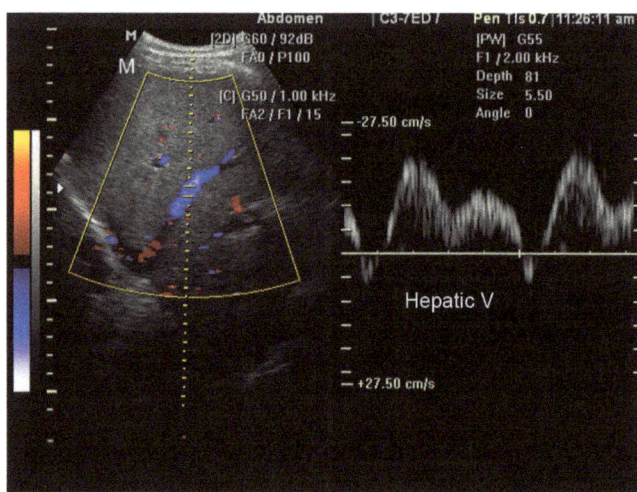

Fig. 9.2: Pulsed Doppler tracing of right hepatic vein in a normal subject showing the characteristic three-phase profile according to the phases of the cardiac cycle.

increase flow in both splanchnic arteries and veins has been reported. This is attributed to increase in mean flow velocity caused mostly by the increase in the diastolic component of the mesenteric arterial flow.[5]
5. *Humoral variations:* Significant increase in portal velocity and flow has been noted after glucagon and secretin administration.[6]

PORTAL HYPERTENSION

Real time sonography has become increasingly useful in the examination of patients with long standing liver disease and/or portal hypertension.

Portal hypertension develops when increased resistance to portal flow and/or increased portal blood flow occur. Recent evidence suggests that both the mechanisms are involved in the maintenance of chronic portal hypertension that result in enlargement of the extrahepatic portal vessels, the development of spontaneous portosystemic collaterals and slow portal vein flow.

Sonographic Findings in Portal HT

Portal vein diameter is measured in basal conditions (quiet respiration, supine, and fasting). In patients with advanced cirrhosis and portal hypertension, a threshold of 13 mm is used. Dilatation of portal vein greater than 13 mm occurs in 56% of patients (Figs. 9.3 and 9.4). Some authors have demonstrated that presence of esophageal varices is correlated with dilatation of portal vein, a caliber over 17 mm is 100% predictive for large varices. A normal caliber of portal vein does not, however, exclude portal hypertension. The main intrahepatic portal branches are normally also dilated.

Varying degrees of dilatation of splenic and superior mesenteric veins also occur in portal hypertension. The upper limit of normal splenic and superior mesenteric veins range from 10 to 12 mm. Splenomegaly is usually associated with dilatation of splenic vein (Fig. 9.5), possible because of increased splenic blood flow. Ascites and hepatomegaly with altered liver architecture are indicators of steatosis and cirrhosis. Opening up of vessels between high pressure portal venous system and low pressure systemic circulation is usually seen with portal hypertension. Occasionally, collaterals may be seen in gallbladder wall. Direct visualization of esophageal varices is often difficult or impossible, though their presence may be inferred by demonstrating thickening of the esophageal wall, irregularity of the lumen and variation of esophageal wall thickness with respiration.

Doppler Findings in Portal Hypertension

The clinical applications of Doppler studies of the splanchnic vessels include the assessment of the presence, direction and characteristics of blood flow. The hemodynamic parameters provided by Doppler ultrasound (US) can be classified as qualitative, semiquantitative, and quantitative. The qualitative data include evaluation of the presence, the direction and the characteristics of the blood flow and their alterations. Semiquantitative measurements include vascular impedance which is calculated by means of pulsatility and resistance indices. Quantitative data include calculation of the maximum and mean flow velocity and of the flow volume in larger diameter veins.

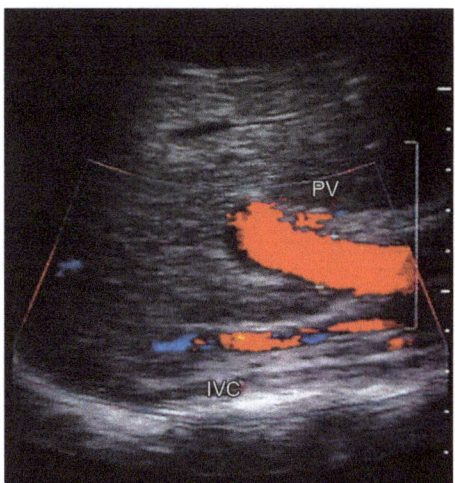

Fig. 9.3: Dilated portal vein in a case of portal hypertension.

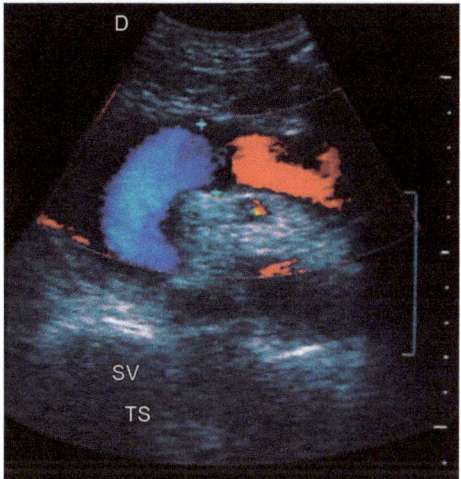

Fig. 9.4: Grossly dilated splenoportal axis with normal direction of flow.

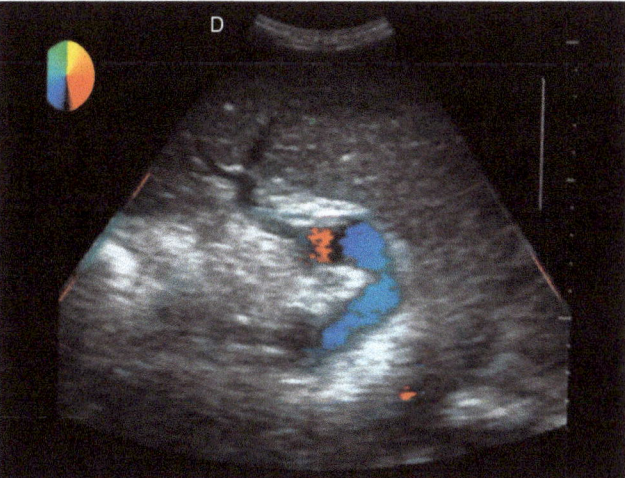

Fig. 9.5: Dilated and tortuous splenic vein with splenomegaly.

The earliest sign of portal hypertension is loss of normal respiratory/cardiac variations in portal venous flow. In severe cases, hepatofugal flow may be noted with reversal of color flow.

QUALITATIVE FINDINGS

Portal System Thrombosis

Establishing the presence of blood flow within the portal veins is the simplest Doppler finding and is usually easy to perform. Color Doppler directly shows the blood flow inside the vein, distinguishing the portal vein from other channel like structures such as dilated biliary ducts at porta hepatis.

In cases of chronic portal thrombosis, when ultrasound shows the portal vein to be small and hyperechogenic, (Fig. 9.6). Doppler flowmetry at porta hepatis shows no blood flow. An indirect sign of thrombosis of the portal vein consists of presence of high frequency arterial signals in both porta hepatis and the intrahepatic branches, due to the increase in arterial circulation in the attempt to compensate for portal thrombosis. When cavernous transformation takes place, color Doppler shows turbulent flow inside the small serpentine vessels which cross the thrombosed veins (Fig. 9.7A).

Partial thrombus appears as an absence of color signal and this can equally be identified when the thrombus is anechoic. Neovascularization within the thrombus, a pathognomonic sign of tumor thrombus, may be identified as arterial signals within the thrombus (Fig. 9.7B). Given its reliability, sensitivity and noninvasiveness, Doppler is considered as the most suitable technique to assess the prevalence of portal thrombosis in cirrhosis.

Directions of Blood Flow

Flow direction is another unequivocal qualitative finding provided by Doppler ultrasound. Kawasaki et al. reported a prevalence of spontaneous hepatofugal flow of 6.1% in liver cirrhosis.[7] Hepatofugal portal flow is associated with a decreased risk of variceal bleeding, while it does not predict survival.[8] Reversed portal flow is generally associated with a significant reduction in the diameter of the portal vein. A close correlation was demonstrated between hepatofugal flow of the splenic vein and hepatic encephalopathy, probably in relation to the drainage of a great deal of

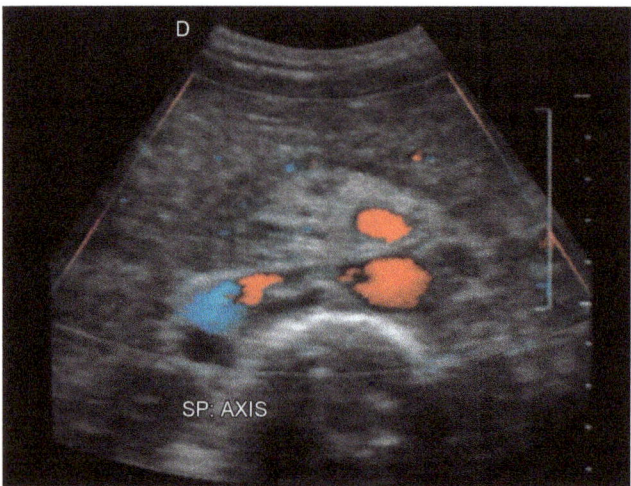

Fig. 9.6: Chronically thrombosed splenoportal axis showing thin lumen with no flow.

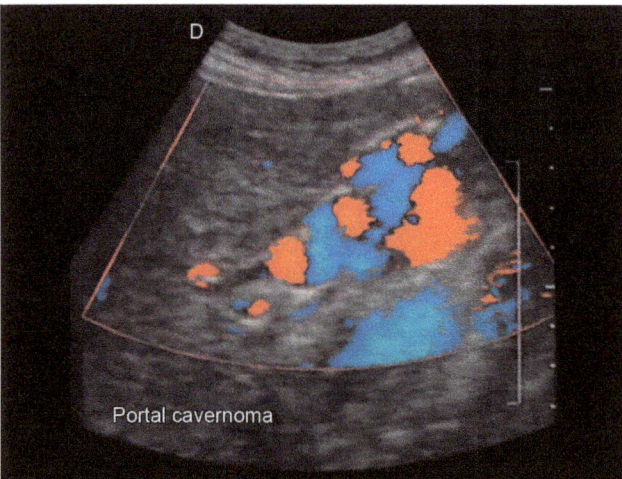

Fig. 9.7A: Portal cavernoma formation in main portal vein thrombosis.

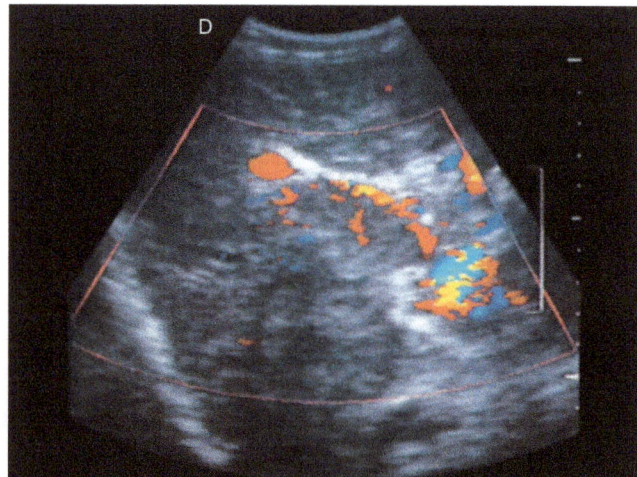

Fig. 9.7B: Color Doppler flow image shows an echogenic tumor thrombus partially occluding the portal vein. The thrombus is contiguous with a heterogeneous mass lesion in the adjacent color flow is also seen within the tumor thrombus.

blood in the large splenorenal lienorenal collaterals. Color Doppler clearly shows flow inversion which shows the color opposite to that of the arterial branches, in which the blood flow increases to compensate for the inversion of portal flow. These intrahepatic flow inversions are probably determined by arterioportal shunts where the signal becomes turbulent and rapid.[9]

Portosystemic Collaterals

The diagnosis of portal hypertension must include search for collateral beds. Real time US and Doppler can explore the paraumbilical veins and the lienorenal collaterals and those of left gastric vein and of the gastroesophageal plexus. Doppler flowmetry though cannot provide precise measurement of the collateral bed flow rate, however, contributes to provide an approximate idea of the hemodynamic importance of collateral vascular bed.

Paraumbilical veins are generally quite large and run in a straight line towards the umbilical region (Figs. 9.8A and B). On other occasions, the paraumbilical vascular bed appears as one or more irregular vessels which cross hepatic parenchyma. The presence of a high velocity venous flow makes it possible to differentiate between these beds and peripheral portal branches in which the venous flow is much slower, the paraumbilical bed flow is rarely hepatopetal.

The collateral vascular beds of the left gastric vein are often difficult to study due to obesity, especially in patients in whom the left lobe of the liver is not greatly enlarged. Moreover, the origins and the course of the left gastric vein are variable hence, makes it difficult to study. These may be seen as dilated and tortuous vessels in epigastrium or left gastric vein may be visualized at its origins, running towards the diaphragms with hepatofugal flow (Figs. 9.9 and 9.10).

At level of lower splenic pole, the lienorenal collaterals (Fig. 9.11) appear as tortuous vessels with a high velocity Doppler signal and a broadspectrum of frequencies due to turbulence. Their presence is often associated with flow reversal in the splenic vein.

Other collateral vessels may occasionally be identified at the level of the gastric fundus, in the pancreatic region or in the pericholecystic area (Figs. 9.12 to 9.14).

Flow Characteristics

The characteristics of the tracing and of the spectral distribution of the frequencies are directly consequent to the vessel hemodynamics. Each vessel has its own characteristic tracing which leads to its recognition.

Hepatic veins in normal conditions show a three-phase tracing dependent on the cardiac cycle and particularly on the pressure variations in the right atrium. This phasic fluctuation of the flow is either notably reduced or completely abolished in case of liver cirrhosis with portal hypertension.

The impedance changes in the splanchnic vessels have been studied in the three main arterial beds: the superior mesenteric, splenic, and hepatic.

The superior mesenteric artery supplies a large part of the intestine and subsequently the portal system. Elevated sinusoidal pressure triggers a reduction of mesenteric arterial resistance leading to a hyperdynamic

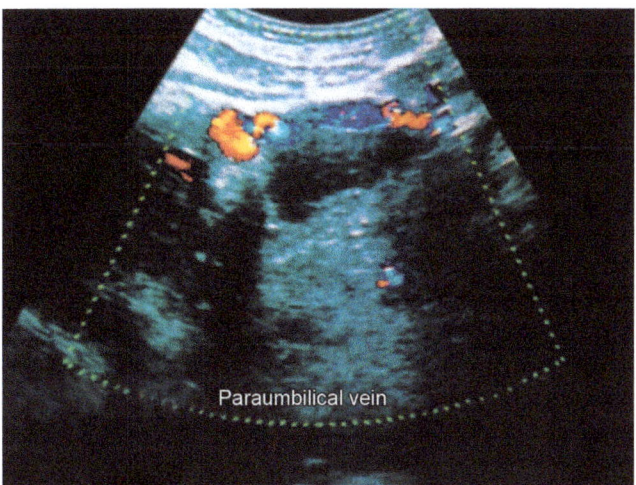

Fig. 9.8A: Patent paraumbilical vein in a case of advanced cirrhosis.

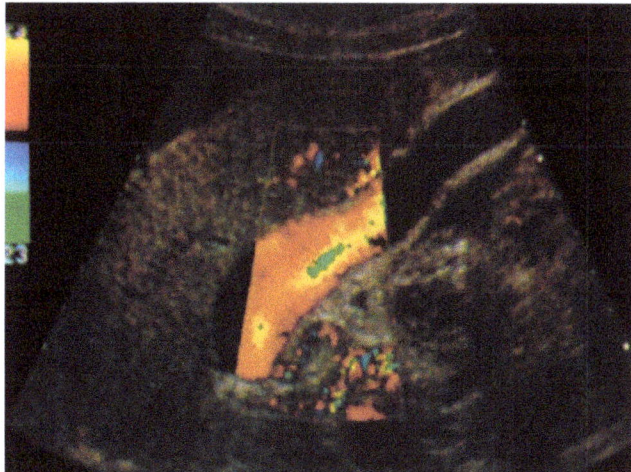

Fig. 9.8B: Color Doppler imaging in patient with advanced cirrhosis. Enlarged paraumbilical vein flow gradients, increased parenchymal vascularity and turbulent hepatic arterial flow are all present.

78 | Textbook of Color Doppler Imaging

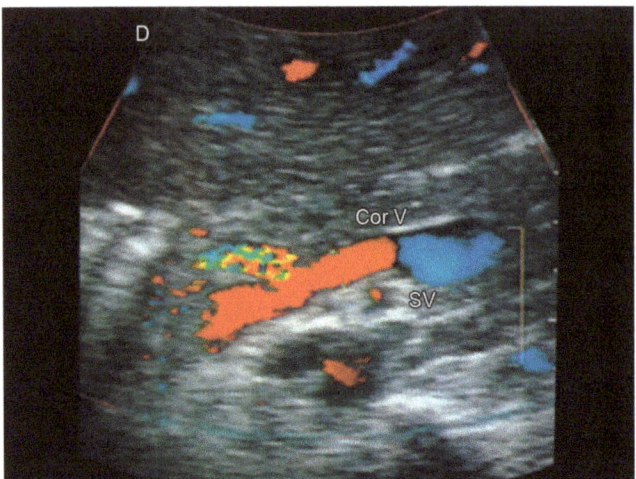

Fig. 9.9: Dilated coronary vein in a patient of portal hypertension with history of repeated variceal bleeding.

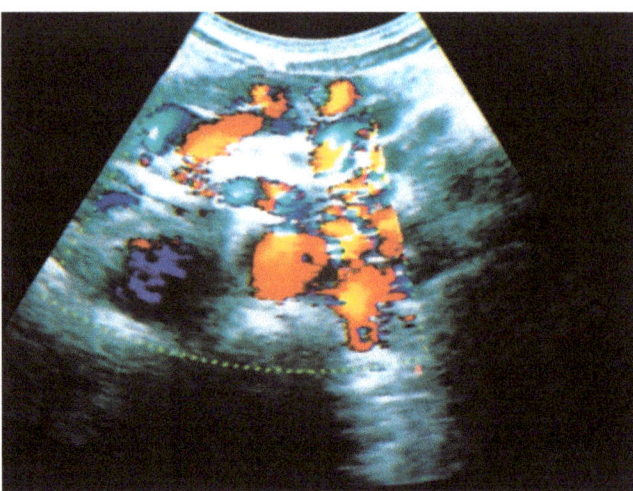

Fig. 9.12: Voluminous collaterals at gastroesophageal junction and at fundus of stomach.

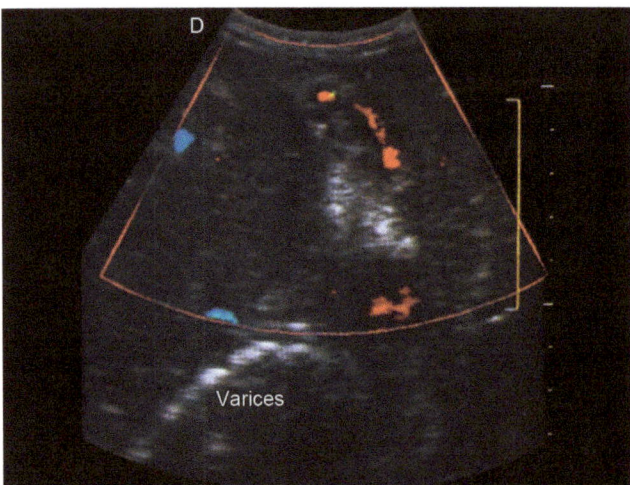

Fig. 9.10: Tortuous varices at gastroesophageal junction.

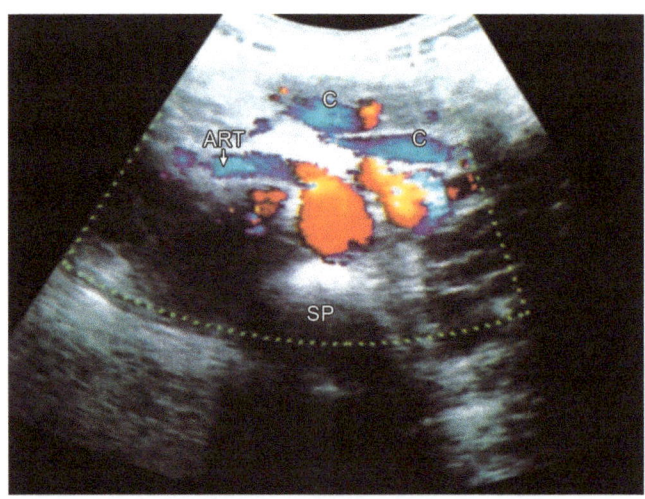

Fig. 9.13: Peripancreatic collaterals.

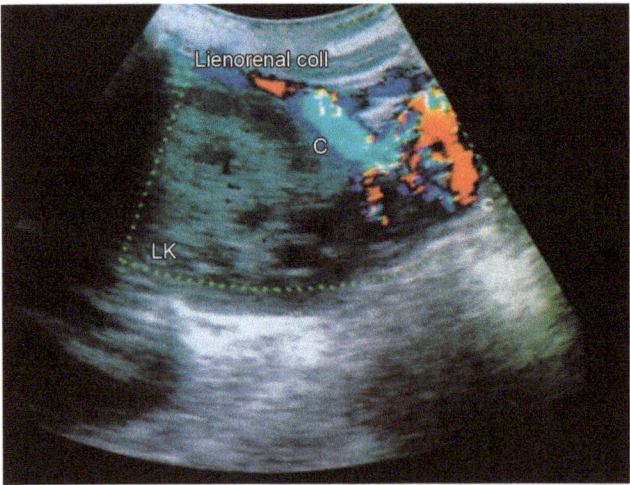

Fig. 9.11: Lienorenal collaterals.

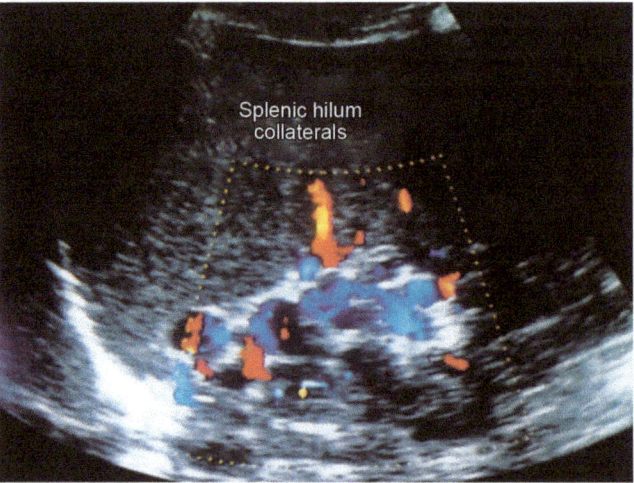

Fig. 9.14: Splenic hilar collaterals.

splanchnic circulation. Thus, the portal vein flow is increased and this contributes to the maintenance of portal hypertension.[10] This dilatation of intestinal arterioles decrease the impedance indices in the superior mesenteric artery.[11] A decrease in pulsatility index is seen to accompany worsening liver function and development of esophageal varices.

Doppler impedance indices measured in the intraparenchymal branches of the splenic artery were found to be increased in patients with cirrhosis, and they correlate closely with lienorenal vascular resistance.[12]

Hepatic arterial impedance indexes are increased in patients with liver cirrhosis. This increase becomes even more pronounced if portal vein thrombosis occurs.[13]

SEMIQUANTITATIVE FINDINGS

Evaluation of the flow alteration can also be performed by semiquantitative methods based on the analysis of the velocity profile and on calculation of the relations between maximum, minimum and mean spectrum frequency. Numerous indices have been proposed to describe the characteristics of arterial flow:

$$\text{Pulsatility index (PI)} = \frac{A - B}{\text{mean}}$$

A = Peak systolic velocity
B = Peak diastolic velocity
Mean = Mean of velocity in a set interval of time

$$\text{Resistance index (RI)} = \frac{A - B}{A}$$

PI of the superior mesenteric artery was significantly reduced in patients affected by liver cirrhosis.

QUANTITATIVE FINDINGS

A complete hemodynamic evaluation of the portal venous system in portal hypertension should include measurements of:
a. The volume of portal venous flow (Qpv).
b. The portal perfusion pressure (pressure gradients between the portal vein and the hepatic veins (Ppv – Phv)
c. The portal vascular resistance (Pvr)[14]

$$Pvr = Ppv - \frac{Phv}{Qpv}$$

Noninvasive measurements using Doppler ultrasound presupposes uniform insonation in which the entire volume of blood in a cross-section of the vessel is exposed to uniform ultrasonic beams. The time-averaged mean velocity (V), calculated from the mean Doppler shift, is multiplied by the cross-sectional area (A) of the vessel to give the volume flow (Q)

$$Q = VA$$

Sources of error include the nonuniform insonation, measurement of the cross-sectional area of the vessel and the assessment of the beam angle.[15]

A further critical point is the calculation of the mean velocity. Both direct calculation by the software of the instrument and its estimation as a fixed fractions of the maximal velocity may be inaccurate. Estimates of the average peak velocity have been found to be reasonably reproducible, particularly after a preliminary training program standardize methodology[16] (Table 9.1).

Ultrasound cannot directly measure portal pressure, however, an indirect assessment can be made using the 'congestion index'. The 'congestion index' is the ratio between the cross-sectional area and the mean flow velocity of the portal trunk. It takes into account the fact that in portal hypertension the portal vein tends to dilate and the blood velocity to decrease, so that higher values are found in patients with more severe portal resistance, pressure and larger varices.[17]

For the portal vein, its straight course for 3-4 cm, relatively long diameter and the oblique course with respect to the abdominal wall are factors which make the Doppler study easy to perform. Measurement of the flow velocity should be made according to the reported guidelines (Table 9.1).

Quantitative measurements of the portal flow can serve as a contributor not only to the diagnosis of portal hypertension but also for the evaluation of hemorrhage risk

TABLE 9.1: Guidelines for Doppler measurements of portal vein (from Sabba et al. 1995[16]).

1. Measure in suspended normal respiration
2. Longitudinal scan of the portal vein
3. Sample volume in the center of the vessel, at the level of the hepatic artery, covering 50% of the vessel diameter
4. Doppler angle of 55° or less
5. Pulse repetitions frequency (PRF) = 4 kHz, wall filter = 100 Hz
6. Doppler and B-mode tracings recorded simultaneously
7. Average maximum velocity obtained by manual tracing of the envelope of the Doppler waveform
8. Doppler waveform calculation obtained by covering two cardiac cycles between three arterial wall artifacts
9. Portal vein diameter measured from the inner anterior to the inner posterior wall
10. Values result from the mean of three consistent measurements.

and the efficacy of pharmacological therapy and surgical portosystemic anastomosis.

EVALUATION OF MEDICAL TREATMENT IN PORTAL HYPERTENSION

Many drugs which are effective on the systemic circulation also influence the splanchnic hemodynamics and have been proposed for the treatment of portal hypertension. Doppler flowmetry is a reliable method of evaluating flow changes after the administration of these drugs.

Bru et al. reported a net reduction in portal flow and portal pressure as a consequence of IV administration of vasopressin.[18] Transesophageal Doppler probe showed a reduction of 55% in portal flow and 15% in azygos vein flow.[19]

Using real time US and Doppler flowmetry to determine the diameter, the velocity and flow volume in the portal vein after administration of propranolol, a significant reduction in flow velocity and volume was found.[20]

Evaluation of Portosystemic Surgical Shunts

Ultrasonography is a useful method in the follow-up of patients after portosystemic shunt surgery, allowing assessment of patency in 75% of cases. The shunt is deemed patent when a direct confluence between portal vein and IVC or between the splenic and left renal vein is demonstrated (Fig. 9.15).

When the shunt itself is not displayed, indirect signs of patency may be used. In portocaval shunts, a decrease in caliber of the portal vein and widening of the IVC above the level of anastomosis is a useful sign of patency.[21] Dilatation of the left renal vein is consistent with a patent distal lienorenal shunt, while reversed flow in the superior mesenteric vein indicates a patent mesocaval shunt.

Doppler has proved useful in preoperative evaluation of patients as well as postoperative follow-up. Provided preoperative baseline studies have been performed, it is possible within certain limits to assess flow through the shunt and to gauge changes in portal perfusion.

Indirect signs of patency can be found in patients by examining the direction of flow in the portal vein or characteristics of flow towards the shunt. Presence of hepatofugal flow in the intrahepatic portal branches is side-to-side portocaval shunt is a reliable indicator of patency of the shunt.[22] Conversely, hepatopetal portal flow detected is a late postoperative study raises the suspicion of thrombosis of the shunt, especially if flow was hepatofugal at a previous examination.

In end-to-side portocaval shunts, portal flow is usually absent or hepatofugal in the intrahepatic branches. Demonstration of reversal of flow in the splenic and sometimes portal veins is proof of patency of a conventional lienorenal shunt (Fig. 9.16). Distal lienorenal shunts which are performed to decompress gastroesophageal varices while maintaining hepatopetal flow in the mesoportal venous bed are not always visualised on real time ultrasound. However, splenic vein displays phasic flow synchronous with caval pulsatility indicating shunt patency.[23]

Transjugular Intrahepatic Portosystemic Shunt (TIPS)

A minimally invasive option for complications of portal hypertension including variceal bleeding and refractory ascites has been developed: Positioning a metallic stent

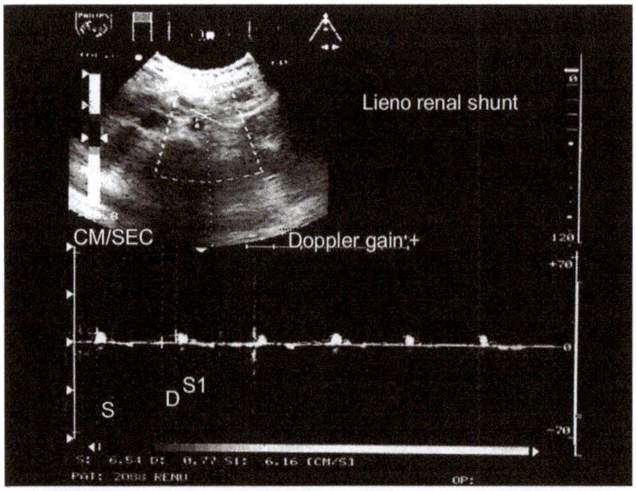

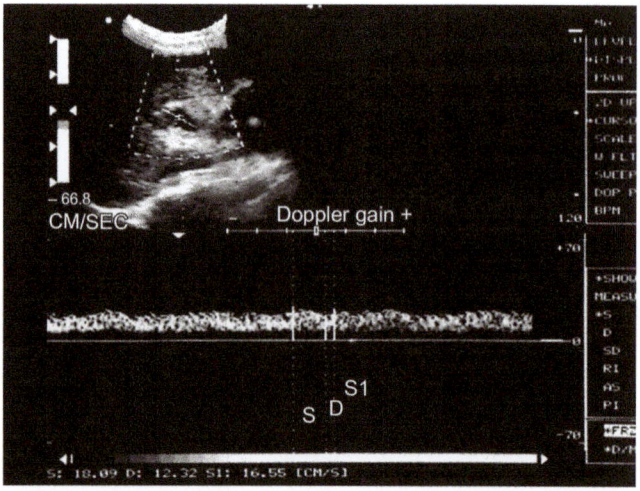

Fig. 9.15: Duplex Doppler of lienorenal shunt showing low velocity turbulent flow.

Fig. 9.16: Right portal vein branch demonstrates hepatofugal flow in the same patient.

between a hepatic vein and an intrahepatic portal vein branch (usually the right) by a percutaneous transjugular approach. This avoids open surgery and is safe for patients with severe liver failure. A major problem of tips is stenosis or occlusion of the shunt. While occlusion is irreversible, early diagnosis of stent stenosis allows angioplasty. Follow-up by repeated venography is the most reliable approach but is an expensive and invasive procedure. Routine follow-up is therefore by repeated sequential doppler examinations.

Immediately after TIPS placement, both portal vein diameter and velocity have been reported to increase resulting in a marked increase in portal vein flow volume.[24]

Blood flow in the main portal vein is hepatopetal but flows towards the shunt in the intrahepatic segments in patient with well functioning TIPS. Flow in other collaterals such as left gastric, paraumbilical veins may decrease, cease or reverse. Mean flow velocity in the shunt is high after tips placement.[25]

Duplex Doppler is accepted as a reliable technique in the long-term surveillance for complications such as stent thrombosis or stenosis and hepatic vein stenosis. The absence of detectable flow within a stent by doppler sonography has proved to be sensitive and specific for occlusion.[26] A stent velocity less than 50 cm(s) achieved a sensitivity of 100 percent and a specificity of 93% in the diagnosis of hepatic vein stenosis. Other diagnostic criteria are progressive reduction of peak velocity in the stent and a stent velocity less than 60 cm/s.[27] Localized acceleration of flow suggests stent stenosis while high flow velocity throughout the stent simply represents high volume flow without pathological significance. Contrast-enhanced power Doppler sonography has been reported to improve sensitivity and specificity in the diagnosis of stent dysfunction.[28]

Endoscopic Doppler Ultrasound

The recent introduction of endocavitary Duplex transducers has opened new perspectives for hemodynamic investigation. More recently, endocavitary Duplex transducers have been connected with fiberoptic endoscopes and are capable of providing an endoscopic visualization at the same time as the real time imaging and Doppler flowmetry. This has made it possible to obtain hemodynamic data for the esophageal and gastric varices, the periesophageal vascular beds and the azygos vein with a relatively noninvasive and innovative method.[29]

The instruments, currently available for endocavitary Doppler flowmetry are based on 7.5 MHz convex transducers with a 100° visual angle, incorporated longitudinally in an optical fiber endoscope. The sonographic scanning direction is longitudinal along the greater axis of the esophagus. The periesophageal collateral vascular bed

KEY POINTS

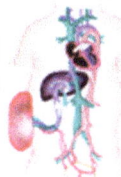

- Normal portal vein—hepatopetal, monophasic flow with some fluctuations.
- In PHT
  - Dilated splenoportal axis, hepatofugal flow.
  - Portosystemic collaterals, high velocity signals with broad spectrum of frequencies.
  - Cirrhosis with PHT—phasic variation of hepatic vein is reduced or absent.
  - SMA shows, decrease pulsatility index.
  - Doppler flowmetry evaluates success of medical and surgical treatment.

is visualized as echopoor channel like structures with a longitudinal course, often tortuous and irregular the study of the azygos vein is performed by using the reference points provided by the US images obtained when the transducer is in contact with the esophageal wall.

Budd-Chiari Syndrome (BCS)

It is a syndrome with clinical features of ascites, abdominal pain, hepatomegaly and jaundice that follows obstruction of the hepatic veins. If the inferior vena cava is also involved, distended superficial veins and edema of the lower extremities may be present.[30]

The Budd-Chiari syndrome includes hepatic veno-occlusive diseases, hepatic veins thrombosis, secondary obstruction of the inferior vena cava and the hepatic veins due to tumor or trauma (secondary Budd-Chiari syndrome) and primary membranous or segmental obstruction of the hepatic portion of the inferior vena cava (primary Budd-Chiari syndrome).[31]

The cause, clinical features and treatment depend on the site of the hepatic vein obstruction, at level of the small centrilobular veins, major hepatic veins or IVC.

Obstruction at the level of the central and sublobular veins may be due to toxins, particularly only pyrrolidine alkaloids. These effects are potentiated by protein-deficient diets.[32]

Obstruction of the major hepatic veins occurs most frequently in patients with coagulation abnormalities particularly polycythemia rubra vera and paroxysmal nocturnal hemoglobinuria.[33] It is also seen in Egyptian children from poor rural areas.[34] It may also be secondary to obstruction at the level of the hepatic venous ostia or within the IVC. The treatment of hepatic venous thrombosis is anticoagulant medication.[35]

Obstruction of the IVC which can extend into the orifice of the hepatic veins may be due to thrombosis, tumor extension, external compression, displacement or an obstructing membrane.

The necessity for an initial, often extensive radiologic evaluation is not surprising given the broad-spectrum of anatomic abnormalities associated with Budd-Chiari syndrome.[36] After the diagnosis is established, most patients with Budd-Chiari syndrome require a decompressive shunt which is constructed to divert blood away from a congested liver via the portal vein. The frequency of complications in these complex decompressive shunts is relatively high and adds further to the overall radiographic procedures.[37]

Since the 1950s, angiography has been the mainstay of diagnosis in patients with Budd-Chiari syndrome, both before and after surgery. Angiography in fact, remains the definitive technique. Unfortunately, angiography is invasive and frequently the hepatic veins cannot be opacified beyond their ostia. Numerous less invasive technique, including nuclear medicine, sonography and more recently MR imaging have had various degrees of success in characterizing the underlying vascular lesions in Budd-Chiari syndrome.[38]

Doppler imaging is an appealing technique in patients with Budd-Chiari syndrome. Duplex sonography can be used to assess the presence, direction and characteristics of flow within the hepatic veins and the IVC. Figure 9.17 shows power Doppler image of the normal hepatic veins confluence with the IVC.

Doppler Findings in Budd-Chiari Syndrome

1. *Hepatic veins:* Color Doppler images showed absence of flow in the hepatic veins. Direction of flow, if present and

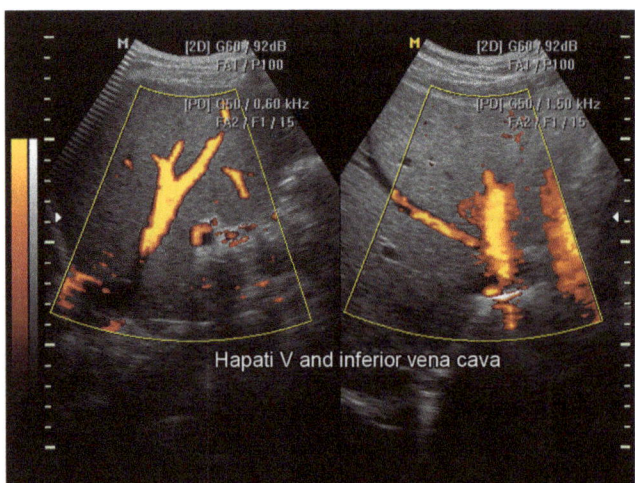

Fig. 9.17: Power Doppler image: Hepatic veins draining into inferior vena cava (IVC).

KEY POINTS

⇒ **BCS**
- HV—absent or reversed flow lacking phasic variation.
- IVC—No flow, reversed flat flow, very slow flow, or in partial obstruction-turbulent high velocity flow without phasic variation.
- Intrahepatic collaterals present.
- Focal liver lesions.

areas of occlusion can be clearly visualized. Reversed flow can be detected in the hepatic veins. A flat hepatic vein waveform lacking normal phasic fluctuation indicates distal compression and supports diagnosis of BCS.[39]

2. *Intrahepatic collaterals:* Intrahepatic venous collaterals typical of Budd-Chiari syndrome are either intrahepatic veins that communicate or collateral vessels that shunted blood from occluded veins to non-occluded veins or to enlarged inferior right hepatic veins or caudate lobe veins.

3. *Portal vein:* Evaluation of portal vein is essential in patients with Budd-Chiari syndrome because portal vein thrombosis precludes decompression of liver via a portosystemic shunt.

4. *Inferior vena cava:* The diagnosis of Budd-Chiari syndrome is based on an analysis of the flow direction and of the wave profile in the IVC. Abnormalities seen in IVC include no flow, reversed flow, very slow flow, visualization of echogenic thrombus, compressions by caudate lobe, long segment narrowing without associated enlargement of caudate lobe and localised marked narrowing consistent with a web.[40]

Obstruction of the IVC at the opening of the hepatic veins is seen as a reversed and flat flow in the lower section of the IVC. In cases of partial obstruction, the tracing of IVC loses its phasic oscillations and become turbulent with high velocity.

This flat wave profile was found in all the intrahepatic vessels resembling the hepatic veins. This aspect has been defined as a major criterion for the diagnosis of Budd-Chiari syndrome with Doppler US.[41]

Role of Color Doppler in Decompressive Shunts

Color-flow Doppler with either 5.0 or 3.0 MHz transducer showed the patency of the shunts dramatically. The anastomosis with the native vessel is visualized clearly in patients with patent graft. Duplex scanning with a 5 MHz transducer clearly showed appropriately directed flow in all cases. Spectral analysis showed a triphasic pattern in all of the shunts which is a reflection of right atrial contractility.[42]

COLOR DOPPLER IN HEPATIC LESIONS

The detection of a primary or metastatic liver tumor is a common clinical problem in which sonography, computerized sonography and magnetic resonance imaging are used for optimal detection. Benign pathological processes occur frequently in the liver and need to be differentiated from malignant tumors. Color flow and Duplex Doppler can help in this regard.[43] The incidental finding of a liver mass may result in a major dilemma of patient management.[44]

Echogenic focal areas of the liver are found in focal fatty infiltration, hemangiomas and a number of rare benign or tumor like conditions such as liver cell adenoma or focal nodular hyperplasia as well in malignant tumors. Commonly encountered echogenic malignant tumors include a primary hepatocellular carcinoma as well as common metastases such as those from gastrointestinal primaries, particularly from colonic primaries.

A vessel passing through an echogenic area without deviation suggests that the parenchymal abnormality is due to focal fatty infiltration, this condition should be considered especially in diabetes or alcoholics. Focal fatty infiltration may change rapidly with time.

Focal nodular hyperplasia (FNH) is a benign tumor of the liver. It is characterized pathologically by a cholangiolar proliferations associated with hyperplastic hepatocytes, blood vessels, and fibrosis.[45] The favored pathogenetic concept for FNH is that it develops from a focal excess of arterial blood flow from a pre-existing arterial malformation. Sonography is a reliable noninvasive method for evaluating focal liver lesions. Gray scale sonography has failed to distinguish between benign and malignant liver lesions. In this respect, a halo sign, i.e. a hypoechoic rim around lesions is usually considered to be a sonographic sign suggestive of malignancy.[46] However, recent studies have shown this interpretation to be misleading because the halo sign is frequently detectable in benign liver lesions such as in FNH, benign liver adenoma, liver abscess or atypical hemangioma. Color Doppler sonography has shown to be a reliable noninvasive method for evaluation of blood flow in liver lesions. In 71% of patients with FNH blood flow was detected within the halo zone (hypoechoic rim), spectral analysis of the blood flow indicated that the blood flow was arterial in all patients.[47] However, comparable blood flow in hypoechoic rim is also mentioned even in hepatocellular carcinoma (HCC) by some investigators.[48] There findings indicate that color Doppler sonography is not helpful in distinguishing FNH from HCC. In cases of risk factors for HCC or liver metastases, malignancy has to be ruled out by other investigations. Demonstration of blood flow in a hypoechoic rim of a focal liver lesion in patients without clinical suspicion of HCC or metastases suggest the diagnosis of FNH.

Hemangiomas are essentially large sinusoidal spaces which are full of slowly moving red cells. The Doppler frequency shift is small and is generally too low to be detected by Doppler systems utilizing conventional wall filters of 100 Hz or less. Thus, hemangiomas are well circumscribed echogenic focal masses which demonstrate little or no detectable flow. A 'spot pattern' is considered to the indication towards hemangioma and is seen in about 50% cases.[48] Color Doppler and Duplex sonography are also very useful in characterization of solid liver lesions. Several studies using vascular distribution criteria with color Doppler have attempted to make a histological characterization of liver lesions with different results. In a study conducted by M Gonzalez-Anon et al, it was postulated that the intratumoral venous color and pulsed Doppler signal regardless of other Doppler findings, is very suggestive of benignancy, with 70% sensitivity and 89% specificity. All lesions were benign when the only finding was venous color intratumoral Doppler Duplex signal (specificity 100%).[50]

The occurrence of detour venous pattern has been reported in metastases by Nino-Muncia et al.[49] and Tanaka et al.[48] Although it shows low sensitivity it is of great importance to objectify this vascular pattern because its specificity for malignancy in metastatic lesions is very high.

The simultaneous occurrence of both intra and peritumoral arterial flow in the same lesion strongly suggests malignancy.[50]

Tanaka et al. described four patterns of vascularity in focal liver lesions on color doppler flow imaging (CDFI). A basket pattern of peritumoral flow and a 'vessel-in-tumor' pattern was regarded as being very specific for hepatocellular carcinomas as seen in 75% and 65% of HCC respectively, while a spot pattern and a detour pattern were described for hemangiomas and metastases respectively.[51] The color pattern of the lesion is recorded as basket when a fine blood flow network surrounding the tumor is seen, VT (vessel within tumor) when blood flow entering into and branching within the tumor, Detour when a dilated portal vein is seen meandering around the tumor, or spot when color stained dots or patches seen in the central region of the tumor. HCC is seen to have a basket or VT pattern and hence color flow patterns can help in distinguishing them from metastases and hemangioma. Patients with lesions measuring less than 3 cm with detectable Doppler signals are likely to have HCC. Peak-systolic shifts greater than 3 kHz were found in few patients with HCC greater than 4 cm.[51] The use of highly sensitive color flow demonstrates neovascularization in virtually all hepatocellular carcinomas. Utilizing transducer insonating to optimize the Doppler shift, a Doppler shift greater than 2.5 kHz (at an insonating frequency of 3 MHz) or with an angle-corrected velocity greater than the main hepatic artery is highly suggestive of malignancy. These patients usually have elevated alpha-fetoprotein (AFP) levels.[52]

Power Doppler sonography is thought to be three to five times more sensitive than color Doppler sonography. The advantages of power Doppler sonography are that it detects lower velocity flows than color Doppler sonography, it decreases the noise background, it does not produce aliasing and it is independent of angle. Detection of the color signals in HCC was significantly more sensitive with power Doppler sonography than with color Doppler sonography. Power Doppler sonography however does not reveal the flow speed or direction of the color signals. Another disadvantage of power Doppler sonography is that it is sensitive to motion.[53]

Role of Contrast-enhanced Color Doppler Sonography in Liver Tumors

Duplex sonography and color Doppler imaging of liver tumors have shown characteristic vascular patterns that reflect the vascular anatomy of specific types of hepatic lesions. Although color Doppler sonography has opened up new diagnostic possibilities, it is limited in its ability to evaluate low velocity blood flow is very small intratumoral vessels particularly in small hepatic lesions and lesions located deep within the liver parenchyma because of the low intensity of Doppler signals or an insufficient Doppler shift. The use of ultrasound contrast agents has received increasing attention. Intravascular contrast agents improve the detection of low velocity blood flow because they increase the signal-to-noise ratio, allowing a more complete display of the vascular pattern of the tumor. In a study by D Strobel et al. sonographic contrast medium used was SHu 508A (Levovist; Schering, Berlin, Germany) a suspension of galactose based microbubbles.[54] The study demonstrated that the use of a galactose-based contrast agent improves the detection of intratumoral vascularity. An improvement of 20-86% was seen in the detection rate of intratumoral vascularity using a contrast agent in HCCs by Tanaka et al.[55] Contrast enhanced color Doppler sonography demonstrated intratumoral vascularity in 71% of metastases compared to 35% using conventional color Doppler sonography.

Color and pulsed Doppler sonography also has a role in detecting transient flow disturbance in early stage of hepatic abscesses. Chinami et al.[56] observed transient reversal of portal flow at the periphery of the abscesses during the active stage, which normalized after treatment (Figs. 9.18 and 9.19). Analysis of Doppler signal shows a decrease in RI and an increase in flow velocity in the hepatic artery followed by a decrease in the flow velocity and an increase in RI after normalization of flow in the branch of portal vein running parallel to it. The reversal of portal flow is usually seen in abscesses measuring greater than 6 cm.[57] However, a study in our institution showed this phenomenon in abscesses measuring more than 10 cm.[58] Thus, a differential diagnosis of hepatic tumors with reversal of portal flow should also include early stage hepatic abscesses.

KEY POINTS

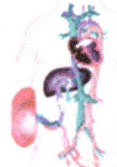

Duplex Doppler findings:

- Arterial flow within halo zone—malignant lesion not excluded.
- 50% hemangioma—spot pattern.
- Intratumoral venous signals—highly specific for benign lesions.

Criteria for malignant lesions

- Detour venous pattern (metastases).
- Intra and peritumoral arterial signals.
- Basket pattern of 6 peritumoral flow and vessel in tumor (HCC).
- Angle corrected velocity more than main hepatic artery velocity.
- GB malignant mass—high velocity blood flow signals.

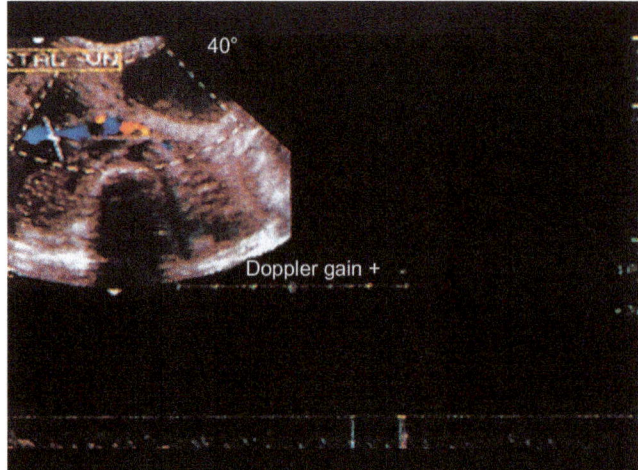

Fig. 9.18: Duplex Doppler US in a case of hepatic abscess before treatment showing reversal of portal flow in the anterior branch of the right portal vein.

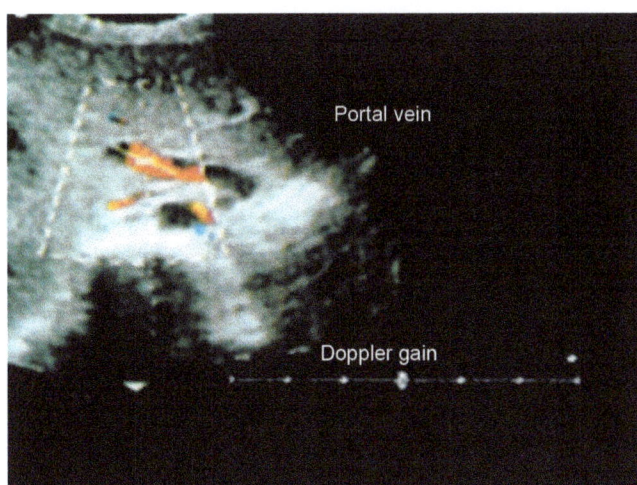

Fig. 9.19: Duplex Doppler US of the same case after treatment showing normalization of portal flow.

Gallbladder Carcinoma

Gallbladder carcinoma is a common gastrointestinal tumor and is three times more common in women than in men. It occurs most often in elderly patients. The lesion on gray scale sonography is imaged as (a) a solid mass occupying the whole gallbladder, (b) a focal polypoid mass or (c) diffuse wall thickening. Type (a) and (b) constitute the majority of cases and in these cases differentiation between gallbladder carcinoma and tumefactive biliary sludge is needed. It is important diagnostic problem because former should be treated surgically and the latter should be managed medically. Conventional gray scale US provides very little if any useful information for differentiation. The addition of color Doppler sonography offers a definite advantage for this purpose. Blood flow signals are seen in majority of cases of gallbladder carcinoma (Fig. 9.20). However, no significant correlation is seen between the tumor and the maximal flow velocity. Cystic artery can also be visualised in few of the tumors. In the tumefactive biliary sludge group, color Doppler sonography detected no blood signals in the mass. High velocity flow is considered to be an important sign suggestive of malignant nature of the tumor. Although benign tumors show a lower rate of detection of blood signals compared with gallbladder carcinoma and the presence or absence of blood flow signals seem to be a useful sign for differentiating benign from malignant tumors.

LIVER TRANSPLANTATION

Since the first hepatic transplant was performed in 1963, this procedure has become an accepted method of treatment for fulminant and subfulminant hepatic failure, cirrhosis, Budd-Chiari syndrome, biliary atresia and tumor. Successful transplantation requires careful selection of recipients to avoid conditions that would significantly reduce the success of the procedure. After transplantation, careful monitoring of the recipient is required to identify complications of the procedure and adverse effects of immunosuppression required to prevent rejection. Diagnostic ultrasound augmented with Duplex and color Doppler plays an important role in both preoperative and postoperative evaluation of the patient undergoing hepatic transplantation.

Preoperative Assessment

Prior to hepatic transplantation, significant hepatic parenchymal and vascular abnormalities must be identified to aid the surgeon in planning the operation. Ultrasound, aided by Doppler, is used to document the anatomy, and patency of the inferior vena cava, hepatic veins and portal vein. In children with biliary atresia, anatomic mapping is of particular importance because approximately 25% of patients with biliary atresia have portal vein or inferior vena cava anomalies. If transplantation is being performed for treatment of hepatic malignancy, ultrasound may aid in defining the extent of the tumor and determining the presence of vascular invasion or biliary obstruction.

Portal Vein Patency

Successful liver transplantation depends upon several factors, but among the most important is successful vascular anastomosis. Portal vein occlusion is a recognized sequel of long-standing liver disease and causes rapid hepatic decompensation, it is therefore important for the status of portal vein to be assessed pre-operatively. Patency of portal vein is an essential prerequisite for liver transplantation.

The extrahepatic components of the portal venous system can be assessed via subcostal scans, combination of imaging and color flow Doppler usually rapidly confirms their patency.

Both imaging and color Doppler studies of the intrahepatic portal venous system are best achieved via right lateral intercostal scans, which allow visualization of the main and right portal veins even in the smallest of livers. Flow within the intrahepatic portal vein does not necessarily imply patency of the extrahepatic venous system. Low velocity forward intrahepatic flow can occur in patients in whom splenic and superior mesenteric venous occlusion has been proved. Both components of the portal system must be examined. If color flow and power Doppler studies fail to detect flow within the portal vein the equipment control settings must be optimised to detect

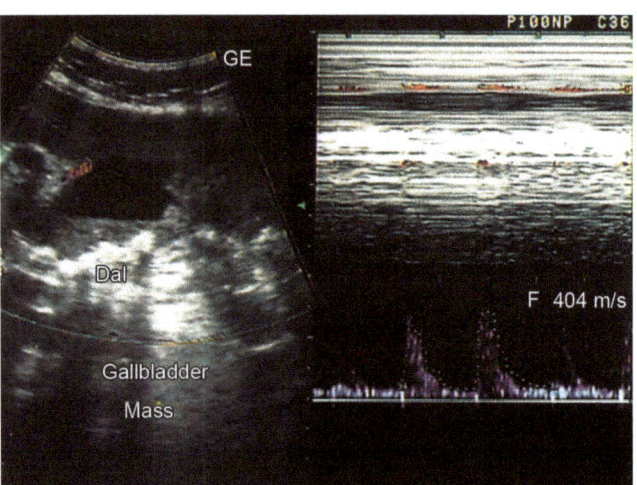

Fig. 9.20: Color Doppler flow mapping in a case of cholelithiasis associated with carcinoma of gallbladder: Poorly defined anatomical boundary of gallbladder. Multiple calculi in the lumen associated with mass lesion in fundus and body of gallbladder. Anterior wall is irregularly thickened due to neoplasia and vascular study show pulsatility and Resistive Index 2.153 and 0.865 respectively; suggestive of increased neovascularization.

low velocity flow. In addition, the Doppler shift frequency must be optimized by minimizing the beam/vessel angle, particularly by using lateral intercostal scans. If no flow is found, the examination should be repeated after an interval or after a meal. If doubt persists after a second or subsequent examination, the use of ultrasound contrast agents may be helpful by increasing the signal intensity from any blood within the portal vein.[59]

If little or no flow is detected in the intrahepatic portal veins, and if there is imaging evidence of either fresh or old thrombosis in the intrahepatic portal system. The superior mesenteric vein must be assessed. If the superior mesenteric vein remains patent at the level of the splenic vein confluence the surgeon may be able to use this as a source of portal supply to the grafted liver.

A further source of error in the diagnosis of portal vein occlusion is cavernous transformation of the portal vein which develops as a long-term sequel to portal vein thrombosis. Imaging alone may suggest the diagnosis by detecting numerous serpiginous channels replacing the portal veins at the porta hepatis. In the majority of patients with cavernous transformation, the intrahepatic portal vein branches are either abnormally small or absent and therefore the assessment should include both the intra and extrahepatic components of the portal vein.

The final component of portal assessment is the detection of periportal collaterals.

It is customary to measure the maximum diameter of the spleen when assessing patients with liver disease, this should always be recorded prior to liver transplantation. Progressive splenic enlargement in the postoperative period may be the first indication of portal vein stenosis or occlusion, recurrent liver disease or rejection. A preoperative baseline measurement is therefore important.

Preoperative Donor Assessment

Usually a relative, mother, father, uncle or aunt is used as the donor. Prior to removal of the segments it is important to exclude the presence of liver disease is the donor and to assess the presence of any vascular anomalies.

Preoperative Scanning

Intraoperative ultrasound is not an accepted technique and may fulfill a number of notes in the transplant patient.

Prehepatectomy intraoperative ultrasound may be helpful to confirm the number and extent of neoplasms and to assess vascular invasion.

After successful transplantation intra-operative Doppler studies are invaluable in confirming good flow through the vascular anastomosis.[60]

Postoperative Scanning

The role of ultrasound in postoperative period varies according to the time lapsed since the operation. If circumstances permit, it is probably ideal to perform routine examinations on days 1, 3, 5 and 7, and weekly thereafter, unless otherwise indicated by clinical or biochemical findings.[61]

Before undertaking postoperative examinations it is important to be conversant with the surgical details. Detailed information concerning the hepatic artery, portal vein, IVC and biliary anastomosis is important. The operator should follow a predetermined protocol to ensure that all aspects of the transplant anatomy are carefully assessed and that all possible sites for fluid collections are evaluated.

Hepatic Artery

Problems related to hepatic artery anastomosis are the most common vascular complications after liver transplantation.[62] In adults early arterial occlusion occurs in 1–3 percent of patients but is more common in paediatric age group, especially in patients under one year of age. Early arterial occlusion is almost always a catastrophic event, with rapid and irreversible liver cell death.

Postoperative occlusion of the hepatic artery most commonly occurs at the site of the vascular anastomosis but may occur elsewhere in the main vessel. Ideally all segments including the extrahepatic and intrahepatic main hepatic artery and right and left intrahepatic branches should be studied. A spectral trace from the hepatic artery must be obtained before its patency can be confirmed.[63] The flow velocity waveform obtained from the hepatic artery in the acute post-transplant phase is variable. However, if the velocity is formed to be extremely low or the waveforms very damped, this strongly raises the suspicion of a significant stenosis. If the Doppler studies show a progressive reduction in arterial velocity or a fall-off in diastolic flow in the absence of obvious parenchymal abnormality, the possibility of a progressive arterial obstructive lesions should be considered and angiography must be advised.[64] Doppler studies of the hepatic artery are important but in any patient in whom the Doppler findings do not concur with the clinical context angiography must be performed.

A further complication of hepatic artery occlusion is the increased risk of intrahepatic abscess formation. The whole volume of liver must be scanned in patient with known or suspected arterial occlusions.

If the arterial stenosis is treated by transluminal angioplasty, serial Doppler studies are invaluable for confirming improvements in the arterial flow and for monitoring the patient's subsequent progress.

Portal Vein

Early postoperative occlusion of the portal vein is rare in adults and uncommon in children. However, early occlusion may have catastrophic consequences with early graft dysfunction or variceal bleeding. Color flow imaging is almost always sufficient for confirmation of patency. Patients with Budd-Chiari syndrome, abnormal portal vein anatomy, portal vein conduit or who have had an operative thrombectomy are all at increased risk or portal vein thrombosis.

The flow characteristics within the transplanted portal vein are often abnormal. There may be severe flow disturbances beyond the anastomosis and a relatively high velocity jet may be found at the anastomosis. Spectral Doppler studies should be attempted using color flow imaging to detect the highest velocity, and a peak velocity estimate must be performed. If this is more than 100 cm/s, the anastomosis is likely to be unacceptably tight and patient must be carefully monitored for portal stenosis and evidence of extrahepatic portal hypertension.

Late stenosis of the portal vein is an uncommon but serious complication[65] and can usually be predicted by detecting a narrow anastomosis on the early postoperative scan.[66] In these patients serial measurements of the jet velocity permit the detection of a progressive stenosis and the spleen is seen to enlarge if the lesions becomes hemodynamically significant.

Late the sudden portal vein occlusion is rare and usually presents with a sudden deterioration in liver function tests, the onset of resistant ascites and rapidly increasing splenomegaly. Any patient with these symptoms should undergo full Doppler assessment.

Hepatic Veins and IVC

Early hepatic veins thrombosis is almost always unheard of except in patients who have been transplanted for Budd-Chiari syndrome. The clinical relevance of hepatic vein Doppler studies in liver transplantation remains uncertain.

Stenosis of IVC is extremely rare and generally presents with ascites and lower limb edema. The diagnosis is established by demonstration of a dilated and pulseless vena cava below the level of the stenosis,[67] but contrast cavography is the definitive diagnostic test (Figs. 9.21A and B).

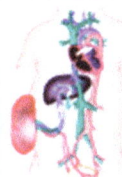

KEY POINTS
- Liver transplantation.
- Duplex Doppler used for establishing PV patency preoperatively.
- In postoperative period—routine US and Doppler done on 1,3,5,7 days and weekly thereafter.
- Hepatic artery occlusion—at site of vascular anastomosis.
- Transplanted portal V—peak velocity > 100 cm/sec-suggests tight stenosis and patient is carefully monitored.

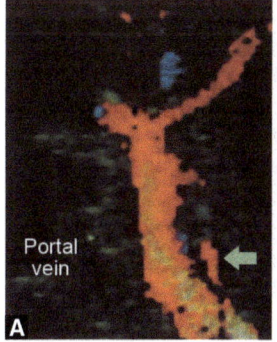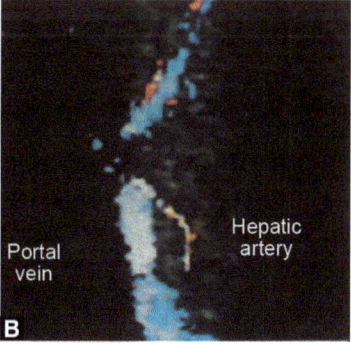

Figs. 9.21A and B: Severe acute hepatic transplant rejection (A) five days after transplant. There is a hepatopetal flow in the portal vein and hepatic artery (⇐). The arterial flow velocity waveform appeared normal and (B) seven days after transplant. There is hepatofugal flow in the portal vein. Increased slow flow sensitivity Doppler signal explain the lighter color hue in both arteries and veins. Pathology demonstrated severe rejection with centrilobular necrosis and periportal inflammation.

REFERENCES

1. Partiquin H, Lofortun M, Peter N, et al. Duplex Doppler exam in portal HT: Technique and anatomy. AJR. 1987;149:171-6.
2. Sutton D. The liver and spleen. Dick R, Julic FC (Eds). Textbook of Radiology and Imaging, 6th edition. Edinburgh Churchill Livingstone.
3. Bolondi L, Gandolfi L, Arienti V, et al. Ultrasonography in the diagnosis of portal HT: Diminished response of portal vessels to respiration. Radiology. 1982;142:167-72.
4. Ohnishi K, Saito M, Nakayama T, et al. Portal venous hemodynamic is chronic liver disease: effect of posture change and exercise. Radiology. 1985;155:757-61.
5. Jacger K, Bollinger A, Valli C, et al. Measurement of mesenteric blood flow by duplex scanning. J Vasc Surg. 1986;3:46-51.
6. Okazaki K, Miyaraki M, Onishi S, et al. Effect of food intake and various extrinsic hormones on portal blood flow in patients with liver cirrhosis demonstrated by pulsed Doppler with Octoron. Scand J Gastroenterol. 1986;21:1029-34.
7. Kawasaki T, Moriyasu F, Nishida O, et al. Analysis of hepatofugal flow in portal venous system using ultrasonic Doppler duplex system. Am J Gastroenteral. 1989;84:937-41.
8. Gaiani S, Bolondi L, Li Bassi S, et al. Prevalence of spontaneous hepatofungal portal flow in liver cirrhosis. Clinical and endoscopic correlations in 228 patients. Gastroenterology. 1991;100:160-67.
9. Nakayama T, Hiyamma Y, Ohniski K, et al. Arterioportal shunts on dynamic computed tomography. AJR. 1983;140:953.
10. Schrier RW, Arroyo V, Bernandi M, et al. Peripheral vasodilatation hypothesis: a proposal for the initiation of renal sodium and water retention in cirrhosis. Hepatology. 1988;8:1151-57.
11. Piscaglia F, Gaiani S, Gramantieri L, et al. Superior mesenteric artery impedance in chronic liver diseases: relationship with disease severity and portal circulation. Am J Gastro enterol. 1998;93(10):1798-99.
12. Bolognesi M, Sacerdoti D, Merkel C, et al. Splenic Doppler impedance indices: influences of different portal hemodynamic conditions. Hepatology. 1996;23:1035-40.
13. Sacerdote D, Merkel C, Bolognesi M, et al. Hepatic arterial resistance indexes in cirrhosis without and with portal vein thrombosis relationships with portal hemodynamics. Gastroenterology. 1995;108:1152-58.
14. Moriyasu F, Nishida O, Bass N, et al. Measurement of portal vascular resistance in patients with portal hypertension. Gastroenterology. 1986;90:710-16.
15. Burns PN. Interpretation and analysis of Doppler signals. In: Taylor KJW, Burns PN, Wells PNT (Eds.). Clinical Application of Doppler Ultrasound. New York: Reven, 1988.
16. Sabba C, Mrkel C, Zoli M, et al. Interobserver and interequipment variability of echo Doppler examination of the portal vein: Effect of a cooperative training programme. Hepatology. 1995;21:428-33.
17. Moriyasu F, Bass N, Nishida O, et al. 'Congestions index' of the portal vein. AJR. 1985;146:735-9.
18. Bru C, Bosch J, Navasa M, et al. Pulsed Doppler measurements of portal blood flow in man: Applications in the noninvasive evaluation of the pharmacological therapy of portal hypertension. In: Bondestam S, Alanen A, Joupplila P (Eds.). Proccedings of the 6th congress of the European Federation of the societies for ultrasound in Medicine and Biology 14-18 June 1987. Finland; Helsinki. 1987;66.
19. Kinura T, Moryiasu F, Kawasaki T, et al. Changes in the azygos venous flow evaluated using transesophageal Doppler ultrasound after vasopressin infusions in portal hypertension. Hepatology. 1989;10:A42.
20. Zoli M, Marchesini G, Brunori A, et al. Portal venous flow in response to acute beta-blocker and vasodilatatory treatment in patients with liver cirrhosis. Hepatology. 1986;6:1248.
21. Holmin T, Alwmark A, Forsberg L. The ultrasonic demonstration of portocaval and interpositions mesocaval shunt. Br J Surg. 1982;69:673-75.
22. Lafortune M, Patriquin H, Pomier G, et al. Haemodynamic changes in portal circulation after portosystemic shunts: Use of duplex sonography in 43 patients. AJR. 1987;149:701-06.
23. Balondi L, Gaiani S, Mazziotti A, et al. Morphological and hemodynamic changes from distal splenorenal shunt: An ultrasound and pulsed doppler study. Hepatology. 1988;8:652-7.
24. Lafortune martenet JP, Denys A, et al. Short and long term hemodynamic effects of transjugular intra hepatic porto systemic shunts: A doppler/manometric correlative study. AJR. 1995;164:997-1002.
25. Feldstein VA, Patel MD, Laberge, JM. Transjugular intrahepatic portosystemic shunts: Accuracy of doppler US in determination of patency and detection of stenosis. Radiology. 1996;200:141-7.
26. Chong WK, Malioch TA, Marer MJ, et al. Transjugular intrahepatic portosystemic shunt: US assessment with maximum flow velocity. Radiology. 1993;189:789-93.
27. Foshager MC, Ferral H, Nazarian GK, et al. Duplex sonography after transjugular intrahepatic portosystemic shunts (TIPS): normal hemodynamic findings and efficacy in predicting shunt patency and stenosis. AJR. 1993;165:1-7.
28. Uggowitren MM, Kugler C, Machan L, et al. Value of echo enhanced doppler sonography in evaluation of transjugular intrahepatic portosystemic shunts. AJR. 1998;170:1041-6.
29. Sukigara M, Komarali T, Yamaraki T, et al. Color flow mapping of the esophageal varices and vessels in and around the liver with real time two-dimensional Doppler echography. Clin radiol. 1987.
30. Parker RGF. Occlusion of the hepatic veins in man. Medicine. 1959;38:369-402.
31. Masatoshi Makuuchi, Hishoshi Hasegava, Suoumu Yamazaki, et al. Primary Budd-Chiari syndrome: Ultrasonic demonstration. Radiology. 1984;152:775.
32. Philip Stanley. Budd-Chiari syndrome. Radiology. 1989;170:625-27.
33. Mitchell MC, Boitnott JK, Kaufman S, et al. Budd-Chiari syndrome: etiology, diagnosis and management. Medicine. 1982;61:199-218.

34. Safouh M, Shehata AH. Hepatic vein occlusion disease of Egyptian children. J Pediatr. 1965;67:415-22.
35. Campbell DA Jr, Rolles K, Jamieson, et al. Hepatic transplantation with perioperative and long term anticoagulation as treatment for Budd-Chiari syndrome. Surg Gynecol Obstet. 1988;166:511-18.
36. Scissors IW. Membranous obstruction of the infection vena cava and hepatocellular carcinoma in South Africa. Gastroenterology. 1982;82:171-78.
37. Longer B, Stone RM, Colapinto RF, et al. Clinical spectrum of the Budd-Chiari syndrome and its surgical managements. Am J Surg. 1975;129:137-45.
38. Stark DD, Hahn PF, Trey C, et al. MRI of the Budd-Chiari syndrome. AJR. 1986;146:1141-48.
39. Rallo PW, Johnson MB, Radin DR, et al. Budd-Chiari syndrome: Detection with color Doppler sonography. AJR 1992;159:113-16.
40. Millener P, Grant EG, Rose S, et al. Color Doppler imaging findings in patients with Budd-Chiari syndrome: correlation with venographic findings. AJR. 1993;161:307-12.
41. Horoki T, Kuroda C, Tokunaga K, et al. Hepatic venous outflow obstruction: Evaluation with pulsed Doppler sonography. Radiology. 1989;170:733.
42. Grant EG, Parrella R, Tessler FN, et al. Budd-Chiari syndrome: The results of duplex and color Doppler imaging. AJR. 1989;152:377-81.
43. Onishi K, Nomura F. Ultrasonic Doppler studies of hepatocellular carcinoma and comparison with other hepatic focal lesions. Gastroenterology. 1989;97:1489-97.
44. Taylor CR, Taylor KJW. Imaging techniques. An incidental hemangioma of the liver: The dilemma of patient management. J Clin Gastroenterol. 1981;3:93-97.
45. Wanless IR, Mawdsley C, Adams R. On the pathogenesis of focal nodular hyperplasia of the liver. Hepatology. 1985;5:1194-200.
46. Yoshida T, Matuse H, Okazaki N, et al. Ultrasonographic differentiation of hepatocellular carcinoma from metastatic liver cancer. J Clin Ultrasound. 1987;15:431-37.
47. Herbay A, Frieling T, Niederau C, et al. Solitary hepatic lesions with a hypoechoic rim: Value of color Doppler sonography. AJR. 1997;169:1539-41.
48. Tanaka S, Kitamura T, Fujita M, et al. Color doppler flow imaging of liver tumors. AJR. 1990;154:509-14.
49. Nino-Murcia M, Ralls PW, Jeffrey RB, et al. Color flow Doppler characterisation of focal liver lesions. AJR. 1992;159:1195-97.
50. M Gonzalez-Anon, et al. Characterisation of solid liver lesions with color and pulsed Doppler imaging. 1999;24:137-43.
51. Srivastava DN, Mahajan Amit, Berry M, et al. Color Doppler flow imaging of focal hepatic lesions. Australasian Radiology 2000;44:285-89.
52. Ebara M, Ohto M, Shiragawa T, et al. Natural history of minute hepatocellular carcinoma smaller than 3 cm complicating cirrhosis. Gastroenterology. 1986;90:289-98.
53. Rubin JM, Bude RO, Carson PL, et al. Power doppler US: A potentially useful alternative to mean frequency-based color Doppler US. Radiology. 1994;190:853-56.
54. Deike Strobel, UDO Krodel, Peter Martus, et al. Clinical evaluation of contrast-enhanced color Doppler sonography in the differential diagnosis of liver tumors. J Clin Ultrasound. 2000;28:1-13.
55. Tanaka S, Kitamra T, Yoshioka F, et al. Effectiveness of galactose based intravenous contrast medium on color Doppler sonography of deeply located hepatocellular carcinoma. Ultrasound Med Biol. 1995;21:157.
56. Chinami. Liver abscess with reversal of portal flow. Ultrasound International. 1997;3:135-38.
57. Linzy, Wang JH, Wang LY. Changes in intrahepatic portal hemodynamics in early stage hepatic abscesses. J Ultrasound Med. 1996;8:595-98.
58. Mehrotra P, Bhargava SK. Reversal of portal flow in liver abscesses. Ind J Radiol Imag. 2000;10:21-23.
59. Teefey SA, Middleton WD, Crowe TM, et al. Doppler sonographic evaluation of the portal vein: Effects of intravenous dodecafluoro-pentane. J Ultrasound Med. 1997;16:641-45.
60. Waldman DL, Lee DE, Bronsther O, et al. Use of intraoperative ultrasonography during hepatic transplantation. J Ultrasound Med. 1998;17:1-6.
61. Hellinger A, Roll C, Stracke A, et al. Impact of color Doppler sonography on detection of thrombus of the hepatic artery and the portal vein after liver transplantation. Langenbecks Arch Chir. 1996;381:182-85.
62. Wozeney P, Zajko AB, Bron KM. Vascular complications after liver transplantation: A five year experience. AJR. 1986;147:657-63.
63. Flint EW, Sunkin JH, Zajko AB. Duplex sonography of hepatic artery thrombosis after liver transplantation. AJR. 1988;147:481-83.
64. Marnjo WC, Langnas AN, Wood RP, et al. Vascular complications following orthotopic liver transplantation: outcome and the role of urgent revascularisation. Transplant Proc. 1991;23:1484-86.
65. Malassagne B, Soubrane O, Dousser B, et al. Extrahepatic portal hypertension following liver transplantation: A rare but challenging problem. HPB Surg. 1998;10:357-63.
66. Lee J, Ben-Ami T, Yousefzadeh D, et al. Extrahepatic portal vein stenosis in recipients of living-donor allografts: Doppler sonography. AJR. 1996;167:85-90.
67. Brouwers MA, De Jong KP, Peeters PM, et al. inferior vena cava obstruction after orthotopic liver transplantation. Clin Transplantation. 1994;8:19-22.

Role of Color Doppler in Splenic Lesions

PORTAL HYPERTENSION

Portal hypertension results in changes in various vessels along with development of multiple portosystemic collaterals.

Along with dilatation of portal vein, varying degrees of dilatation of splenic and superior mesenteric veins and loss of respiratory variations also occur in portal hypertension. A caliber of splenic vein over 12 mm should be regarded as suspicious whereas splenic vein over 20 mm diameter or greater should be considered a specific sign of portal hypertension. Dilatation of superior mesenteric vein is a more specific marker for portal hypertension. Splenomegaly, usually associated with portal hypertension, is also responsible for dilatation of splenic vein possibly because of increased splenic blood flow (Fig. 10.1).

Dilatation of splenic artery was also found to accompany splenomegaly which is required to supply a more extensive capillary bed. Splenic artery dilatation was also found to occur more frequently in cirrhosis caused by chronic viral hepatitis than in alcohol abuse. A ratio between the diameter of the hepatic and splenic arteries above 0.9, measured at 1.5-3 cm from their origins, suggests an alcoholic cause for cirrhosis, whereas a lower ratio is indicative of an infectious cause.

Another important sign of portal hypertension is the lack of variations in caliber with respiration in the splenic and superior mesenteric veins (Fig. 10.2).

Along with hepatofugal portal flow, splenic vein also shows hepatofugal flow which has proved to be closely correlated with hepatic encephalopathy.

At level of lower splenic pole, lienorenal collaterals appear as tortuous vessels with a high velocity Doppler

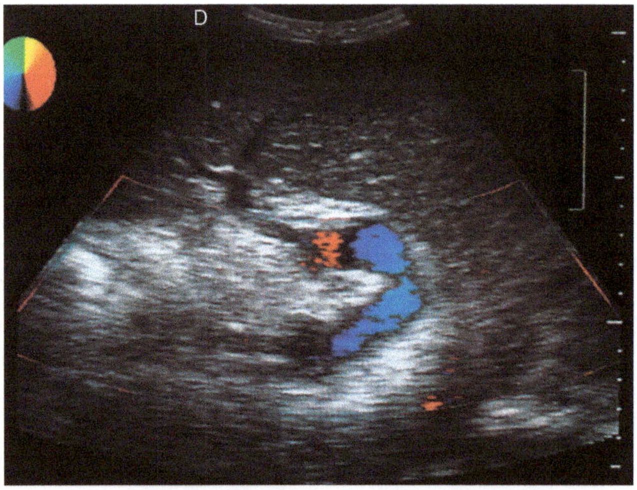

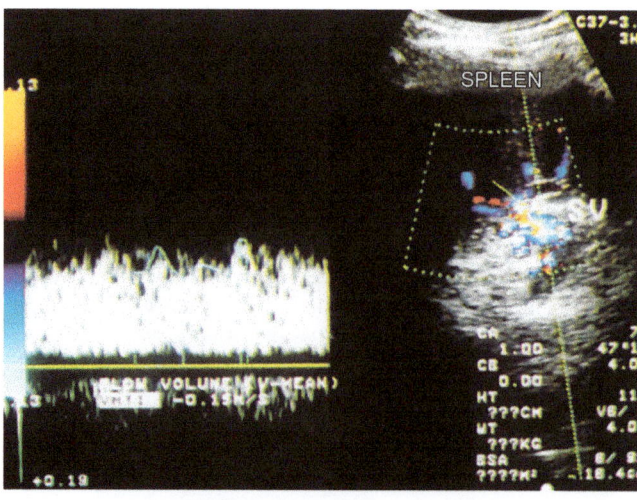

Fig. 10.1: Dilated and tortuous splenic vein with splenomegaly.

Fig. 10.2: Splenic venous flow pattern in a portal hypertensive.

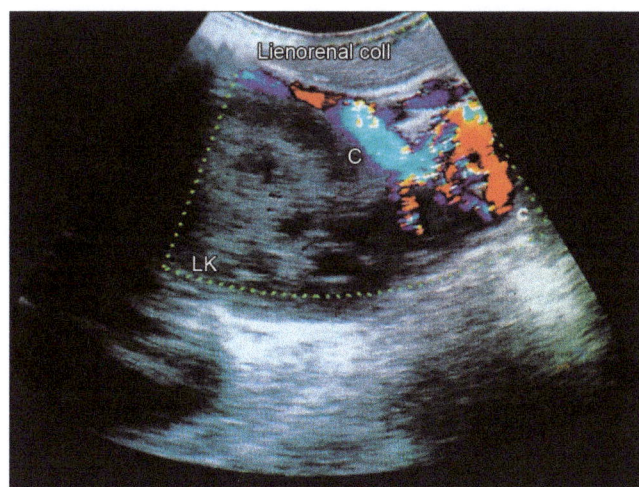

Fig. 10.3: Voluminous lienorenal collaterals.

Flowchart 10.1: Characteristics and complications of splenic infarction.

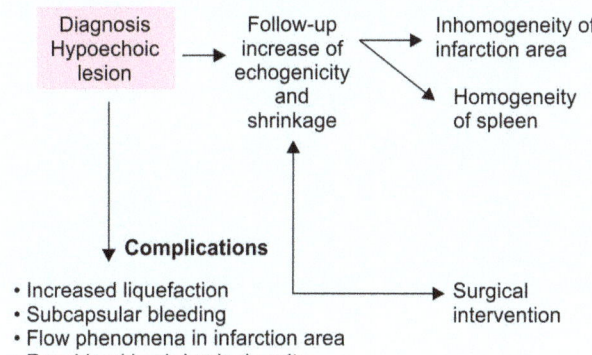

signal and a broad spectrum of frequencies due to turbulence (Fig. 10.3). Their presence is often associated with flow reversal in the splenic vein.

SPLENIC INFARCTION

Splenic infarcts occur in patients with myeloproliferative syndromes, hemolytic anemias and sepsis especially in sepsis associated with endocarditis. The striking clinical feature is sudden onset of pain in the upper left abdomen, occasionally associated with a painful restriction of the respiratory excursion or local pain on palpation. However, clinical diagnosis can be difficult because pain can be associated with almost all cases of splenomegaly and infarct may be silent.

Splenic infarcts can be visualized at ultrasound scanning and B-mode pulsed Doppler US can identify infarct related complications (Flowchart 10.1).

For the imaging diagnosis of splenic infarction, a wide range of ultrasound appearances have been observed. About 24 hours after therapeutic embolization of the splenic artery for treatment of portal hypertension, splenic infarcts appear as wedge-shaped, hypoechoic and well-demarcated lesions at sonography. This is the typical US appearance of acute stage without complications. Scar stage of infarction may be seen as in homogeneity of splenic texture months later.

Severe infarct related complications might develop in the course of disease that can be detected by follow-up US and Doppler scanning. The findings that require surgical intervention are the following:
1. Increasing subcapsular hemorrhage
2. Extravasation of blood into peritoneal cavity
3. Flow phenomena in the area of infarction as seen at B-mode pulsed Doppler US.

In patients demonstrating arterial signals within the infarction area, histological examination revealed superinfection of the splenic infarcts. The presence of arterial signals and increasing subcapsular hemorrhage were signs of occurrence of spontaneous splenic rupture. Hence, with clear sonographic signs of life-threatening splenic rupture, splenectomy should be recommended.

INTRASPLENIC PSEUDOANEURYSM

Post-traumatic pseudoaneurysm involving splanchnic arteries are very rare in the pediatric age group and affect mostly the splenic artery or intrasplenic arterial branches. Because of the potential life-threatening complications, intrasplenic pseudoaneurysm must be diagnosed and treated immediately. Although, the trend in the management of blunt splenic injuries has been towards conservative treatment, formation of a pseudoaneurysm at the site of a splenic hematoma may cause delayed splenic rupture requiring splenectomy. This has necessitated routine follow-up of blunt splenic injuries by color Doppler sonography or CT to detect pseudoaneurysm at an early stage when selective embolization might prevent expansions of the hematoma and rupture of the spleen.

Intrasplenic pseudoaneurysm is formed by active bleeding from injured intrasplenic arterial branches. Although, spontaneous thrombosis is possible, the usual evolution of the lesions is gradual expansion of the hematoma with eventual rupture of the splenic capsule. This unpredictable ominous complications necessitates a meticulous search for there lesions in all cases of blunt splenic trauma.

Initial scanning in patients who have experienced blunt splenic trauma may be performed with color Doppler sonography or contrast-enhanced CT. Intrasplenic

KEY POINTS

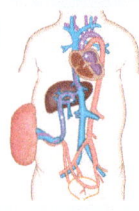

Spleen

- **PHT**
  - Dilated splenic vein (>12 mm), lack respiratory variation, hepatofugal flow lienorenal collaterals.
- Complications of splenic infarction.
  - Doppler detects—arterial signals in infarct—superinfection.
  - Arterial signals in infarct and increasing sub-capsular hemorrhage suggests possibility of spontaneous splenic rupture.

pseudoaneurysm appears on gray scale sonography as nonspecific anechoic lesions. Their aneurysmal nature can be revealed by the demonstration of arterial flow on color Doppler sonography. Turbulent arterial flow within the lesion suggests a diagnosis of pseudoaneurysm. Not all intrasplenic pseudoaneurysm develop at the time of initial trauma. Some lesions develop in a delayed fashion presumably because of gradual lysis of the clot sealing the injured arterial wall. Thus, conservative management of blunt splenic trauma should include periodic follow-up with color Doppler sonography or CT even if admission scans are negative. Coil embolization of splenic artery is the preferred method for hemostasis of intrasplenic pseudoaneurysm.

Color Doppler in Pancreas

Color Doppler sonography displays blood flow information on the morphologic data obtained from the gray scale sonogram and becomes a useful imaging modality for the evaluation of patients with abdominal tumors.[1]

Although the use of angiography and computed tomography (CT) in the preoperative evaluation of pancreatic tumors has been well-documented, it is highly desirable to obtain the most accurate diagnostic information possible with more noninvasive and cost-effective technique such as color Doppler sonography. Color Doppler sonography has been found to be more sensitive than angiography in depicting vascular involvement of carcinoma. Hence, a preoperative assessment in suspected pancreatic carcinoma patients with initial color Doppler sonography helps in improved patient management.

To look for vascular involvement in patients with pancreatic carcinoma, all the peripancreatic mesenteric vessels, i.e. celiac artery, superior mesenteric artery, hepatic artery, splenic artery, splenic vein, superior mesenteric vein and main portal vein are to be examined. Color Doppler sonographic criteria used for staging vascular involvement are normal (no contact between tumour and vessel), abutment (tumor adjacent to vessel and no clear in growth), encasement (circumferential narrowing of the vessel lumen) and occlusion (sudden interruption of the vessel). A vessel if normal or showed abutment favored resectability whereas encasement or occlusions of vessel favor non-resectability. This is important because pancreatic carcinoma is one of the leading causes of adult cancer death.[2]

Only patients whose tumors are completely resected can expect to survive. Unnecessary surgical exploration may result in increased postoperative morbidity and a prolonged recovery. Hence, precise preoperative staging is rapidly increasing. Patients showing signs of peripancreatic vessel involvement are considered to be unresectable.[3]

In a study conducted by H Ishida et al., accuracy of color Doppler sonography in the staging of 26 patients with pancreatic carcinoma and compared with accuracy of angiography. The study showed that color Doppler sonography was more sensitive than angiography in the diagnosis of vascular involvement. This tendency was more obvious in the arteries than in the veins. Hence, it was concluded that in predicting the unresectability of pancreatic carcinoma rarely requiring additional confirmatory studies. In contrast in prediction of resectability, it is sometimes inaccurate and additional examinations are needed for more accurately unresectable pancreatic carcinoma patients.[4]

PANCREATIC TRANSPLANTATION

First segmental pancreatic transplant was performed in 1966. It has now become an increasingly important option for the management of type I diabetes mellitus. Technical features and graft rejection were the major causes of high graft failure rates and recipients' mortality. With recent technical success and improvements in immuno-suppression, there has been an increase in the number of patients undergoing pancreatic transplant. With improvement in immuno-suppression causing better control of graft rejection, the major cause of transplant failure in early post-transplant period is graft ischemia due to arterial or venous thrombosis or stenosis. As in other organ transplants, arterial and venous integrity is critical in pancreatic transplantation. Color and Duplex Doppler are commonly used to monitor blood flow postoperatively to the pancreas.[5]

Procedure

The transplanted pancreas is superficially located and is easily accessible for examinations with ultrasound imaging with high-frequency transducers (5-7.5 MHz) is possible and major vessels can be readily examined with Duplex or color Doppler interrogation. The arterial supply of the pancreatic allograft is from the coeliac and superior mesenteric arteries. These vessels are anastomosed to the iliac artery. The portal veins are anastomosed to the external iliac vein to provide venous drainage. Pancreatic secretions are drained by a variety of procedures, frequently by duodenocystostomy.

Complications

Common complications of pancreatic transplantation are vascular thrombosis, intra-abdominal infections, rejection, anastomotic leaks and pancreatitis. Imaging techniques include ultrasound, Doppler ultrasonography, CT and radionuclide imaging. Sonography with Doppler is the procedure of choice in detecting fluid collections and identifying pancreatitis, vascular thrombosis and rejection to some extent.

Postoperative Evaluation

Postoperative evaluation of the pancreas transplant should include careful inspection of the pancreas, the surrounding structures and the transplant vessels. The normal pancreatic transplant appears sonographically as a homogeneous structure of low-to-moderate echogenicity lying medial to iliac vessels. The normal anteroposterior dimension of the pancreatic allograft ranges from 1.5-2.0 cm. Pancreatic enlargement though nonspecific, may accompany infarction, pancreatitis and rejection.[6] Peritransplant fluid collections indicating pseudocyst, abscess, hematoma, serum or lymphocele can be seen in over 50% of patients with transplantation.[7]

With Doppler ultrasound, arterial flow to the transplant is characterized by a low-resistance waveform with flow continuing throughout the diastole. Duplex and color Doppler ultrasound aid in the early identification of mechanical problems with arterial and venous anastomosis and are important in transplant evaluation.[8]

Confirmation of flow within the body of the pancreas is easily performed with visualization of the splenic artery and vein along the posterior aspect of the allograft. The iliac artery and vein are examined to identify the anastomosis of the coeliac and superior mesenteric arteries and portal vein. Thrombosis of the veins draining the pancreatic transplant is a particularly important for the graft loss.[9]

Venous thrombosis is most common during first week following transplantation, if untreated. Duplex Doppler findings associated with venous thrombosis include absence of demonstrable flow in the transplant veins and abnormalities in the transplant coeliac and splenic arteries with a blunted systolic peak and reversal of flow in diastole. This waveform is indicative of high vascular resistance and when present should suggest the possibility of venous outflow obstruction.

The role of Doppler in transplant rejection is non-specific. Some studies have suggested relation of transplant arterial resistive index (RI) with signs of rejection. An RI of more than 0.70% was a pointer towards rejection.[10] However, the utility of RI measurements in predicting rejections is not confirmed. However, when rejection is suspected, biopsy is usually necessary. Biopsy guidance with ultrasound and color Doppler can be done and reduces the possibility of inadvertent vascular damage during biopsy.

KEY POINTS

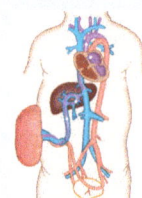

Pancreas
- Color Doppler sensitive than angiography—detecting vascular involvement by pancreatic carcinomas, encasement/occlusion—nonresectibility.
- Pancreatic transplant postoperative evaluation
  - A low resistance arterial waveform with forward diastolic flow.
  - 1st week-venous thrombosis m/c complication—RI > 0.7-pointer towards rejection.

REFERENCES

1. Mrerton DA, Golberg BB. Abdominal applications of color flow imaging. In: Goldberg BB, Merton DA, Deane Cr (Eds). An Atlas of Ultrasound Color Flow Imaging. Martin Dunitz, London. 1997. pp.67-142.
2. Weill FS. Pancreatic tumours and overview of pancreatic disease. In: Weill FS (Ed). Ultrasound Diagnosis of Digestive Disease. Springer, New York. 1996.pp.481-510.
3. Raijman I, Levin B. Exocrine tumours of the pancreas. In: Haubrich WS, Schaffner F, Berk JFB (Eds). Gastroenterology. WB Saunders, Philadelphia. 1995.pp.3002-04.
4. Ishida H, Konno K, Hamashina Y, et al. Assessment of resectability of pancreatic carcinoma by color Doppler sonography. Abdom Imaging. 1999;24:295-98.

5. Yang HC, Neumyer MM, Thicle BL, et al. Evaluation of pancreatic allograft circulation using color Doppler ultrasonography. Transplant Proc. 1990;22:609-11.
6. Letourneau JG, Maile CW, Sutherland DE. et al. Ultrasound and computed tomography in the evaluation of pancreatic transplantation. Radiol Clin North Am. 1987;25:345-55.
7. Patel BK, Garsim PJ, Aridge DL, et al. Fluid collections developing after pancreatic transplantation: Radiologic evaluation and intervention. Radiology. 1991;181:215-20.
8. Kubota K, Billin H, Kelter U, et al. Duplex-Doppler ultrasonography for evaluating pancreatic grafts. Transplant Proc. 1990;22:183.
9. Hanto DW, Sutherland DER. Pancreatic transplantation: Clinical consideration. Radiol Clin North Am. 1987;25:333-43.
10. Patel B, Wolverson MK, Mahanta B. Pancreatic transplant rejection: Assessment with duplex US. Radiology. 1989;173:131-5.

Role of Color Doppler in Urinary System

KIDNEYS

Gray scale ultrasound has greatly increased the morphologic detail that could be displayed within the kidney. Further the addition of pulsed Doppler allowed arterial and venous perfusion to be assessed both qualitatively and quantitatively. Recent addition to color flow and power Doppler imaging now allow superb demonstration of the entire renovascular tree from the main renal arteries and their fine terminal branches (Figs. 12.1A and B).

Technique

The main renal arteries arise from the lateral aspect of aorta just inferior to the superior mesenteric artery and left renal vein. Using these vessels as landmarks, the origin and proximal portion of the main renal arteries are best examined with the patient supine using a 3 MHz transducer and a transverse midline approach. Patients should ideally fast for at least 8 hours prior to examination. In larger patients, decubitus positioning with intercostal scanning may be more helpful.

Approximately 20% of patients will have accessory renal arteries.[1] Visualization of the entire course of the main renal arteries is incomplete in over 30% of adult patients.

The normal waveform (Fig. 12.2) of the main renal artery demonstrates a low impedance pattern with continuous forward diastolic flow reflecting the low resistance of blood flow to the native kidney. When the origins of the main renal arteries can be identified angle corrected velocity estimates can be made. Peak systolic velocity is usually less than 100 cm/sec. The resistive index should be less than 0.7.[2,3]

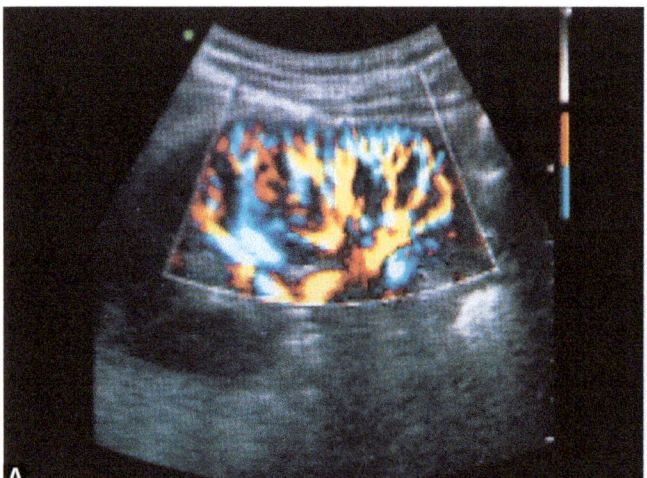 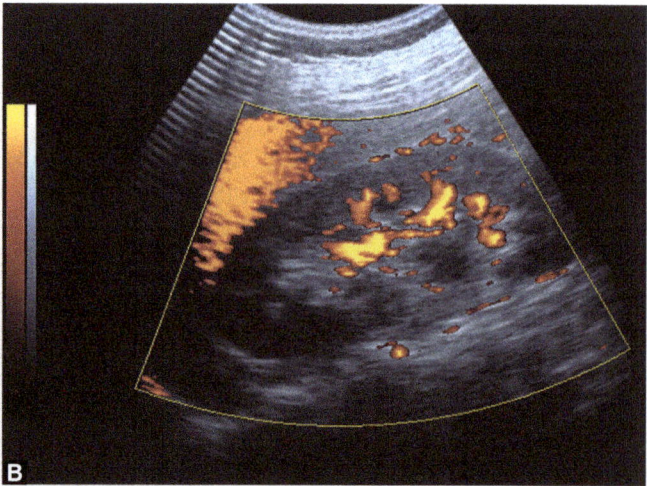

Figs. 12.1A and B: (A) Color Doppler image of native kidney demonstrates intraparenchymal renal arteries and veins; (B) Power Doppler image of native kidney. Blood flow is coded yellow on this color map.

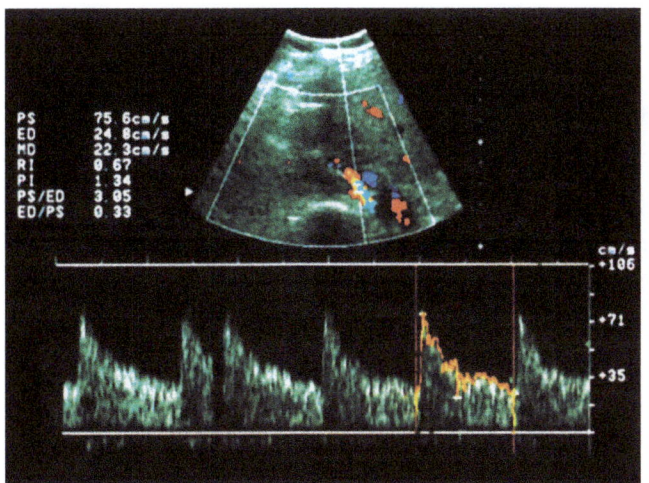

Fig. 12.2: Duplex Doppler image of normal renal artery showing low impedance pattern with continuous forward diastolic flow.

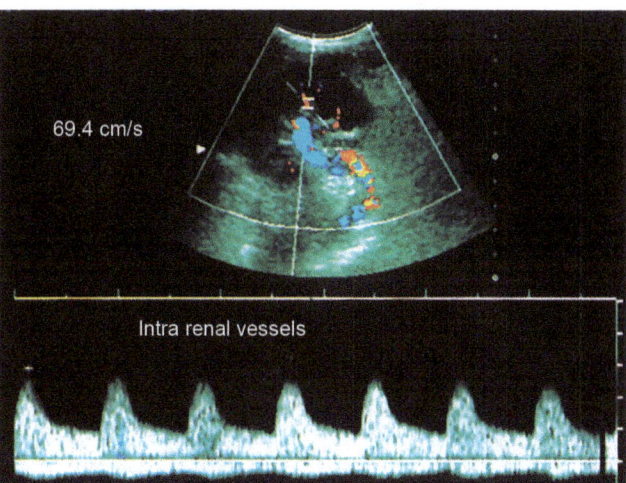

Fig. 12.3: Normal pulse Doppler waveform of intrarenal artery showing low resistance pattern with continuous forward diastolic flow.

KEY POINTS

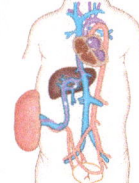

- Renal artery shows low impedance pattern with continuous forward diastolic flow.
- Peak systolic velocity < 100 cm/sec.
- Normal Intrarenal RI < 0.7.

The segmental renal branches which lie within the renal hilum as well as the more distal interlobar and arcuate vessels within the renal cortex are readily identified on color or pulse Doppler examination. Renal parenchymal vessels are best examined from a lateral intercostal approach. Decubitus positioning may be helpful. Most patients can be imaged with a 3 to 5 MHz transducer. The Doppler sample volume should be kept small (2-5 mm) and the wall filter should be set as low as possible (<50 Hz). In order to minimize the relative error the Doppler tracing should be maximized by using minimum frequency range (pulse repetition frequency) possible before aliasing occurs. With this technique the deflection of the Doppler spectrum from the baseline is maximized, thus filling as much of the scale as possible. The larger the spectrum the smaller will be the relative error produced by any fault when positioning cursors or placing calipers. A spectrum is considered optimal if three to five consecutive similar appearing waveforms are noted. Both kidneys are always examined even if renal disease in unilateral.

Pulsed Doppler interrogation of the intrarenal vessel reveals a low resistance waveform with decreasing peak systolic velocities as the vessels are traced distally (Fig. 12.3). To characterize intrarenal Doppler waveform, most investigators have used the resistive index (RI). This parameter is defined as peak systolic shift-minimum diastolic shift/peak systolic shift. Increase in downstream resistance results in a relative reduction of diastolic flow compared with systolic. Hence, RI can be used as an estimate of state of renal arterial resistance.

The RI of intrarenal vessels in normal adult kidney has been reported to range from 0.58 to 0.64 + 0.05,[2,3] and an intrarenal RI of 0.7.

Children and neonates will have RIs of higher value. In premature infants, neonates and toddlers RI of 0.7-1.0 may be normal. The RI in children decreases with age and after age 4-5 years it stabilizes in the adult-range.[4,5]

Doppler signals from parenchyma or main renal veins demonstrates continuous flow in the opposite direction that of arterial flow. Respiratory and cardiac variations are typically present.

As the RI values and PSV of the various arteries are dependent on multiple factors including Doppler machine, hence it has been proven beyond doubt that using the ratios of PSV of various arteries is more useful than utilizing the absolute PSV of the arteries. Renal artery to aortic PSV ration (RAR) of more than 3.5 is highly suggestive of renal hypertension. Similarly, the renal artery to interlobular artery PSV ratio (RIR) of more than five has been advocated as a sensitive indicator of renal hypertension.

Intrarenal Duplex Doppler Sonography of the Dilated Collection System

Conventional sonography is indeed quite sensitive for diagnosing renal obstruction by detecting dilatation of the collection system. However, the converse is not true, as pyelocaliectasis identified by sonography is certainly not synonymous with true obstruction.[6] This clinically important distinction of true renal obstruction from non-obstructive dilatation cannot be resolved by gray scale sonography and often requires the use of invasive procedures and tests. Intrarenal Doppler has a great potential value in identifying true renal obstruction.

The non-obstructive causes of a dilated collecting system include a distended urinary bladder, overhydration, mediation, diabetes insipidus, congenital megacalyces, post-obstructive dilatation, chronic reflux, and acute pyelonephritis.

Complete or Nearly Complete Obstruction

The hemodynamic changes that occur with renal obstruction must be understood to explain the observed Doppler changes. Most studies have described a triphasic renal vascular and ureteral pressure response to obstruction.[7]

The initial phase occurring in the first 1-2 hours after obstruction is characterized by a transient rise in renal blood flow and prostaglandin mediated vasodilation.[7] Although this very stage would rarely be relevant in the clinical setting, one would except a normal RI immediately after the onset of obstruction.

The second phase begins after 2 hours of obstruction and last approximately 3 hours. This phase is characterized by elevated post-glomerular renovascular resistance, decreased renal blood flow and elevated ureteral pressure. This is the only stage in which renal vascular resistance and ureteral pressure one both elevating at the same time.

The third phase, beginning after 5 hours of obstruction is characterized by decreasing and often normalized ureteral pressure at a time when renal vascular resistance is markedly rising.[7]

This phase is characterized by an elevation in preglomerular resistance with ureteral pressure appearing to be less important. In this phase marked elevation of renal vascular resistance and hence RI elevation would be expected.

Currently many researchers believe that renal vascular resistance changes observed with obstruction may be due to locally acting circulating vasoactive factors and hormones.[8]

Recently investigators have evaluated the ability of Doppler to detect these renal vascular changes.[2,3,9] These studies have defined a reasonably discriminatory RI value of 0.7 to differentiate obstructive from nonobstructive pyelocaliectasis. That is, in a kidney with a dilated collecting system an RI value of 0.70 or more is suggestive of obstruction, while RI values less than 0.70 are suggestive of nonobstructive dilatation.

Acute Renal Obstruction

Although conventional US is sensitive though not specific in detection of the collecting system dilatation that accompanies established obstruction, previous researchers have shown conflicting results in evaluation of the suspected but early renal obstruction.[55,56] These studies demonstrated a key limitation of conventional US. Acutely obstructed kidneys may demonstrate only mild pyelocaliectasis or none. Laing et al.[55] in a previous study found that 35% of acutely obstructed kidneys exhibited no pyelocaliectasis. Previous animal research indicates that acute obstruction elevates renal arterial resistance within a few hours[7,8] Platt et al.[56] found an elevated mean RI of 0.77 is acutely obstructed kidney. Elevation of RI occurs after as few as 6 hours of clinical obstruction.[56] Kidneys obstructed for a somewhat longer period of time (12-36 hours) did not have significantly higher RI than those with shorter duration <12 hours. One potential limitation of Doppler analysis is the patient with intermittent very acute renal colic. If the obstruction is present for a few hours only and then is relieved theoretical considerations would suggest that the RI may not increase even of this pattern of intermittent obstruction and relief persists for days.

In conclusion analysis with intrarenal duplex Doppler US is a valuable addition to the standard sonographic examination in patients with acute renal colic. The Doppler study enables detection of marked elevation in renal arterial resistance by 6 hours of clinical obstruction at a time when conventional US often reveals little pyelocaliectasis or none. Because obstruction of less than 6 hours duration or pyelosinus extravasation may cause normal RI in obstruction a knowledge of clinical history and identification of perirenal fluid on real time US scan are crucial.

Release of Significant Obstruction

Animal data indicates that duration of obstruction prior to relief is crucial for predicting what types of vascular changes will be observed.[10]

If obstruction is relieved within the first two phases (by 5 hours), then renal vascular resistance may normalize within few hours. However, if the obstruction is present for at least 18-24 hours, the normalization of renal vascular resistance may not be immediate and may take days or even weeks to return to baseline levels. This continued elevation in RI is presumably due to renal vasoconstriction caused by persisting local factors such as thromboxane.[10]

Partial or Mild Obstruction

Unlike significant obstruction, which appears mediated by vasoconstriction such as TXA_2, mild partial obstruction is characterized by prostaglandin mediated vasodilation.[10,11] Studies[11] also have found that the presence or degree of pyelocaliectasis does not predict or correlate with renal atrophy and nephron loss. Clearly, the use of pyelocaliectasis as the gold standard for significant partial obstruction is not correct. Renal vascular resistance should only be elevated in partial obstruction significant enough to result in renal vasoconstriction. Milder degree of partial obstruction mediated by renal vasodilators produce no elevation in renal vascular resistance and a normal RI would be expected.

Partial obstruction highlights the fact that Doppler analysis attempts to provide physiologic rather than anatomic information while a normal RI argues against significant physiologic obstruction it does not imply that a ureter is free of any mild region of narrowing or structures, the renal Doppler examination alone does not suffice if precise anatomic information is required. The clinical utility of an elevated RI value in a child with a dilated urinary tract is less well defined. In a child over age 5 years an RI >0.70 is suggestive of obstruction. However, RI values that are elevated by adult standards are frequently observed in children under age 5 years. When there is unilateral collecting system dilatation a resistive index ratio RIR, which is defined as the RI of the dilated kidney divided by RI of the contralateral nonobstructive kidney of 1.1 or greater is suggestive of obstruction.[57] However, an RIR between 1.0 and 1.1 may be found in children with obstructive dilatation if the child is not hydrated. Therefore, a fluid and/or diuretic challenges may be needed to unmask the obstruction. Nonetheless the lasixrenogram remains the gold standard for evaluation of renal obstruction in children and relative glomerular filtration rates are very helpful when deciding if a child needs surgical repair.

Pitfalls in Resistive Index Analysis of Obstruction

A few potential pitfalls in Doppler evaluation of the dilated collecting system are useful to consider.

One potential pitfall that generally can be avoided is very acute obstruction of less than 8 hours in which the RI may not have had sufficient time to reach 0.70. However, in these early obstructed cases the difference in RI between the obstructed and the contralateral normal kidney is 0.10 or more. Therefore the accuracy of the RI discriminator value (0.70) can be improved by evaluation of contralateral kidney.

A theoretical limitation of RI analysis is severe chronic obstruction with marked parenchymal loss. It is possible that interstitial infiltrate thought to lead to circulating renal vasoconstrictors is lost in these cases with less elevation of renal vascular resistance (RI). Such cases of end stage obstruction will generally not be clinically problematic as the presence of obstruction will be known.

One very important potential limitation in the case of Doppler in the evaluation of obstruction is in imaging children. Elevated RI values (by adult standards) are commonly observed in children. Available animal data suggest the altered renal blood flow with obstruction involves the outer portions (cortex) of the kidney to a greater degree than the medulla, so the vessels interrogated may be an important factor especially in children.[7,8]

One of unavoidable limitation of Doppler analysis of possible obstruction is that RI is a non-specific parameter. Obstruction is not the only cause of an elevated RI.[3,12] Therefore, in the setting of known renal medical disease (RMD) and pyelocaliectasis an elevated RI could be due either to true obstruction or to renal medical disease with coexistent nonobstructive dilatation. If the dilatation is unilateral, the examinee can study the contralateral non-dilated kidney and look for significant difference in RI (>0.1) to suggest obstruction superimposed on renal medical disease. The specific setting where Doppler imaging is truly limited is in the patient with bilateral pyelocaliectasis known and usually severe renal medical disease and an elevated RI.

Color Doppler of Vesicoureteric Junction

Color Doppler evaluation of ureteric jets within the bladder may also be useful is diagnosing ureteric obstruction. Color Doppler examination of the bladder demonstrates ureteric jet. If a ureteric jet is not seen after 15 minutes of continuous observation the ureter is obstructed.

Hemolytic Uremic Syndrome

The hemolytic uremic syndrome comprised of the clinical triad of hemolytic anemia, thrombocytopenia and renal failure, most frequently presents in children less than two years of age following a bout of gastroenteritis. The associated renal microangiopathy is characterized by endothelial swelling and thrombus formation. In children vascular obstruction typically occurs at the level of the glomerulus whereas in adults, arteries or arterioles are primarily involved.

KEY POINTS

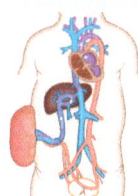

- Obstructive uropathy
  – US and Duplex Doppler findings
- Hydronephrosis, RI ≥ 0.7
- Acute cases (≥ 6 hrs). No pyelo-caliectasis, elevated RI
  RI (obstructed kidney)-RI (Normal kidney) ≥ 0.1
- Unilateral pyelocaliectasis
  $$\frac{RI\,(Obstructed\,kidney)}{RI\,(Non\text{-}obstructed\,kidney)} \geq 1.1$$

Decreased arterial renal parenchymal blood flow has been documented on renal scintigraphy. The resultant oliguria or anuria frequently requires dialysis. A diuretic phase generally precedes recovery which typically occurs within 1-2 week. Recovery is more common in children than in adults. Using pulse Doppler in children aged 1-7 years Patriquin[13] have demonstrated abnormal renal parenchymal arterial waveform characterized by abnormal diastolic flow (absent, reversed or markedly reduced) and elevated intrarenal RI > 0.9 during the oliguric phase. These Doppler changes reflect increased arteriolar resistance most likely as a direct result of narrowing of arteriolar lumen or loss of arteriolar elasticity due to endothelial swelling and intraluminal thrombus formation. Furthermore in their series the reappearance of normal diastole blood flow and drop of RI normal (0.65-0.70) in children accurately predicted recovery of renal function and urine output allowing dialysis to be terminated. Improved end diastolic flow or decreased RI usually preceded the diuretics phase by 24-48 hours.[13] The authors hypothesize that if normal Doppler signal are present in the oliguric patient with hemolytic uremic syndrome, the disease will have a mild course and dialysis will not be required.

Hepatorenal Syndrome

It is defined as unexplained kidney failure in a patient with liver disease who does not have clinical laboratory or anatomic evidence of other known cause of kidney failure. The progressive kidney dysfunction that accompanies liver disease is generally considered to be functional because consistent pathologic changes are absent because the kidney failure can be reversed with liver transplantation and because kidneys in patients with hepatorenal syndrome can be successfully transplanted into patients with normal liver.[17]

Renal hemodynamic changes begin early in the course of liver disease related functional kidney failure even before changes in serum creatinine concentration are detectable. The hallmark change is intrarenal vasoconstriction.[18]

Duplex Doppler sonography can be used to assess vascular resistance in small renal intraparenchymal vessels by measuring RI. An elevated RI reflecting intrarenal vasoconstriction has been observed in various condition associated with elevated renal vascular resistance such as kidney obstruction, acute tubular necrosis, renal vein thrombosis and hemolytic uremic syndrome and should be detectable in liver disease related functional kidney failure. Patt et al.[19] have found renal RI to be useful new non-invasive predictor of subsequent kidney states in non-azotemic patients with liver disease. An abnormal renal RI predicts an increased chance for development of hepatorenal syndrome by presumably detecting renal vasoconstriction. When an elevated RI is obtained, a formal evaluation for hepatorenal syndrome including fluid challenge should be considered. A normal renal Doppler study would indicate that hepatorenal syndrome is very unlikely. Doppler will be useful for prognosis and in the management of liver disease whenever they require paracentesis, diuretic therapy potentially nephrotoxic medicine or radiographic contrast examination.[19]

Renal Masses

The most common use of ultrasound in the evaluation of renal mass is to differentiate a cyst from a solid neoplasm.

Pulse and color Doppler examination can be useful for further evaluation of solid renal masses. Most renal cell carcinomas are hypervascular and contain numerous arteriovenous shunts. Increased vascularity can be readily demonstrated on color Doppler imaging. On pulse Doppler imaging arteriovenous shunting will lead to high peak systolic frequency shifts secondary to the rapid drop in pressure gradient across the anastomosis. Several authors have demonstrated significantly elevated peak systolic frequency shift on pulse Doppler in renal cell carcinoma.[14,15] Kier[14] in their series reported that 83 percent of untreated renal cell carcinoma demonstrated peak systolic frequency shifts greater than 2.5 KHz and above those in the main renal artery. Renal cell carcinoma have a propensity to invade renal veins (20-30% of cases) and the tumor thrombus may extend into IVC (5-10%) occasionally growing into right atrium. Accurate diagnosis of venous extension is important both for prognosis and patient management. The presence and extent of tumor thrombus within these veins can be easily detected by color Doppler examination as a filling defect within distended veins. Tumor thrombosis is typically isoechoic with the primary neoplasm and the renal vein is often distended. In addition, unlike hemorrhagic thrombus, tumor thrombus will demonstrate neovascularity which can be detected on Doppler examination. Even if main renal vein cannot be visualized pulse Doppler examination may suggest renal vein thrombosis. In three patients with renal cell carcinoma and angiographically confirmed renal vein extension Dubbins and Wills[16] documented high impedance intrarenal arterial waveforms characterized by little or no forward flow in end diastole (Figs. 12.4 and 12.5A to C).

Renal Vein Thrombosis

Acute renal vein thrombosis (RVT) most often presents in adults with flank pain, macroscopic hematuria and deteriorating renal function characterized by proteinuria.

In adults, acute, RVT occurs most frequently as a result of dehydration, vascular congestion, hypercoagulopathies,

Role of Color Doppler in Urinary System | 101

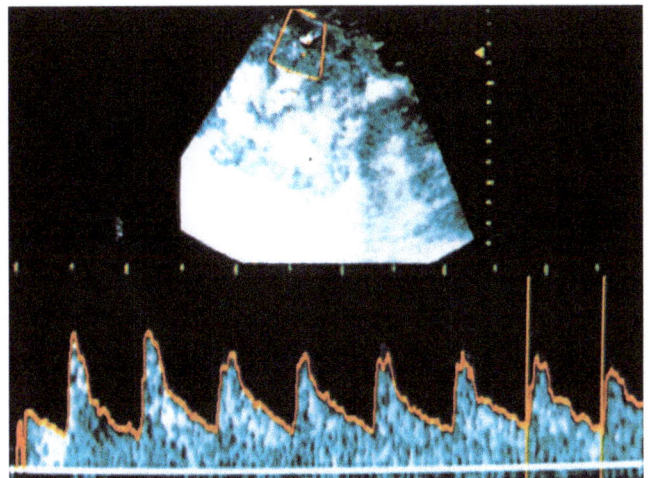

Fig. 12.4: Duplex Doppler showing high velocity flow signals in Wilm's tumor.

malignancy or trauma. Patients usually improve following thrombolytic therapy.

In neonates and children, the mortality rate is higher and acute RVT occurs most commonly in the clinical setting of severe dehydration secondary to diarrhea, sepsis, birth trauma, maternal diabetes, or maternal hypertension.

Conventional sonographic findings of altered renal size and echogenicity are nonspecific. Duplex Doppler sonography of the kidney with the study of the main renal vein is often used in the non-invasive evaluation of this condition. Typical findings include the presence of thrombosis and the absence of a Doppler signal in the renal vein. Because thrombus often is not seen and because lack of renal venous signal can be due to technical consideration (e.g. the patient's condition or body habitus) rather than true renal venous thrombosis, ancillary sonographic sign are useful. Prior experience in transplanted kidneys suggests that absent or reversed end diastolic flow in intraparenchymal arteries is highly suggestive of renal vein thrombosis.[20]

Acute RVT may result in increased renal vascular impedance secondary either to compromise of venous drainage or to intrarenal edema. Increased renal vascular impedance will result is diminished or reversed diastolic flow and elevation of RI.[23] Laplarte et al.[24] have recently reported that intrarenal venous flow may often be present in children with renal vein thrombosis due to collateral circulation. They note however that the normally transmitted cardiac pulsatility may be absent in these collateral vein and that the RI of segmental arteries may be 10% higher than in contralateral normal kidney.

However, in a study by Platt et al.[21] intrarenal arterial Doppler analysis is neither sensitive nor specific for

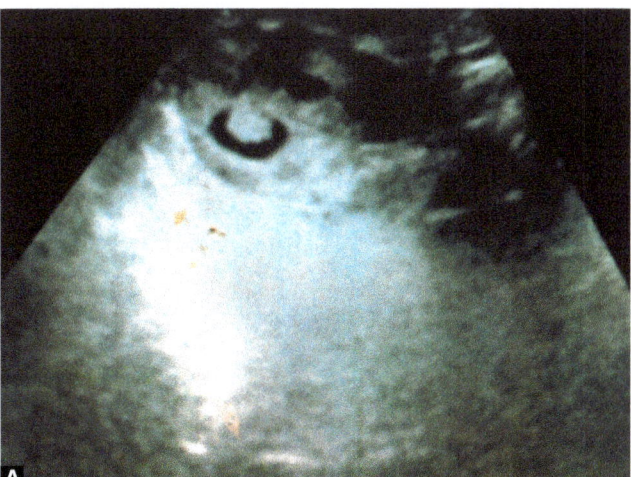
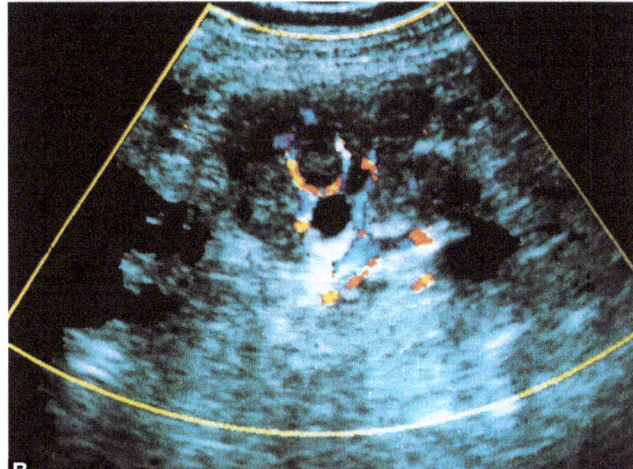
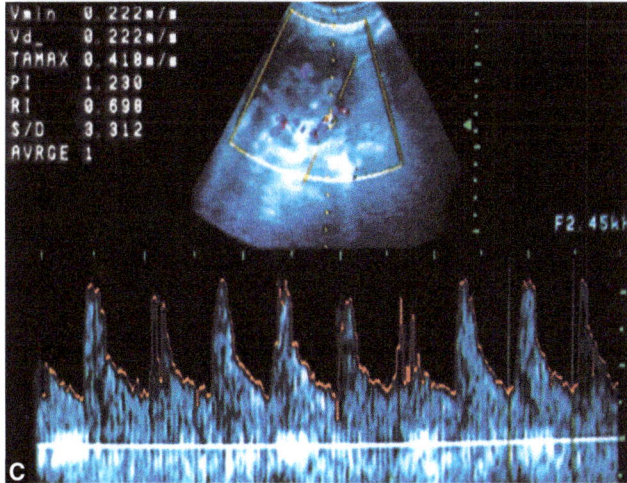

Figs. 12.5A to C: (A) Renal cell carcinoma: Gray scale sonography showing well-defined heterogeneous mass with cystic areas; (B) Renal cell carcinoma: Color Doppler showing moderate vascular signals (C) Renal cell carcinoma: Duplex Doppler in another patient showing high velocity low resistance waveform.

renal vein thrombosis in native kidneys. This is probably secondary to the development of venous collaterals in the native kidneys which allows a decrease in renal resistance and normalization of arterial RI. Extensive venous collaterals can develop in native kidney but not in transplanted kidneys which lack capsular venous anastomosis.[22]

Chronic RVT is more difficult to diagnosis both clinically and radiographically. Patients with nephrotic syndrome have an increased incidence of RVT. Criteria are same as for diagnosis of acute RVT. However, the kidney may not be enlarged, renal vein may not be dilated. Development of venous collateral which is more common in chronic DVT than in acute DVT may reduce renal impedance such that secondary sign of RVT namely diminished diastolic arterial flow and increased RI will not be present.

Renal Artery Stenosis

Hypertension is a significant risk factor for the development of cardiovascular disease, renal failure and stroke and renovascular hypertension is the most common surgically curable cause of hypertension. Estimates of prevalence of renovascular hypertension among the general hypertensive population range from 0.5% to 5%.[25]

Because renovascular hypertension has such a low prevalence in the large hypertensive population, effective low cost screening for the disease remains a problem, clinicians have relied on the clinical history and on new or changing physical findings to identify patients at higher risk for RVH. Atherosclerotic RAS as a cause of RVH should he suspected under the following circumstances:
- Onset of hypertension in a patient over 60 years of age
- Worsening hypertension that is difficult to control
- Associated peripheral vascular disease, coronary, artery disease or cerebrovascular disease
- Cigarette smoking more than 25 pack years
- Abdominal bruit
- Of white race
- Concomitant renal dysfunction is a patient with new hypertension. A therosclerosis tends to involve the proximal 1 cm of the main renal artery or branch points (Figs. 12.6 and 12.7).

One should suspect the fibromuscular group of abnormalities as cause for hypertension in women less than 30 years of age and in young patients with abdominal bruit. Typically the disease involves middle of the main renal artery and other arteries including carotid are involved. Once patients are suspected of having RVH the question of how to proceed with their evaluation becomes somewhat controversial. The imaging modalities that have had the greatest clinical impact in recent years include intravenous and intra-arterial digital subtraction

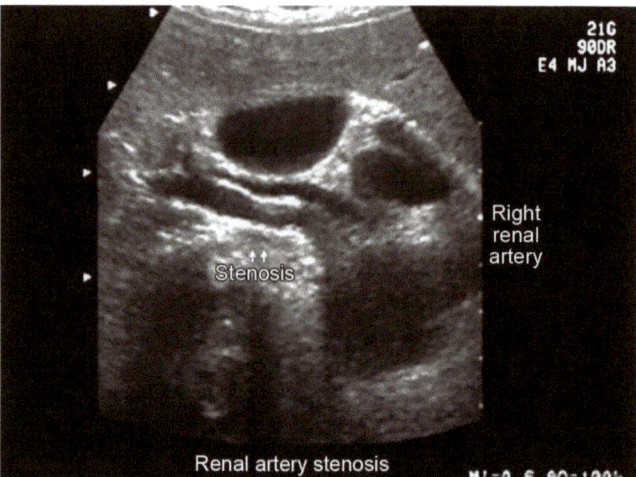

Fig. 12.6: Gray scale sonogram shows a plaque at the origin of right renal artery.

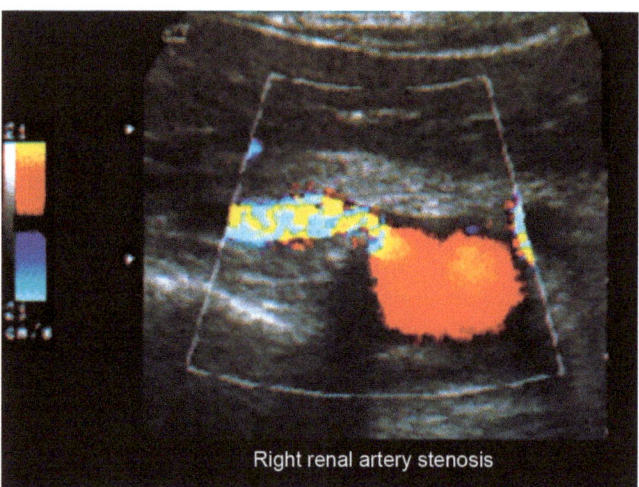

Fig. 12.7: Color Doppler flow image in another patient showing narrowing of right renal artery at its origin.

angiography and captopril renal scintigraphy. The newer modalities including MR angiography and color Doppler sonography continue to be investigated as to their role in RVH. Angiography is the gold standard for diagnosing RAS. However, there are several factors which limit the use of angiography as a screening technique. Angiography is costly and invasive. As many patients with renovascular hypertension have borderline or frankly impaired renal function, the use of potentially nephrotoxic intravenous contrast is to be avoided if possible.

Further the demonstration of an anastomotic stenosis in a patient with atherosclerotic disease does not necessarily establish a causal relationship with hypertension.

Therefore, an imaging modality providing physiologic data and/or anatomic detail would be a more ideal screening technique. IVP and nuclear medicine renal scans have been abandoned as screening test for RVH due to their low sensitivity (74-86%) and specificity (86% or less).[25,26]

Recently captopril scintigraphy has been demonstrated to have a very high sensitivity (91%) and specificity (93%) for diagnosis renovascular hypertension.[27] This physiologic study roughly measures the glomerular filtration rate which will decrease when the kidney is ischemic. However, no anatomic detail other than renal size is provided by captopril renogram.

During the 1980s the potential of pulse Doppler US as a screening method for diagnosing RAS was explored at numerous institutions. As a screening method pulse Doppler US has many attractive features. It is noninvasive and relatively inexpensive. There is no nephrotoxicity. Further more analysis of the pulse Doppler waveform has the ability to suggest physiological information whereas real-time US provides anatomic detail often identifying the stenotic lesion.

There are two basic approaches to the Doppler US diagnosis of RAS. The first depends on the ability of both real time and Doppler US to identify a focal area of increased peak systolic velocity (PSV) at the anatomic site of stenosis and the second involves demonstrating a decrease in the rate of systolic acceleration distal to a stenosis. A hemodynamically significant arterial stenosis leads to a focal increase in peak systolic velocity at the anatomic site of stenosis (Fig. 12.8). Compensation for individual variation in cardiac output can be made by comparing the PSV of main renal artery to the PSV of the aorta at the level of renal artery.

Studies have suggested that a PSV > 100 cm/sec and or RAR > 3.5 (ratio of peak systolic renal artery velocity to peak systolic aortic velocity) have sensitivities of 79-91% and specificities of 73-92% for hemodynamically significant RAS (>50-60% diameter reduction).[28,29]

However, despite initial enthusiasm experiences have shown that pulse Doppler evaluation of the main renal arteries has limited practical application as a screening technique.

The examination is very operator dependent and time consuming often requiring 1.2 hours or repeat examinations. It may be impossible to visualize the main renal arteries completely in up to 42% of patients due to presence of bowel gas, obesity, surgically incision, and/or aortic calcification.[30]

Tortuousity of the main renal artery may make it impossible to obtain accurate angle corrected velocity calculations. In addition accessory renal arteries have been reported in up to 14-26% of patients[30] but the detection rate by US for accessory renal arteries is very low near zero. Detection of renal artery occlusion may be difficult because collateral vessels may be inadvertently sampled. Finally, it is also unlikely that stenosis in branches of the main renal artery would be detected via this technique.

Virtually all these technical limitations result from the need to visualize the main (plus accessory) renal arteries along their entire course in order to document a focal increase in peak systolic velocity at the exact site of an anatomic stenosis.

However, on the basis of high technical success rate, high sensitivity and specificity and short examination time waveform analysis of the segmental renal arteries has been recommended as an alternative to direct examination of the main renal arteries for evaluation of RAS by various studies.[31,32]

Hemodynamically significant arterial stenosis cause changes in velocity waveforms that can be detected with Duplex sonography in distal contiguous arteries. Kotval reported such changes in peripheral arteries and called them tardus and parvus.[33,34]

Tardus refers to delayed or prolonged early acceleration and parvus to the diminished amplitude and rounding of the systolic peak. In continuation the two changes cause prolonged acceleration time (AT) and diminished acceleration index (AI).

The AI is the systolic slope of the time velocity waveform per unit time adjusted for the transmitted frequency [systolic frequency MHz after 1 sec/transmitted US frequency (MHz)]. The AI is the length of time in second from onset of systolic to peak systoles.[32]

Renal artery stenosis induced AT and AI abnormalities are detectable with Duplex sonography in the distal main renal artery and segmental renal arterial branches.[32] RAS may also cause an additional morphologic abnormality of

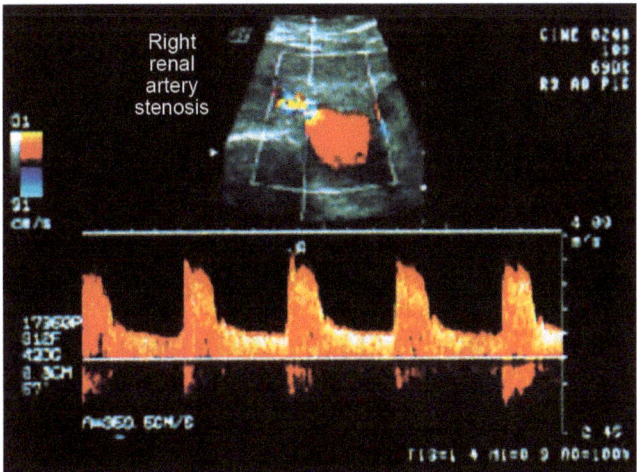

Fig. 12.8: Pulse Doppler tracing at the point of narrowing shows high peak systolic velocity in renal artery.

velocity waveforms obtained from these arteries and loss of normal early systolic compliance peak/reflective wave complex ESP.

In their study Handa et al.[32] an AI of <3.78 had an accuracy of 95%, sensitivity of 100% and specificity of 93% for RAS defined as a 50% diameter reduction by angiography. An AT of >0.07 seconds had an overall accuracy of 87%, a sensitivity of 100% and a specificity of 83% for diagnosing RAS. Furthermore because these measurements were made in segmental renal arteries within the renal hilum is distal to stenosis. Doppler interrogation could be performed via the translumbar approach with a technical success rate of 98% Starvos et al.[31] in their study have reported that while an AT of 0.07 seconds or longer and an AI less than 3.0 m/sec or less were each effective simple pattern recognition for loss of early systolic peak (ESP) had better sensitivity (95%) and specificity (97%) than either of the semi-quantitative parameter. The normal waveform morphology in 0 to 59% RAS is shown in Figure 12.9A. AT and AR are measured from beginning of early systolic rise to the ESP. The normal ESP is defined as follows: (a) The leading edge is continuous with and has the same slope as early systole, (b) The peak has an acute angle and rises above the second part of systole (c) It is completed by angle less than 180° between it and the second part of systole. Figure 12.9B waveform corresponding to 60–79% RAS. An abrupt change in slope still exists between early systole and middle systole but ESP is absent. AT and AI are measured from the start of early systole to the point of slope change. Figure 12.9C shows waveform corresponding to critical 80% or more RAS or occlusion of the renal artery. No point of abrupt change in slope exists between early and late systole.

Accurate assessment of AT and AI and for absence of ESP requires large crisp spectral waveforms. Proper chance of patient position, sonographic window, Doppler probe carrier frequency PRF or velocity scale setting scope speed and Doppler power settings are all necessary to achieve this goal.[31] In addition variations in the size of the normal ESP relative to the second part of systolic wave must be recognized.[31] Small and ill-defined spectral waveforms obtained without proper attention to detail will cause false positive tardusparvus appearance. Few terminal criteria have been set to ensure that the apparent tardus and parvus waveform are real and not artifacts of poor technique and suboptimal Doppler sensitivity.[31] These include:

- No liver or spleen visible between skin window and kidney. This ensures that the approach has been sufficiently posterior or lateral to minimize the depth of the segmental arteries and the angle of incidence
- Highest frequency probe possible (3.5 MHz or high). The signal from segmental arteries is stronger and the waveforms larger and more well-defined in higher Doppler carrier frequency
- Lowest spectral display velocity scale or PRF setting possible. Improper use of higher velocity scales than necessary is the most common cause of waveforms that are too small and ill-defined to interpret or are falsely interpreted as normal
- Standard or full pulsed Doppler power settings segmental arterial waveforms obtained with low pulsed Doppler power settings are frequently too ill-defined to measure accurately or to evaluate for absence of ESP.

Limitations

Because tardus and parvus waveforms may be seen distal to slight stenosis or occlusion with collateral arteries, indirect Doppler studies cannot enable distinction between these two conditions.

Stenosis of only one of multiple renal arteries or of segmental renal arteries may cause false negative finding with this techniques. However, obtaining sample from both the upper pole and another from the lower pole improves changes of detecting stenosis in an accessory renal artery or segmental renal artery.[31]

Color Doppler imaging is even more helpful in the setting of RAS because in the presence of RAS fewer vessels have blood flow that is detectable by means of Duplex sonography alone. Color Doppler imaging indicates which segmental arteries have the strongest signals and blood flow at optimum angles, thus providing guidance for pulsed Doppler in the pediatric population. Patriquinn et al.[36] reported an AI <4.0 measured in segmental or interlobar arteries had a sensitivity and specificity of 100% detection of severe RAS (>75% stenosis). However, moderate stenosis which may nonetheless be of clinical significance. In addition narrowing of aorta upstream to the intrarenal arteries for example in patients with aortic abdominal coarctation produces a similar decrease in AI.

Renal Transplant

Renal transplantation is the most commonly performed abdominal organ transplant worldwide. Over 10,000 patients receive renal transplants each year.

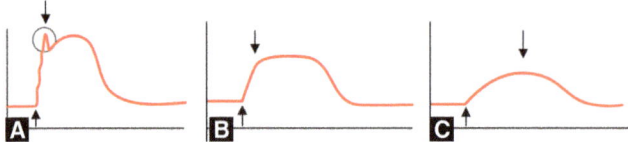

Figs. 12.9A to C: The renal artery waveform morphology is RAS (A) 0 to 59% RAS; (B) 60 to 79% RAS; and (C) 80% or more RAS. *Note:* Top arrow: early systolic peak (ESP) and Bottom arrow: beginning of early systolic

KEY POINT

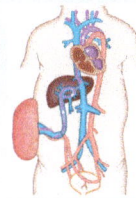

Renal cell carcinoma
- Peak systolic frequency shift > 2.5 kHz, or above main renal artery.
- Tumor extension into renal vein—thrombus with neovascularity.

Renal vein thrombosis
- Acute cases—no renal venous signal.
- Ancillary signs—absent or reversed end diastolic flow in intraparenchymal arteries.
- Elevated RI.
- In chronic cases. Venous collaterals present.
- Ancillary signs absent.

RAS
- Pulse Doppler—noninvasive screening method.
- Hemodynamically significant stenosis (50–60%).
- PSV >100 cm/sec (renal artery at site of stenosis).
- RAR >3.5.
- Alternatively segmental renal arteries-tardusparvus waveform.
- AT >0.07 sec, AI <3.78.

Most often the indication for transplantation is the presence of irreversible chronic renal failure.

Effective evaluation following transplantation requires familiarity with the surgical technique used for transplantation. These are two main types of arterial anastomosis, the choice of which is guided by the type of allograft available for transplantation. Cadaver kidneys are usually harvested with an intact main renal artery and an attached portion of aorta. The piece of aorta is trimmed to a circular or oval configuration (Carrel patch) and then sutured end to side to the external iliac artery of the recipient's external iliac artery or sometimes end to end to the recipient's internal iliac artery. Venous anastomosis is one almost always performed end to side to the recipient external iliac vein.[35]

In case of multiple donor renal arteries or veins patch grafts to the recipient external iliac vessel are performed. When pediatric kidneys are transplanted to an adult recipient a segment of donor aorta with both kidneys is patched to the iliac artery. Ureteric drainage is usually established by ureteroneocystomy or occasionally by pyeloureterostomy using the recipient's native ureter. Following transplantation a variety of immunosuppressive regimen are used to prevent rejection.[36]

Pretransplant work up includes evaluation of the recipient general medical condition and diagnostic studies to exclude conditions that are contraindications to transplantation including presence of outflow tract obstruction, active infection, and severe debilitating systemic disease or disseminated malignancy. Ultrasound is of value in the pretransplant evaluating of recipient's native urinary tract for evidence of obstruction calculi and neoplasm.

The sonographic evaluation of the transplanted kidney combines imaging and Doppler because transplant dysfunction arises from both vascular and non-vascular causes.

Protocol for ultrasound of renal transplant includes:[36]
- Documentation of renal size and position
- Presence or absence of dilatation of collecting system
- Presence, location, dimension of any extrarenal fluid collection.

Imaging examination also documents corticomedullary contrast, the appearance of renal parenchyma and the presence of renal in masses or calcification. The size and configuration of urinary bladder and urinary anastomosis are also recorded.

Transplant dysfunction may result from vascular complication such as vessel stenosis or occlusion or parenchymal changes secondary to rejection, tubular necrosis, or drug toxicity.

Vascular Complications

Vascular complications are reported to occur in up to 10% of transplantation patients with the most types being arterial and venous stenosis and thrombosis and intrarenal and extrarenalarteriovenous fistula (AVF) and pseudoaneurysm.[37] If detected early, many are amenable to graft sparing surgical or radiologic intervention. However, clinical presentation of these lesions is often ambiguous and imaging is required to differentiate them from the more common nonvascular causes of dysfunction.

For most transplant vascular application, both color and Duplex Doppler imaging should be performed with the lowest filter setting maximal gain without background noise and smallest scale that will accommodate the highest normal peak velocities without aliasing. Gate size should be between 3 and 5 mm and angle connection which should be adjusted when quantifying peak flow.[35]

Renal Artery Stenosis

Arterial stenosis with a reported prevalence of approximately 10% are the most common vascular complication of renal transplants.[38] They usually occur within the first three years after transplantation and are more common in grafts from cadavers especially those of young donors than in grafts from living donors.[38] The hallmark of significant stenosis is hypertension. However, up to 80% of transplant recipients may exhibit hypertension unrelated to arterial stenosis. Therefore, suspicion of stenosis is reversed for patients with specific hypertensive profiles such as newly developed or progressive hypertension, marked hypertension resistant to medical therapy hypertension with graft dysfunction in the absence of rejecting or hypertension in the presence of a systolic bruit over the graft.[35] Three main types of stenosis have been described: anastomotic, distal donor, and recipient artery. Anastomotic stenosis occurs more frequently in end to end anastomosis; distal stenosis occurs more frequently in end to side anastomosis and recipient artery stenosis occurs equally in both types. Anastomotic lesions are primarily short segment stenosis composed of variable amounts of intimal fibrosis and calcium that have been ascribed to surgical difficulties such as tight sutures, incomplete intimal approximation, excessive vessel length, twisting of vascular pedicle and large discrepancies in donor and recipient arterial size. Distal donor stenosis are single or multiple long segment stenosis composed primarily of diffuse intimal hyperplasia that is caused by hemodynamic turbulence distal to anastomosis intimal injury caused by graft perfusion catheter or excessive dissection around the main renal artery that results in destruction of vasa vasorum. Both anastomotic and distal donor stenosis may also be caused by rejection. Recipient stenosis are uncommon and usually due to either native atherosclerotic disease or intraoperative clamp injury.[38,39]

The combination of color and Duplex Doppler sonography provides a very sensitive method for the detection of arterial stenosis.

The vessels of interest are insolated throughout their extent looking for abnormally elevated peak systolic velocities and turbulent flow indicative of stenosis.

The most reproducible criteria for renal transplants were published by Taylor et al.[40] Using a 3 MHz transducer they found that significant stenosis (those requiring intervention) were associated with peak Doppler shifts greater than 7.5 MHz (2 m/sec) at the stenosis and turbulence in the immediate post-stenotic segment. As stenosis occurs in different locations in both the main and segmental renal arteries, these vessels must be insolated throughout their entirety. Unfortunately visualization of these vessels is often quite difficult. Thus, the Duplex Doppler examination is commonly a prolonged and tedious procedure in which the arteries are located by a trial and error method.

Color Doppler sonography with its larger field of view and ability to detect vessels invisible to gray scale sonography is both faster and less likely to miss a stenosis than is Duplex Doppler with properly adjusted color controls the abnormally increased velocities associated with stenosis appear as regions of focal aliasing. Once located, these regions can be examined with Duplex Doppler sonography to determine the nature and severity of flow disturbances. If a Doppler study is of reasonable quality and no significant flow abnormalities have been identified then significant stenosis can be excluded with a relatively high degree of confidence. If a strong clinical suggestion of stenosis persists, then angiography should be performed to exclude an undetected stenosis of a segmental or accessory renal artery.

Gottilibe et al.[41] have suggested that the use of intrarenal waveform parameter substantially improves the accuracy of detecting a hemodynamically significant proximal arterial stenosis compared with the use of the peak systolic velocity measured from the main renal artery as the sole criterion.

An acceleration index > 0.1 sec or a subjective assessment of dampening of the waveforms results in greater accuracy of detecting proximal arterial stenosis.

Renal Artery Thrombosis

Thrombosis of the main renal artery occurs in less than 1% of renal transplantation patients.[35] It is usually an acute event in the early postoperative period (<1 month) and invariably results in graft loss. Hyperacute and acute rejection are by far its most common causes. However, intraoperative intimal trauma, faulty intimal approximation, wide disparity in vessel size, and its end anastomosis, vascular kidney hypotension, hypercoagulable states, cyclosporine and atherosclerotic emboli have all been cited as precipitators of thrombosis.[42] Segmental renal artery thrombosis is clinically less obvious than is main renal artery thrombosis symptoms may be absent or consists of graft tenderness, decreased function or hematuria. Most limited infarcts result in a focal scar rather than complete graft loss.[35] In the presence of an occlusive arterial thrombus, neither Duplex nor color Doppler sonography will detect flow in the arterial branches distal to the occlusion.[40] Venous flow likewise will be absent. As long as Doppler equipment is functioning properly these findings are highly specific for renal artery thrombosis.

However, false positive reading may occur if the Doppler equipment is poorly calibrated, or in rare cases with high grade stenosis and minimal flow. Color Doppler sonography because of its larger field of insonation is more likely to detect segmental infarcts than is Duplex Doppler sonography.[35]

Intrarenal Arteriovenous Fistulas and Pseudoaneurysms

Intrarenal AVFs and pseudoaneurysms are almost exclusively the result of trauma induced during percutaneous needle biopsy. AVFs occur with simultaneous laceration of adjacent arteries and vein whereas pseudoaneurysm result from isolated laceration. Most AVFs are small and resolve simultaneously. AVFs that produce symptoms do so when they become large enough to cause decreased renal perfusion via marked arteriovenous shunting or when they communicate with calyceal system and produce hematuria.

Pseudoaneurysm cause symptoms when they rupture into the perinephric space or renal collecting system.[43] Majority of these lesions can be treated effectively by percutaneous transcatheter embolization.[43]

The Duplex Doppler findings of both AVFs and pseudoaneurysms are fairly specific. AVFs exhibit high velocity low impedance arterial waveforms with associated arterialized venous tracings. Pseudoaneurysms show highly turbulent pulsatile flow in their central lumen with classic to and fro flow at their neck.[40]

The spectral aberration of both AVFs and pseudoaneurysm are always localized to a portion of the kidney with normal hemodynamics in the remaining parenchymal vessels.

Color Doppler owing to its wide field full of view greatly increases the detection for AVF.[44]

The color appearance of AVFs depends on their size. Small lesions appear as focal areas of color abasing that reflect increased arterial velocities. Larger produce considerable perifistula tissue vibration that causes a focal flurry of disorganized color at normal Doppler setting.[44] Regardless of size AVFs detected by color Doppler sonography should be verified with Duplex Doppler sonography to exclude confusion with similar color aberrations that may be caused by segmental stenosis or focally prominent vessels.[44]

The color appearance of pseudoaneurysm consists of disorganized color flow within an apparent cyst with the same surrounding parenchymal vibration color as in seen with AVFs.[44] Close interrogation may reveal the communicating neck which appears as alternating jets of forward and reverse flow.[44]

Extrarenal Arteriovenous Fistulas and Pseudoaneurysms

Extrarenal AVFs and pseudoaneurysms are less common and usually have a different cause and work prognosis than their intrarenal counterparts do. They are commonly asymptomatic. Occasionally they cause renal dysfunction by excessive arteriovenous shunting or direct compression of the main renal artery. The most serious complication of these lesions is exsanguination due to spontaneous rupture of the pseudoaneurysm. The severity of this complication makes extrarenal pseudoaneurysms a relative clinical emergency requiring timely intervention.[45]

Extrarenal pseudoaneurysm appears as predominantly anechoic spherical paranephric fluid collections that exhibit Doppler characteristics identical to those of intrarenal pseudoaneurysm. However, recognition of the external lesions is more difficult because of involvement of larger common vessels. In the main renal arteries the increased velocity and turbulence that occur in AVF feeding arteries may be mistaken for abnormal hemodynamics of the more common arterial stenosis.

Recognition of associated increased diastolic flow will suggest the correct diagnosis. Presence of arterialized vein will help in confirmation. However, the arterialization will be diffuse rather than focal as occur with intrarenal AVFs. This diffuse venous pulsation can be confusing because it also occurs in normal transplanted kidney. Thus, diagnosis of extrarenal AVF requires careful evaluation of both arterial and venous Doppler spectra.[35]

Renal Vein Thrombosis and Stenosis

Renal vein thrombosis is a rare complication of transplantation that occurs mostly in the early postoperative period. Symptoms are usually abrupt in onset and consist of graft tenderness, swelling, oliguria, proteinuria, and decreased renal function. Predisposing factors include hypovolemia, faulty surgical technique, propagation of ipsilateral common femoral or iliac deep venous thrombosis and renal vein compression by postoperative fluid collections (hematoma, lymphocele, urinoma, and abscess).[35]

Renal vein thrombosis is rarely visualized by gray scale sonography. Instead the allograft can appear normal or enlarged with decreased parenchymal echogenicity and non-visualized renal veins. The Duplex Doppler findings of renal vein thrombosis consist of absent renal venous flow and reversed plateauing diastolic arterial flow.[46] Venous stenosis is readily detected by color Doppler sonography as region of focal aliasing that reflects the increased velocities associated with stenosis.[40]

ATN, Rejection, and Drug Toxicity

Important causes of altered renal blood flow resulting in transplant dysfunction are ATN, acute and chronic rejection, and drug toxicity.

In the normal transplant flow in the segmental interlobar and diastole and RI values range from 0.50–0.70 in the segmental and interlobar arteries.[36] In patients with rejection, ATN and drug toxicity elevation of RI values may be observed. High RI values have also been associated with renal vein thrombosis, renal compression, pyelonephritis, and obstruction. Conversely it is possible to have acute transplant rejection without RI elevation. The value of using

RI measurements to predict rejections has been extensively studied, however most workers now acknowledge the nonspecific nature of mild to moderate RI elevation.[47] This limits the use of this measurement in differentiation of causes of renal transplant dysfunction and when the clinical setting does not permit differentiation, renal biopsy is required. ATN is a result of ischemia and is common following transplantation, particularly of cadaveric kidneys where the incidence may be as high as 50%.[48] Doppler abnormalities including significant elevation of RI (0.9) or greater may accompany ATN but differentiation of ATN from acute rejection is not possible.[47,49]

Transplant rejection, a major complication of renal transplantation results in impaired renal function. Two forms of rejection are recognized. Acute vascular rejection and cellular or interstitial rejection.[36]

In acute vascular rejection, a proliferative endovasculitis narrows the vessel lumen leading to vascular occlusion and ischemia. In cellular or interstitial rejection perivascular edema and infiltrate cause impaired circulation. Pure vascular rejection is uncommon and in most cases interstitial changes predominate. In either case an increase in peripheral renal arterial resistance frequently results in elevation of RI. This may be detected by spectral waveform analysis and can also be seen with Doppler color imaging (DCI). DCI shows reduced duration of systolic arterial flow and reduction or loss of antegrade diastolic flow as the RI in the renal artery increases (Figs. 12.10A and B).

Nishioka et al.[50] have correlated visualization of segmental and parenchymal branches of the renal artery using DCI with transplant function, nothing more pronounced changes in parenchymal vessels.

A comparison of DCI and Duplex Doppler in evaluation of 50 renal allografts performed by Mostbeek et al.[51] has revealed a good correlation of measurement of RI and DCI findings. Allografts with pathologic RI measurements greater than or equal to 0.9 showed abnormal color flow characterized by absence of flow in arcuate and/or interlobar arteries. In children RI has also been shown to be of little value in the identification of rejection with Doppler induce less than 0.7 reported in acute and chronic rejection as well as in cases of ATN and cyclosporine toxicity.[52] The function of renal transplant requires a balance between the beneficial effects of immunosuppressive agents in prevention of rejection and the toxic side-effects of these agents. Cyclosporine is routinely used as an immunosuppressive agent following renal transplantation. Impaired renal function and transplant loss may result from the nephrotoxic effects of cyclosporine. Although changes in vascular impedance in patients with cyclosporine toxicity may be normal, elevation of RI with cyclosporine toxicity may occur, making differentiation from rejection difficult or impossible.

Perella et al.[54] have summarized that RI measurements do not appear capable of differentiating between these major causes of renal transplant dysfunction, i.e. acute rejection, acute tubular necrosis, and cyclosporine. A nephrotoxicity specifically the RI, at any threshold cannot distinguish between acute rejection and acute tubular necrosis. Because of the very different therapy regimens for acute rejection versus acute tubular necrosis and the significant number of cases of acute rejection that can occur in the low RI ranges a biopsy must be performed in all cases.

Differentiation between vascular rejection and cellular rejection as it relates to the RI is of questionable value. However, Duplex and color Doppler ultrasound remain valuable tools for assessing response to therapy and for evaluating the allograft for other vascular abnormalities such as acute venous and arterial thrombosis, arterial stenosis or arteriovenous fistulas.

Renal Transplant Pyelocaliectasis

Urinary obstruction is an infrequent but serious complication of renal transplantation. Obstruction is a common cause of an elevated RI > 0.75 in a transplanted kidney with pyelocaliectasis.[53] In the setting of renal transplant dysfunction and a collecting system seen at US to be dilated an abnormal RI is not conclusive for obstruction but reinforces that obstruction should be strongly considered and its presence excluded. An abnormal Doppler waveforms (increased RI) may also be helpful in the setting of a high clinical suspicion of obstruction but only mild dilatation on the real time US examination.

In conclusion, the importance of correlation of Doppler spectral analysis, imaging and clinical observation in determining the most likely cause of transplant dysfunction

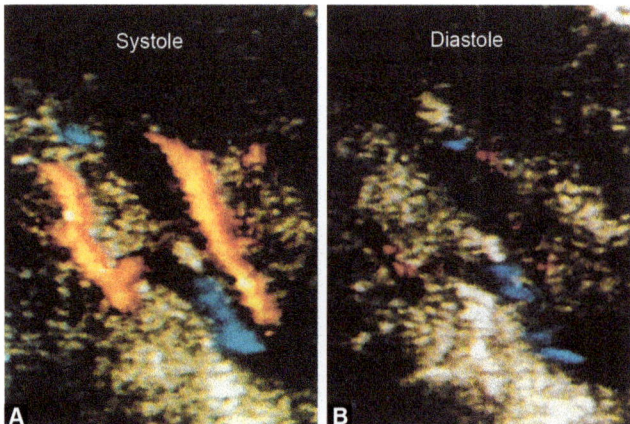

Figs. 12.10A and B: Renal transplant rejection: Color Doppler showing a forward flow during systole (A) while no flow in diastole (B).

deserves emphasis. Abnormal Doppler indices although not specific usually signal pathologic changes in an allograft. Biopsy remains the only definitive procedure for establishing the cause of dysfunction in many cases.

COLOR DOPPLER SONOGRAPHY IN DETECTION OF VESICOURETERIC REFLUX

Vesicoureteric reflux is an important condition leading to renal scarring and deterioration of renal failure and hypertension. To date the most accurate and sensitive investigation has been voiding cystourethrography.[58] Radionuclide cystography is considered to be a sensitive alternative investigation of reflux.[59] Color flow Doppler sonography is an attractive alternative to these imaging modalities as it eliminates the danger of ionizing radiation and the need for urethral catheterization and contrast agent.

Doppler study in conjunction with conventional sonography can evaluate the kidneys for echotexture, parenchymal thickness and scars while dilatation of the pelvicalyceal system helps is grading VUR (Fig. 12.11).

Color Doppler examination is carried out using 3 and 5 MHz phase array convex sector probes. Color gain settings and filters should be optimized for slow flow sensitivity, color map selected is red towards the probe and blue away from probe.

The patients are asked to drink water and hold their urine until they have a strong sensation of bladder fullness or to the point of reflex voiding in infants. Doppler examination is carried out in supine position. Both ureterovesical junctions (UVJ) are identified on a transverse scan and the ureteric jets are easily detected and depicted in red. Bilateral UVJs and distal ureters are scanned in sagittal and oblique sections.

Dilated distal ureter is seen as an anechoic tubular structure posterior to the urinary bladder and entering it at the vesicoureteric junction. The presence of reflux of urine into the ureter is seen as a color jet in blue (Figs. 12.12 and 12.13).

In cases of doubt these color jets were differentiated from nearly vascular structures by combining pulsed Doppler and color Doppler. Color Doppler examination is also carried out during straining and later while voiding.

VUR is graded on color flow Doppler sonography as:[60]

Grade I = Low grade reflux present
Grade II = Reflux present and lower ureteral filling. US does not show pelvicalyceal system dilatation
Grade III = Reflux ± mild dilatation of ureter and pelvis on ultrasound

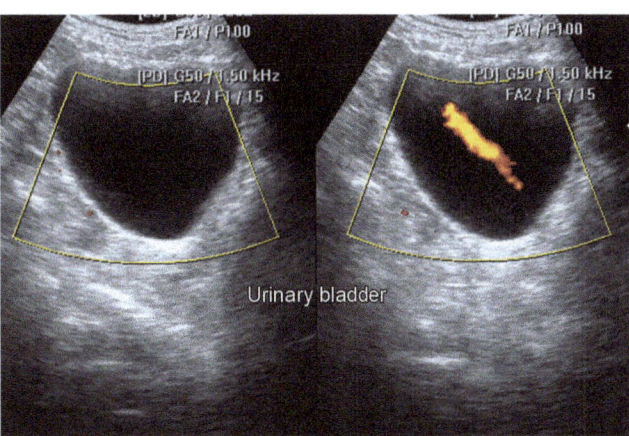

Fig. 12.11: Power Doppler shows color flow produced by normal jet of urine in the urinary bladders.

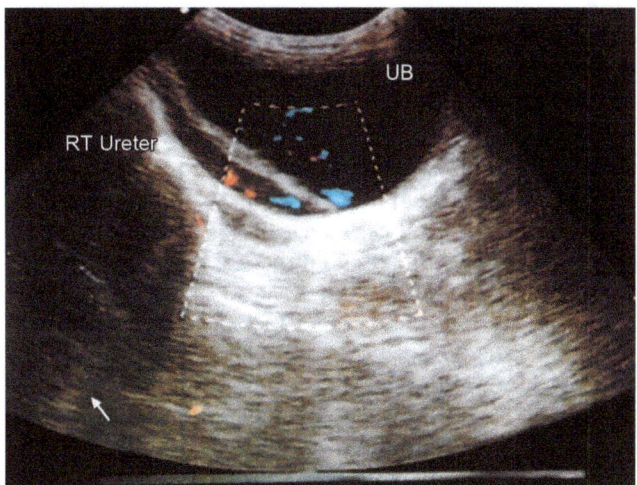

Fig. 12.12: Sagittal scan CDFI showing dilated right lower ureter with VUR seen as blue color.

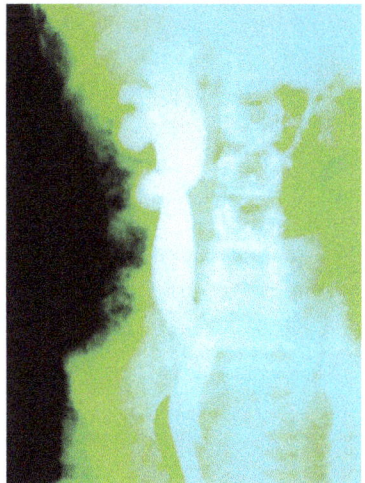

Fig. 12.13: Voiding cystourethrogram (VCUG) of the same patient showing grade V reflux.

Grade IV = Reflux with moderate dilatation of pelvis on USG
Grade V = Reflux with massive dilatation of pelvis and ureter on USG.

Since it is not possible to differentiate Grade I from Grade II VUR on combined and conventional color flow Doppler sonography both are appropriately grouped under low grade reflux.

Studies have demonstrated low sensitivity of CFDS in detecting grade I and II reflux.[61]

However, asymptomatic grade I and II reflux may be a physiological condition in children and CFDS can be used as a possible alternative to standard cystourethrography for the screening and follow-up of low grade reflux.

Patient found to have higher grades (Grade III to V) can be accurately graded by performing color Doppler sonography study.[61]

The major limitation of CFDS is suboptimal imaging of the posterior urethra, an important point to be evaluated is a male child with VUR. However, a trabeculated bladder with bilateral hydronephrosis and hydroureters and a partially seen dilated posterior urethra can suggest distal obstruction.

The result of CFDS depends upon patient compliance and therefore is unsuitable in very young patients below two years of age.

DOPPLER EVALUATION OF THE PROSTATE

Anatomy

The prostate is histologically composed of glandular cancer and non-glandular elements. The non-glandular elements are the prostatic urethra and the anterior fibromuscularstroma.

The glandular prostate consists of outer and inner components.[62] Both the outer and inner prostate are subdivided, the inner prostate consists of periurethral glandular tissue and transition zone and outer prostate consists of central and peripheral zones.

In total, zonal anatomy recognises five components to the prostate (1) anterior fibromuscularstroma, (2) periurethral glandular tissue, (3) transition zone, (4) central zone, and (5) peripheral zone.

From a radiologic view point, there are two important subdivisions of the glandular prostate—the peripheral zone and central gland.[63] Central gland collectively refers to periurethral, transitional, and central zone.

The transitional and central zones are in variable proportion depending on the degree of benign prostate hyperplasia. In young men central gland is composed mainly of central zone whereas in older men with benign prostatic hyperplasia the central gland is composed mainly of transition zone.

Imaging

The prostate can be visualized from a suprapubic position with trans-abdominal transducers but detailed assessment of the zonal anatomy is performed using a transrectal approach. In normal young men, the zones of prostate are not sonographically evident.[62,63] With the development of benign prostate hypertrophy the central gland becomes distinguishable as a well demarcated area of heterogeneity which may contain visible nodules cysts or calcification.[63,64]

The surgical or pseudocapsule may be evident as discrete change in echogenicity or a hypoechoic rim. The peripheral zone forms an area of uniform echogenicity surrounding the central gland. The anterior fibromuscularstroma forms a less echogenic band at the anterior aspect of the prostate.

The seminal vesicles can be seen superolaterally encased in hyperechoic fat that is continuous with fat surrounding the prostate.

Doppler Imaging

Doppler evaluation of the prostate has undergone rapid and continuous development over the last few years. The sensitivity of power Doppler is acknowledged to be superior for detection of blood flow because it relates primarily to the amplitude of Doppler signal and not direction of flow.

Standard color Doppler however may provide some additional information in flow velocity.

Regardless of which technique is used some important scanning techniques should be emphasized following initial gray scale evaluation.

Any focal hypoechoic area or region of mass effect should be interrogated by Doppler. The initial axial scan is performed with the Doppler sample window covering the entire prostate to allow easy bilateral comparison. Any region of increased flow should be assessed further by placing that region within the center of the image. This is particularly important for the bases of the prostate which can have normal increased capsular vessels from adjacent neurovascular bundles. The superior neurovascular bundles provide more prominent capsular flow than the inferior neurovascular bundles at the apex. Therefore, documenting intraparenchymal components to the flow at the bases helps decrease false positives from normal increased capsular flow.[65] Because the mid-gland is less prone to these capsular flow artefacts from the adjacent neurovascular bundles, even subtle increased intra-parenchymal flow in the mid-peripheral zone should be considered more suspicious.

Regions of increased flow need to be taken in context with gray-scale findings and other risks assessment.

Littrup and Bailey[65] have attempted to categorize increased flow patterns to normal, mildly increased or distinctly increased foci.

Normal vascularity is categorized as minimal intraparenchymal flow with symmetric capsular vessels. Subtle vascularity constitutes regions with mild increased intraparenchymal flow or asymmetric capsular vessels that show minimal penetration into adjacent parenchyma. Distinct vascularity includes areas of focal intraparenchymal flow or prominent asymmetric capsular vessels which penetrate well into adjacent parenchyma.

Distinct increased intraparenchymal flow can relate to normal vessels which are clustered together frequently in areas of atrophy where the intervening parenchyma has receded. Intraparenchymal flow is more suspicious when it has a speckled appearance perhaps suggesting much smaller vessels associated with angiogenesis.

It remains well established that prostatic carcinomas have a much higher number of microvessels per high power field than benign parenchyma.

Prostatic Cancer

Small prostatic cancers are generally hypoechoic because of the nodular cellular appearance of the carcinoma against the background of normal peripheral zone glandular tissue. Hypoechoic lesions in addition tended to be better differentiated with lower Gleason glands.[66]

However, other reports have found that hypoechoic tumors were poorly differentiated and better seen with ultrasound.[67] Hyperechoic cancer although seen infrequently has been identified. This appearance may be caused by a desmoplastic response of the surrounding glandular tissue to the presence of tumor or to infiltration of neoplasm into a background of benign prostatic hyperplasia.[66]

A significant number of prostate cancers are difficult or impossible to detect because they are isoechoic with surrounding prostate. Secondary signs such as glandular asymmetry and capsular bulging may then be helpful in diagnosis.

Color Doppler in conjunction with transrectal ultrasound has increased the sensitivity and specificity of prostate ultrasound and ultrasound guided biopsy.

Initial reports on color Doppler were disappointing, showing only a minimum advantage for adding color Doppler to gray scale but suggesting that in isoechoic areas color Doppler may give additional information.[68]

In a recent study[65,69] Doppler findings were correlated with biopsy findings with the conclusion that color Doppler is a useful adjunct to define areas of neovascularity that correlate with high grade cancers (Fig. 12.14). Color Doppler also helps to guide biopsies in potentially more clinically significant neoplasm.

More recent studies evaluating role of color Doppler in the isoechoic cancer also confirm the ability of color Doppler to identify higher grade cancers in the isoechoic gland.[70]

Importantly investigators are now studying the cause of hypervascular color Doppler images as a function of neovascularity that has been identified in prostate and other cancers. These studies[71,72] indicate that increased microvessel density is higher in cancer than in benign tissue. In addition, angiogenesis associated growth factors have been implicated in angiogenesis seen in malignant tumors. It is further suggested that angiogenesis and its associated hypervascularity seen by color Doppler may have stage and grade implications for prostatic cancer.[72]

About 70% of prostate cancers arise in the peripheral zone, 20% in the transition zone and 10% is the central zone. With ultrasound peripheral zone cancers are the most commonly detected and the clinician must strongly suspect cancer to identify and biopsy lesions outside the peripheral zone with gray scale imaging. With color Doppler any area seen with small irregular vessels should be biopsied.

The contours of both the prostate and the surgical capsule are important morphologic landmarks in the evaluation of neoplastic disease. Any contour bulge of more than 1.5 cm with an associated gray scale or color Doppler finding is suspicious for early extra-capsular extension.

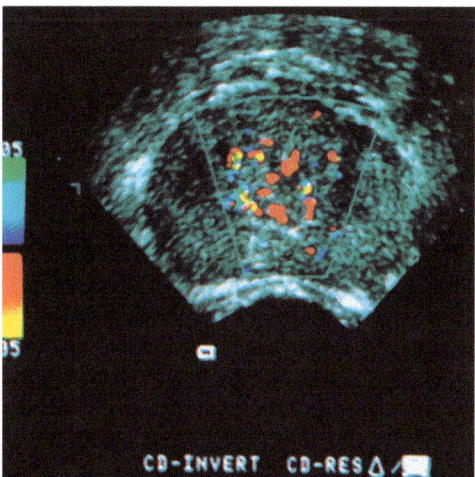

Fig. 12.14: Focal hypoechoic lesion in the prostate showing increased vascularity with haphazard vessels on pulsed Doppler.

KEY POINTS

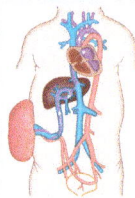

Renal transplant
- US for renal size, PCS dilatation, extrarenal collection.
- Doppler for vascular complications
  - Renal artery stenosis (m/c-10%)/thrombosis (1%).
  - Intrarenal and extrarenal AV fistulas and pseudoaneurysm.
  - Renal vein thrombosis and stenosis.
- Transplant rejection
  - RI > 0.9.
  - Reduced duration of systolic arterial flow.
  - Reduction or loss of antegrade diastolic flow.
- VUR
  - CDFI accurately grades III to V grade VUR.
  - Color jet from bladder into distal ureters.
- Prostatic malignancy
  - Usually hypoechoic with hypervascularity on CDFI.

Contour bulges along the anterior capsule need to be interrogated with color Doppler to confirm increased blood flow differentiating cancer from BPH asymmetry.

Other abnormalities of the prostate can produce focal hypoechoic area and have lead to confusion regarding the significance of this finding. These include ductal ectasia, infarct atrophy, prostatitis and prostatic epithelial neoplasia.[65]

Ductal ectasia is easy to exclude because gray scale images generally demonstrate a parallel pattern of reflective interfaces when viewed in both axial and sagittal projections. Ductal ectasia is also compressible when the probe is pushed anteriorly.

Atrophy generally produces a more vaguehypoechoic appearance without any mass effect and has no distinct vascularity. Granulomatous prostatitis is generally very hypoechoic focal and can produce a palpable nodule. Frequently there is history of prior infection. Granulomatous prostatitis may show increased vascularity if it is in a more active phase, which also corresponds with a recent PSA elevation. Prior or chronic granulomatous prostatitis generally does not have increased Doppler flow.

Prostatic epithelial neoplasia remains difficult to differentiate from focal early neoplasms and requires biopsy confirmation.

REFERENCES

1. Desbergt AL, Paushter DM, Lammert GK, et al. Renal artery stenosis evaluation will color Doppler flow imaging. Radiology. 1990;177:749-53.
2. Platt JF, Rubin JM, Ellis JH. Distinction between obstructive and non obstructive pyelocaliectasis with Duplex Doppler sonography. AIR. 1989;153:997-1006.
3. Platt JF, Rubin JM, ELlis JH, et al. Duplex Doppler US of the kidney differentiation of obstructive from non obstructive dilatation. Radiology. 1989;171:515-17.
4. Buds RO, Dipitro MA, Platt JF. Age dependence of the renal resistive index in healthy children. Radiology. 1992;184:469.
5. Killer MS. Renal Doppler sonography in infants and children. Radiology. 1989;172:603-04.
6. Craonan JJ. Contemporary concepts in imaging urinary from obstruction. Radiol Clin North Am. 1991;29:527-42.
7. Klahr S, Buerkert J, Morrison A. Urinary tract obstruction. In: Brenner BM, Rector FC (Eds). The Kidney 3rd edition Philadelphia, Saunders. 1986.pp.1449-82.
8. Yarger WE, Schocken DD, Harris RH. Obstructive uropathy in the rat. J Clin Invest. 1980;65:400-12.
9. Dodd GD, Kaufman PN, Svachen KB. Duplex Doppler evaluation of urinary obstruction in dogs. J Urol. 1991; 145:644-46.
10. Wilson DR. Pathophysiology of obstructive nephropathy. Kidney Int. 1980;18:281-92.
11. Leahy AL, Ryan PC, Mcentec, GM. Renal injury and recovery in partial ureteric obstruction. J Oral. 1989;142:199-203.
12. Platt JF, Rubin JM, Ellis JH. Acute renal failure: Possible role of Duplex Doppler ultrasound in distinction between acute prerenal failure and acute tubular necrosis. Radiology. 1991;179:419-23.
13. Patriquin HB, O'Regan S, Rabitaille P. Hemolytic uremic syndrome: Intrarenal arterial Doppler Pattern as a useful guide to therapy. Radiology. 1989;172:625-8.
14. Kier R, Taylor KJW Fejock AL. Renal masses: Characterisation with Doppler US. Radiology. 1990;176:703-07.
15. Kuijperi D, Jaspers R. Renal masses: Differential diagnosis with pulsed Doppler US. Radiology. 1989;170:59-60.
16. Dubin PA, Wills I. Renal carcinoma: Duplex Doppler evaluation. Br J Radiol. 1986;59:231-6.
17. Gonwa TA, Poplawski S, Paulsen W. Pathogenesis and outcome of hepatorenal syndrome in patients undergoing orthoptic liver transplant. Transplantation. 1989;47:395-97.
18. Gentiline P, Laffe G, Buzzelli G. Functional renal alteration in chronic liver disease. Digestion. 1980;20:73-78.
19. Platt JF, Ellis JH, Rubin JM. Renal Duplex Doppler ultrasonography: Noninvasive indicator of kidney dysfunction and hepatorenal failure. Liver Disease.Hepatology. 1994;20(2): 362-69.
20. Pozniak MA, Dodd GD, Kelcz F. Ultrasonographic evaluation of renal transplantation. Radiol Clin N Am. 1992;30:1053-66.
21. Platt JF, Ellis JH, Rubin JMA. Intrarenal arterial Doppler sonography in the detection of Renal vein thrombosis of native kidney. AJR. 1994;162:1367-70.

22. Keating MA, ALthausen AF. The clinical spectrum of renal vein thrombosis. J Uroe. 1985;133:938-1045.
23. Parvey HR, Eisenberg RL. Image directed Doppler sonography of intrarenal arteries in acute renal vein thrombosis. J Clin Ultrasound. 1990;8:512-16.
24. Laplante S, Patriguin HB, Robitaille P. Renal vein thrombosis in children: Evidence of early flow recovery with Doppler US. Radiology. 1993;189:37-42.
25. Haber E, Slater EE. High blood pressure. Sci Am i (VII): 1992;1-30.
26. Mann SJ, Pickiring. Detection of renovascular hypertension. Ann Intern Med. 1992;117(10):845-53.
27. Chen CC, Hoffe PB, Vahjen G. Patients at high risk for renal artery stenosis: A simple method of renal scintigraphic analysis with Tc^{99m} DTPA and captopril. Radiology. 1990;176:365-70.
28. Kohler TR, Zierler RE, Martin RL. Non invasive diagnosis of renal artery stenosis by Ultrasonic Duplex scanning. J Vaso Surg. 1986;4:450-56.
29. Taylor DC, Killer MD, Moneta GI. Duplex ultrasound scanning in the diagnosis of renal artery stenosis: A prospective evaluation. J Vase Surg. 1988;7:363-69.
30. Berland LL, Koslin DB, Routh WD. Renal artery stenosis: Prospective evaluation of diagnosis with color Duplex US compared with angiography. Work in progress. Radiology. 1990;174: 421-23.
31. Stavros ATA, Parker SH, Yakes WF. Segmental stenosis of renal artery: Patt recognition of the Tardus and Parvus abnormalities with Duplex sonography. Radiology. 1992;184(2):487-02.
32. Handa N, Fukunaga R, Etani H, et al. Efficacy of echo Doppler examination for the evaluation of renovascular disease. Ultrasound Med Biol. 1988;14:145.
33. Kotval PS. Doppler waveform parvus and tardus. A sign of proximal flow obstruction. J Ultrasound Med. 1989;8:435-40.
34. Patriguin HB, Lafortune M, Jequic JC. Stenosis of renal artery: Assessment showed systole in the downstream circulation with Doppler sonography. Radiology. 1992;184:479-85.
35. Dodd GD, Tublin ME, Shah A, et al. Imaging of vascular complication associated with renal transplants. AJR. 1991;157:449-59.
36. Meerut CRB: Organ Transplants. In: Taylor KJW, Burns PN, WIlls PNJ (Eds). Clinical Application of Doppler Ultrasound, 2nd edition. Raven Press. 1995.pp.203-330.
37. Hohnke C, Abendroth D, Schleibnee S, et al. Vascular complication in 1,200 kidney transplantations. Transplant Proc. 1987;19:3691-92.
38. Roberts JP, Ascher NL, Fryel DS, et al. Transplant renal artery stenosis. Transplantation. 1989;4:580-83.
39. Honto D, Simmons R. Renal transplantation: Clinical considerations in organ transplantation. Radiol Clin North Am. 1987;25:239-48.
40. Taylor KJW, Morse SS, Rigsby CM, et al. Vascular complication in renal allografts: Detection with Duplex Doppler ultrasound. Radiology. 1987;162:31-38.
41. Gottlish RH, Lirberman JC, Pahico RC, et al. Diagnosis of renal artery stenosis in transplanted kidneys value of Doppler waveform analysis of the intrarenal arteries. 1995;165:1441-46.
42. Ahula ND, Greenberg A, Banner BF, et al. Atheroembolic involvement of renal allografts. Am J Med Dis. 1989;12:329-32.
43. Beneit G, Charepntier B, Roche A. Arteriocalyceal fistula after grafted kidney biopsy: Successful management by selective catheter embolisation. Urology. 1984;24:487-90.
44. Middleton WD, Kellran GM, Melson GL. Post biopsy renal transplant arteriovenous fistula: Color Doppler versus US characteristics. Radiology. 1989;171:253-57.
45. Pigott JP, Sharp WV. Arteriovenous fistula involving transplant kidney: Brief communications. Transplantation. 1987;44:1.
46. Kaveggia LP, Parella RR, Grant EG. Duplex Doppler sonography in renal allografts the significance of reversed flow in diastole. AIR. 1990;155:295-98.
47. Taylor KT, marks WH. Use of Doppler imaging for evaluation of dysfunction in renal allografts Comment. AJR. 1990;155:536-37.
48. Tiggeler RG, Berden JH, Hoitsma AI, et al. Prevention of acute tubular necrosis in cadaveric kidney transplantation by the combined use of mannitol and moderate hydration. Ann Surg. 1985;201:246-51.
49. Kelez F, Pozniak MA, Pirsch JD. Pyramidal appearances and resistive and nonspecific sonographic indicators of renal transplant rejection (See Comments). AJR. 1990;155:531-35.
50. Nishioka N, Ikegami M. Imanishim: Renal transplant blood flow evaluation of color Doppler echography. Transplant Proc. 1989;21:1919.
51. Mostbeeh GH, Rachlatter C, Stockenluber F. Comparison of Duplex sonography and color Doppler imaging in renal allograft evaluation: A prospective study: Eur J Radiol. 1990;10:201-07.
52. Drake DG, Day DL, Letourneau JG. Doppler evaluation of renal transplant in children: A prospective analysis with tests pathologic correlation: AJR. 1990;154:785-87.
53. Platt JF, Ellis JH, Rubin JM. Renal transplant pyelocaliectasis: Role of Duplex Doppler US in evaluation Radiology. 1991;179:425-8.
54. Perrella RR, Duerincky A, Tessler FN. Evaluation of renal transplant dysfunction by Duplex Doppler sonography: A prospective study and review of literature. Am J Med Dis. 1990;15(6): 544-50.
55. Laing FC, Jeffrey RB, Wing VW. Ultrasound versus excretory urography in evaluating acute flash plain. Radiology. 1985;154:613-16.
56. Plat JF, Rubin JM, Ellis JH. Acute renal obstruction: Evaluation with intrarenal duplex Doppler and conventional US. Radiology. 1993;186:685-88.
57. Killer MS, Korsvih HE, Weiss RM. Diuretic Doppler sonography with correlative scintigraphy in children with hydronephrosis. Sco Pediatr Radiol. 1992;35:4972.
58. Tremewan RN, Bailey KR, Little PJ. Diagnosis of gross vesicoureteric reflux using ultra-sonography. Br J Urol. 1976;48:431-35.
59. Nasrallah PF, Conway JJ, King LR.Quantitative nuclear cystogram and in determining spontaneous resolution of vesicoureteric reflux. Urology. 1978;12:654-58.
60. Haffman AD, Le Roy AJ. Uroradiology: Procedures and anatomy. In: Kelalils PP, King LR, Belman AB (Eds). Clinical

Pediatric Urology, 3rd edition. Philadelphia WB Saunders: 1992. p.97.
61. Hanburg D, Coulden R, Farman P. Ultrasound cystography in the diagnosis of vesicoureteric reflux. Br J Urol. 1990;65:65-68.
62. Stamey TA, McNeal JE. Adenocarcinoma of the prostate. In: Walsh PC, Retik AB, Stamey TA, Vaughan ED (Eds). Campbells Urology, 6th edition. Philadelphia, WB Saunders. 1992;1:643-58.
63. Older RA, Watson LR. Ultrasound anatomy of the normal male reproductive tract. J Clin Ultrasound. 1996;24:389-409.
64. Rifkin MD, Dahnert W, Kurtz AB. State of the art: Endorectalsonography of the prostate gland. AJR. 1990;154:691-700.
65. Littrup PJ, Bailey SE. Prostate cancer: The role of transrectal ultrasound and its impact on cancer detection and management. Radiol Clinics North Am. 2000;38(1):87-113.
66. Rifkin MD, McGlynn ET, Choi H. Echogenicity of prostatic cancer correlated with histologic grade and stromal fibrosis: endorectal ultrasound studies. J Urol. 1989;170:549-52.
67. Shinohara K, Wheeler TM, Scardino PT. The appearance of prostatic cancer on transrectal ultrasonography: correlation of imaging and pathological examination. J Urol. 1989;142:76-82.
68. Patel V, Rickards D. The diagnostic value of color Doppler flow in the peripheral zone of prostate with histological correlation. Br J Urol. 1994;74:590-95.
69. Brce RC. The prostate. In: Rumach CM, Wilson SR, Charbonean JW (Eds). Diagnostic Ultrasound, 2nd edition Mosby Year Book. 1988;1:399-429.
70. Decarvalho V, Kuligowska E. The role of color Doppler for improving the detection of cancer in the isoechoicprastate gland. Presented at the annual meeting of the American Institute of Ultrasound in Medicine, New York, 1996.
71. Bigler SA, Deering RE, Brawer MK. A quantitative morphometric analysis of the microcirculation in prostate carcinoma. Human Pathol. 1993;24:220-26.
72. MeNeal JE, Redwine EA, Frciha FA. Zonal distribution of prostatic adenocarcinoma. Am J Surg Pathol. 1988;12:897-906.

The Retroperitoneum and Great Vessels

Pulsed Doppler equipment is becoming widely available as an additional facility on many real time scanners whether mechanical, electronic or linear array. The principle on which these instruments rely for the ultrasonic detection of blood flow is described by the Doppler equation. An ultrasonic beam of frequency of scattered by red blood cells moving with a velocity suffers an change in frequency Δf.

$$\Delta f = \frac{2 f \upsilon \cos \theta}{c}$$

where θ is the angle between the axis of beam and direction of flow and c is velocity of ultrasound.

Thus, for a given ultrasonic frequency the Doppler shift is proportional to the blood flow velocity and the cosine of the beam vessel angle. A range of velocities within the vessel lumen will give risk to a range of Doppler shift frequencies. Most instruments provide a real time display of this range of frequencies with time on horizontal axis, Doppler shift frequency on the vertical axis.

A Doppler examination can be made simply to confirm the presence or absence of flow or determine direction. Such a qualitative use of Doppler imaging can be clinically valuable. In patients with cirrhosis, reversed flow in the portal vein may accompany severe portal hypertension. The presence of flow in portal vein or renal vessels can be most helpful in excluding occlusion, while flow signals from solid mass can indicate neovascularization associated with malignancy.

In addition to such qualitative uses of Doppler technique spectral analysis of the signals allows more detailed quantitation. The outline of the maximum Doppler shift frequency corresponds to the time variation of the maximum flow velocity within the vessel. The pulsatility of this waveform is related to the vascular impedance downstream to the point of measurement.[1] In addition the range of frequencies present in the Doppler spectrum yields information about distribution of velocities across the vessel lumen. This provides evidence of the flow conditions, whether there is a plug or parabolic flow profile, whether there are flow disturbances or turbulence related to vessel wall abnormality.

Figure 13.1 for example shows how different velocity profiles in a vessel with laminar flow give rise to different spectral distributions and how this is reflected in the distribution of the gray scale in Doppler display.[1] When all the flow laminae are moving at the same velocity one Doppler shift frequency predominates: this is the plug flow profile typical of the aorta (Fig. 13.1A).

A parabolic velocity profile from a smaller vessel such as hepatic artery results in a more even distribution of power in the Doppler spectrum (Fig. 13.1B).

Intermediate profiles are present in such arteries as the celiac trunk (Fig. 13.1C). These Doppler characteristic which can be quantified using a variety of parameters, enable a description of a signal that is fairly specific to a particular vessel or even vessel site.

AORTA

The abdominal aorta is a compliant tube that supplies blood to the digestive organs, the kidneys, the adrenals, the gonads, the abdominal, paraspinal musculature, the pelvis, and lower limbs. It contributes significantly to the continuous forward flow of blood during diastole by acting as a reservoir of fluid during systole when it has a very pulsatile, inflow. It decreases in size during diastole by discharging blood into rest of the circulation in a much less pulsatile manner.[2] The abdominal aorta tapers from

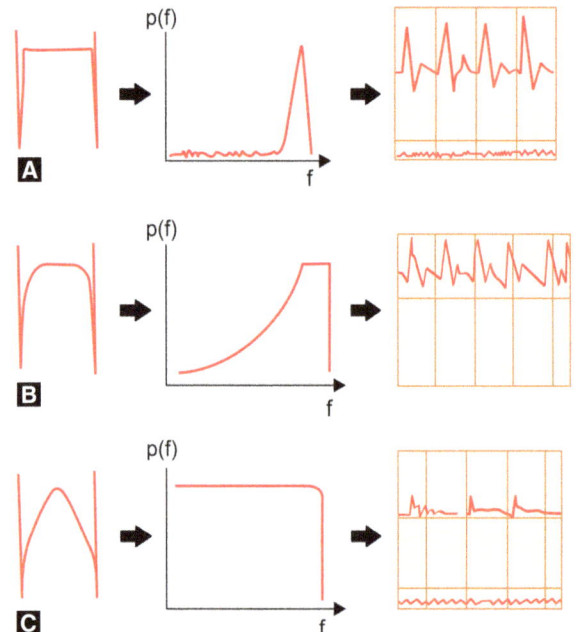

Figs. 13.1A to C: Showing the relationship between differing velocity profiles in a vessel with laminar flow (left column), the Doppler power spectrum (middle), and the resulting spectral display (right).

its cranial to caudal extent in 95% of people and usually measures less than 2.3 cm in diameter for men and 1.9 cm for women.[3] The upper limit of normal for aortic diameter varies with age as the diameter normally increases by up to 25% in the seventh and eighth decades.

The abdominal aorta enters the abdomen through the aortic hiatus of the diaphragm, immediately anterior to the twelfth dorsal vertebra. The upper abdominal aorta lies posterior and slightly to the left of the gastroesophageal junction. The median arcuate ligament of the diaphragm about its anterior surface and it is flanked on either side by the diaphragmatic crura. To the right lies the azygous vein and thoracic duct on its left lies the hemiazygous vein. Below the level of the crura it lies to the left of IVC and posterior to the celiac artery, superior mesenteric artery, inferior mesenteric, left renal vein, gonadal vessels and root of mesentery. At the L4 level, it bifurcates into paired common iliac arteries which are about 5 cm long and generally run slightly anterior to the corresponding veins. The common iliac arteries bifurcate into external and internal iliac arteries. The external iliac artery lies just on the medial aspect of psoas muscle.

The main aortic branches that are frequently seen on ultrasound are the iliac artery the paired renal arteries, the superior mesenteric artery and the common iliac arteries. The celiac artery typically bifurcates into hepatic and splenic arteries within 3 cm of its origin. The left gastric artery is given off superiorly is sometimes seen. The internal iliac arteries have numerous branches immediately after the common iliac artery bifurcation but are rarely seen on routine sonograms. The external iliac artery gives off the inferior epigastric artery and deep circumflex iliac artery before continuing below the inguinal ligament as the common femoral artery.

Other aortic branches not usually identified include paired inferior phrenic, paired middle suprarenal, gonadal arteries, the inferior mesenteric artery and paired first to fourth lumbar artery. At the aortic termination, the middle sacral artery is given off posteroinferiorly.

At sonography aorta is shown as a hypoechoic tubular structure with echogenic walls. It is usually located just to the left of the midline, although it becomes variable in position when it becomes ectatic. The midabdominal aorta at the level of renal arteries is frequently difficult to visualize well because of overlying bowel gas.

The normal flow pattern in the aorta is classified as plug flow, a situation in which most of the blood is moving at the same velocity. In the aorta and iliac arteries, flow is typically of the high resistance type with a sharp increase in antegrade velocity during systole followed by a rapid decrease in velocity and culminating in a brief period of reversed flow (Figs. 13.2A to D). The aortic signals show a clear window below the systolic time velocity pulse implying that most cells are moving at same velocity. During the remainder of diastole there is some low velocity antegrade flow. Of note is the decrease in flow at the end of diastole which begins to reverse in direction at the level of bifurcation.[1] This is due to blood actually rebounding up the aorta as the velocity wave is reflected from high impedance of the peripheral vascular bed of legs. The fact that this flow is found below the renal vessels results in the renal arterial flow being maintained during diastole. Relatively continuous flow in the renal artery may be of importance in renal function.

The main aortic branches supply numerous low resistance areas and as such, these have a lower resistive index and a lower pulsatility index. These smaller vessels show a more variable velocity pattern across the blood vessel and so the thickness of the spectral line is broadened. Good acoustic window for scanning the abdominal aorta includes:
- The midline in the upper abdomen.
- The left flank with patient supine or right lateral decubitus.
- Along the lateral aspect of the lower rectus abdominis muscle for evaluating iliac vessels.

The entire aorta should be visualized in transverse and longitudinal planes and its maximum anteroposterior and transverse diameter measured accurately.

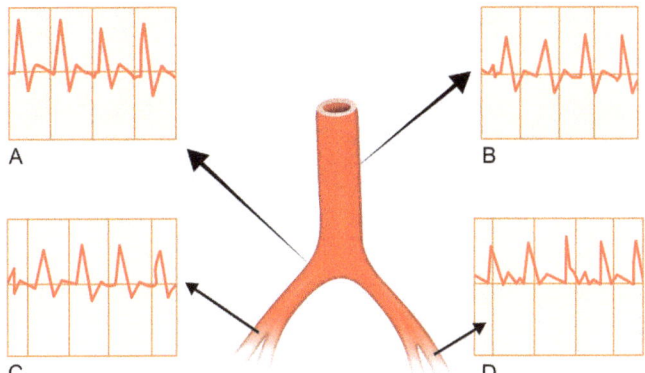

Figs. 13.2A to D: Time velocity spectra in common iliac artery (A), distal aorta (B) external iliac artery (C) and internal iliac artery (D).

AORTIC PATHOLOGY

The abdominal aorta and its main branches are affected by atheroma, aneurysm formation, connective tissue disorders, rupture, thrombosis, infectious, and displacement by and invasion from disease in adjacent structures.

Atheromatous Disease

Atheroma or arteriosclerosis is a vascular wall disorders characterized by the presence of lipid deposits in the intima. Atherosclerotic changes in the aorta are virtually universal beyond the age of 20 years and it affects more men than women. It affects both the aorta, the iliac arteries and the other aortic branch arteries and is most common on the posterior wall in the aorta iliac area.[4] It is associated with cigarette smoking, diabetes mellitus, hypertension, and increased levels of low density lipoprotein (LDL) fraction of serum cholesterol.

If significant lower limb pain is present, it is prudent to assess the entire lower limb arterial tree to rule out emboli and to look for further stenosis. Similarly in down limb analysis the presence of a dampened waveform in the common femoral artery should provoke a search for a stenotic lesion more proximal in arterial tree.[5]

Ultrasound can demonstrate thickening and calcification within the aortic wall (Figs. 13.3A and B). If calcification is extensive, acoustic shadowing may result. In these cases, visualization of the aortic lumen may be limited. Atheromatous plaque is a soft porridge like material which may discharge into the vessel lumen causing a distal embolus or a thrombus or both at the donor site. Thrombus within the vessel usually has a low level echogenicity but may be anechoic (Figs. 13.4A and B). An occluded vessel can appear patent because of echo free lumen but will not pulsate. Plaque cause mural irregularity[6] and frequently narrow the vessel lumen with resulting distal ischemia.

Stenotic or occlusive disease most often occurs in the infrarenal portion of the aorta. Atheroma may also be associated with mural weakening and aneurysm formation.

Patency of the aorta and its branch vessels can be confirmed with color Doppler analysis and where aliasing occurs, a Doppler spectral tracing helps to determine whether a true stenosis is present or not.

Angle corrected spectral Doppler analysis at stenosis typically shows increased pulsatility (increased pulsatility index and resistive index) proximal to stenosis, increased peak systolic and peak diastolic velocity immediately at the stenosis, turbulence immediately poststenosis and dampening of waveform further distal to stenosis.[7]

Several workers[8,9] have classified arterial stenosis. Each arterial segment is graded into five categories of stenosis (i) Normal (ii) 1-19% diameter reduction (iii) 20-49% diameter reduction (iv) 50-99% diameter reduction (v) Total occlusion.

Normal arteries have a triphasic signal and minimal spectral broadening. The spectral band is narrow with a clear area below the systolic peak (systolic window). A diameter reduction of 1-19% causes only spectral broadening and loss of systolic window waveform contour and peak systolic velocity remains normal. In moderate stenosis (20-49% diameter reduction) the peak systolic velocity increases 30-100% with respect to the normal segment immediately proximal to the stenosis and spectral broadening is marked. Stenosis of 50-99% diameter reduction is considered hemodynamically significant. Reverse velocity is absent in these stenosis, the systolic peak is increased by 100% or more and spectral broadening is usually prominent. Occluded arteries have no detectable flow and velocity is markedly decreased in the segments proximal to occlusion.

KEY POINTS

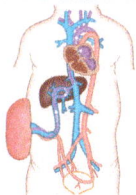

Aorta
- Normal flow pattern—plug flow.
- Atherosclerosis
  - Decreased aortic lumen—aortic wall thickened and calcified.
  - Proximal to stenosis—increased pulsatility and resistive index.
  - At stenosis—increased peak systolic and peak diastolic velocities.
  - Post-stenosis—turbulence.
  - Distally—dampened waveform.
- Significant stenosis of
  SMA (PSV > 275 cm/sec).
  celiac (PSV > 200 cm/sec).

Angiography has long been the definitive test for symptomatic aortic iliac disease. However, this approach provides anatomic rather than functional data and has

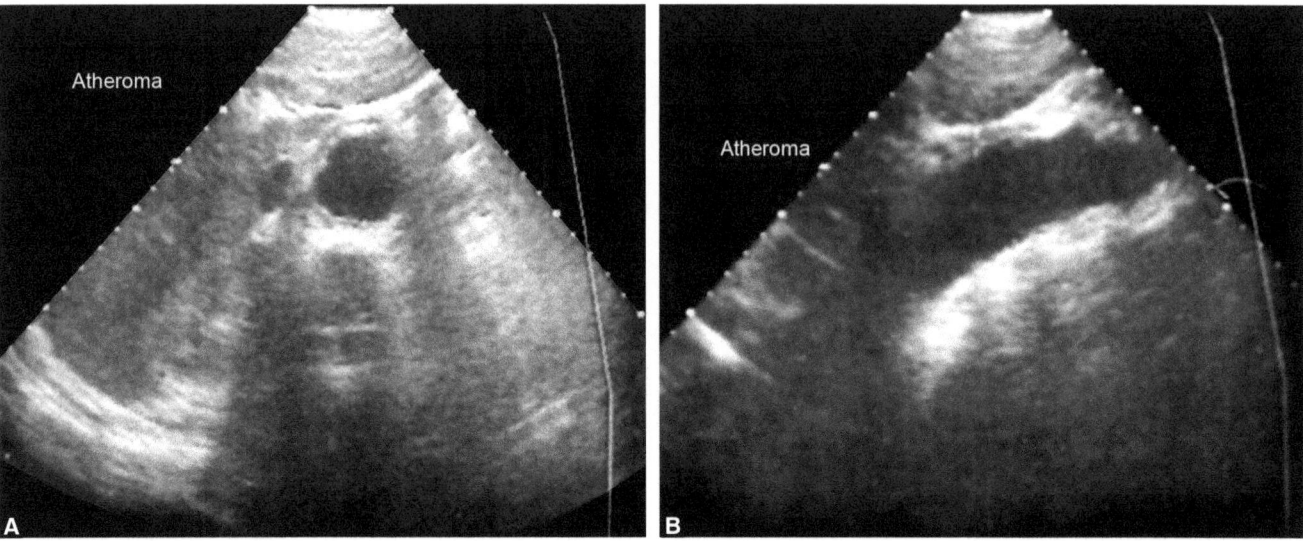

Figs. 13.3A and B: Dilated abdominal aorta in (A) transverse, and (B) longitudinal scan with atherosclerotic plaques.

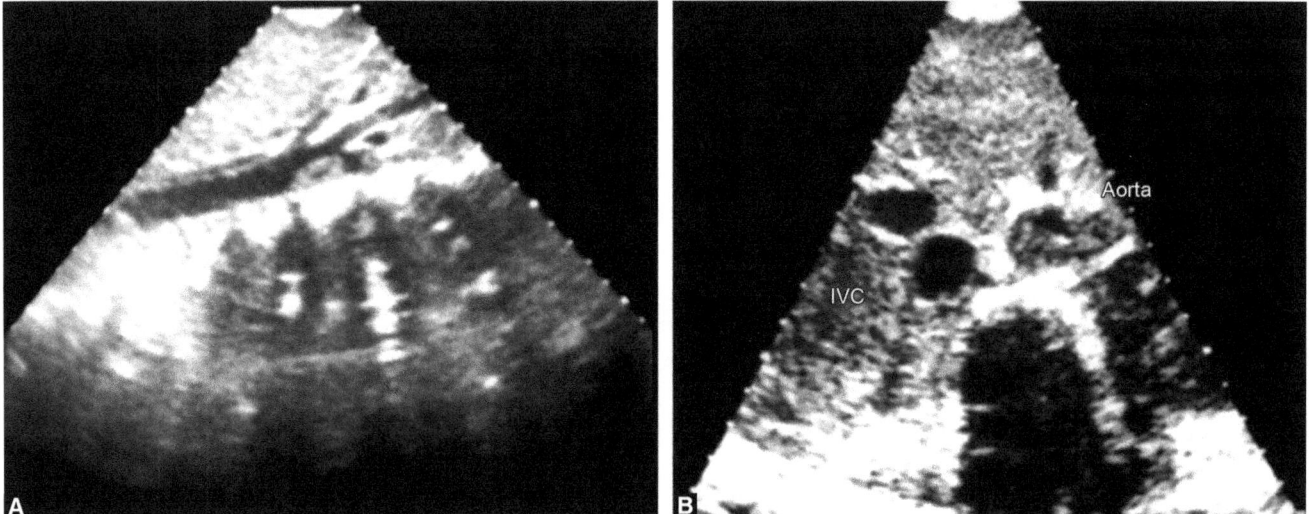

Figs. 13.4A and B: (A) Longitudinal and (B) transverse scans of aorta showing a thrombus in the lumen just at the point of origin of superior mesenteric artery.

many limitations. Because atherosclerotic lesions are often concentric, the angiographic appearance may be misleading, especially if only unipolar views are obtained. The best way to determine the hemodynamic significance of arterial lesion is to measure the pressure gradient at angiography but this is not always practical or anatomically possible. Finally, the invasive nature and relatively high cost of angiography make it unsuitable for screening purpose or routine follow-up.

Duplex scanning can localise and classify peripheral arterial stenosis nearly as well as angiography.[8] A normal Duplex study virtually excludes significant occlusive disease. When the Duplex study localizes the suspected area of disease, it can be helpful to the angiographer who may be able to tailor the angiography technique to fit the needs of patient.

In addition, Duplex scanning provides a baseline for assessing the early and long-term results of PTA. Duplex scanning can detect restenosis of segments dilated by angioplasty or bypass graft stenosis before pressure drops occurs.[8]

Flow velocities less than 40 cm/sec in femoropopliteal bypass[8] grafts are associated with a high rate of graft failure.[18] Thus, the ability of Duplex scanning to distinguish high grade stenosis from occlusion to detect hemodynamically insignificant disease and to localize disease accurately is unique among noninvasive tests and represents the first practical means of documenting arterial disease progression.[18]

Aortic Aneurysms

Abdominal aortic aneurysm is a common disease with potentially catastrophic complications. Untreated, these aneurysms enlarge and eventually rupture with a high mortality of 50-90%. Conversely elective surgical resection has an excellent prognosis and low mortality (2-4%) and currently is the treatment of choice.[10] Because most patients are asymptomatic the diagnosis of abdominal aortic aneurysm is frequently unsuspected. Evaluation of these patients is heavily dependent on imaging and the radiologist is in a unique position to direct the workup.[11]

A true aneurysm of abdominal aorta is a localized dilatation of wall greater than 3 cm in diameter. All these layers of the vessel (intima, media, and adventitia) are involved. A false aneurysm (pseudoaneurysm) is essentially a perforation of the aorta with subsequent hematoma formation limited by adventitial or surrounding vascular tissues (Fig. 13.5).

Most abdominal aortic aneurysms are secondary to atherosclerosis. Other causes include trauma, infection, syphilis, cystic medial necrosis, inflammation, and Marfan's syndrome.

Atherosclerotic plaques cause fibrosis and atrophy of the underlying media of aortic wall. Loss of medial elastic fibers seen with advancing age compounds this insult. The weakened media can no longer adequately support the vessel wall, resulting in aortic dilatation. Increasing dilatation and decreasing wall thickness result in a rapid increase in wall tension (Laplace's law). This leads to progressive dilatation and eventual rupture.[11]

Inflammatory aortic aneurysm is a distinct clinical entity distinguished from uncomplicated atherosclerotic aneurysms by dense perianeurysmal fibrosis and thickened aortic walls of abdominal aortic aneurysms 4-23% are estimated to be inflammatory in origin. They are very difficult to diagnose as they often present with pain and mimic retroperitoneal bleed.[15] While less than 25% of idiopathic abdominal aneurysm present with pain, pain was present in 84% of patients with inflammatory aneurysms.

Surgical repair of these aneurysms is difficult with increased morbidity and mortality compared with simple aneurysm. Abdominal aortic aneurysms 3-6 cm in diameter grow approximately at 4 mm/year. The risk of rupture relates primarily to the size of aneurysm with a clear increase in risk over 5 cm. Even small aneurysms are more likely to rupture and significant enlargement is demonstrated on sequential studies. Consequently it has been proposed that even small asymptomatic aneurysms be re-examined 3-6 months after diagnosis and then at 12 months intervals. Regardless of size symptomatic aneurysm implies rapid growth or rupture. The most common surgical treatment is endoaneurysmorrhaphy which consists of placement of a prosthetic graft within the aneurysm. The aneurysm wall is then wrapped around the graft, providing protection against aortoenteric fistulas. Complete resection of the aneurysm with graft placement can be performed also.

Currently imaging methods for the diagnosis of abdominal aortic aneurysms include US, CT, Conventional angiography or digital subtraction angiography, and MRI.[12]

Ultrasound and color Doppler US[13] are the standard methods in the screening and follow-up of abdominal aortic aneurysm although in many cases they are not able to visualize the renal arteries and can be limited by the extremely variable body weight and bowel gas of the patient.

The CT technique is excellent in both pre and postoperative evaluation of abdominal aortic aneurysms but some controversies exist about the efficiency of CT in evaluating the involvement of renal arteries.[14] Moreover, CT is not always able to discriminate between a thrombus filled aneurysm and a lot within the false lumen of a dissection.[11]

Digital subtraction angiography is the gold standard in the detection of the involvement of increased branches and/or variants of vascular anatomy[11] but it can underestimate both the size and extension of a thrombus filled aneurysm, due to opacification of the lumen alone.

The first MRI reports in the study of abdominal aortic aneurysms, obtained by using spin echo or gradient echo sequences have been encouraging, but more recently by magnetic resonance angiography seems to be the most promising noninvasive method in the assessment of abdominal aortic aneurysms.[12]

Sonography is the standard method for screening and follow-up of aortic aneurysms. It approaches 100% accuracy in detection and measurements correlate within 3 mm of surgical specimen. Sonograms may show thrombus, periaortic abnormalities, dissection its cephalic and caudal extent as well as complication such as hydronephrosis.

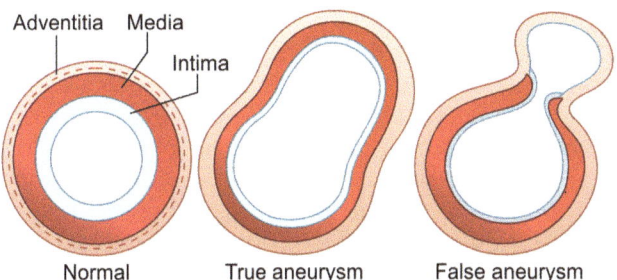

Fig. 13.5: Types of aortic aneurysm.

Sonography is limited in obese patients or those with abundant overlying bowel gas. In addition, the renal arteries are rarely visualized directly and suprarenal extension frequently can only be inferred by the relationship of the aneurysm to the superior mesenteric artery. Availability, cost, noninvasiveness combined with accuracy in detection and measurement make sonography ideal for screening and follow-up of uncomplicated aneurysms.

Diagnosis of an aneurysm is made sonographically by finding a focal dilatation of the aorta or a generalized dilatation bigger than 3 cm. Aneurysms elongate as they grow and as the lower end of aorta rarely moves significantly caudally, most abdominal aortic aneurysms defect to the left side or kink anteriorly or both as they enlarge.[5]

The anterior or posterior borders of the aneurysms are usually better seen than its lateral borders which are indistinct. The adventitia is usually continuous with adjacent fibrofatty tissue and in echogenic. Mural thrombus, which frequently makes up most of the wall, is usually of low to medium echogenicity and it may or may not have a lamellate appearance. The intimal lining may be smooth or irregular and calcification may also be present.

Sonography measurement of these aneurysms may be challenging and it is important to get an accurate outer layer to outer layer measurement in a plane perpendicular to the long axis of the vessel.

Analysis of an aneurysm would include its maximum true length width and transverse dimension, documentation of its shape and also of its location including suprarenal extension or involvement of common iliac vessels. This analysis is of great practical importance, as different surgical approaches are used with the different types of aneurysms. The etiology, complications rate, and post procedure morbidity are also quite distinct. The nature and type of wall thickening should be found and flow pattern characterized. Effort should be made to detect any dissection and to evaluate hypoechoic channels for flow with Doppler. Both kidneys should always be examined, their size measured and pelvic caliectasis excluded.[5]

Following descriptive terms and sonographic criterion as used for abdominal aortic aneurysm:
- Bulbous: Sharp junction between normal and abnormal
- Fusiform: Gradual transition between normal and abnormal
- Saccular: Sharp sudden transition between normal and abnormal
- Dumbbell: Figure eight appearance to the aneurysm
- The decision to operate on an aneurysm is based on[5]:
- Absolute size especially when diameter > 6 cm
- Documented enlargement overtime
- Associated pain or tenderness
- Associated distal emboli
- Renal obstruction or vascular compromise
- Gastrointestinal bleeding
- Suspected rupture.

In a study by Carriero et al.[12] results suggested that MRA together with color Doppler US represented a valid alternative to invasive imaging in the assessment of abdominal aortic aneurysm. In their study color Doppler US proved to be effective in the determination of aneurysm diameter, craniocaudal extension and thrombotic and calcific components. It showed better results than MRA in the evaluation of the relation between aneurysm and main arterial branches (renal and iliac) due to the possibility to detect color encoded flow signals which make it easier to identify the vessel. In particular it always detected the iliac arteries and correctly documented their involvement in 50% of cases. The detection rate of renal arteries proved less satisfactory than MRA due to technical problems.

The recognized complications of abdominal aortic aneurysm include rupture, thrombosis, dissection, distal embolism, infection and obstruction, and invasion of adjacent structures. Most common complications are branch artery occlusions or stenoses which have more to do with atheroma than with aneurysm. They can occur anywhere but are most commonly seen in the inferior mesenteric artery and renal artery.[15]

Aortic Rupture

The most catastrophic of aortic aneurysm complication is aortic rupture which has a mortality rate of at least 50%.[15] Because of the critical nature of problem few of these patients have ultrasound preoperatively. Computed tomography is the test of choice.[16] It is better to detect acute bleeds that is not tampered by bowel gas and provides a greater overall perspective. Some aortic rupture may be contained in the retroperitoneum; they are referred to as chronic ruptures. Ultrasonic appearances those of a pulsating hematoma, a hypoechoic collection in the periaortic region extending to the flanks.[17]

Aortic Dissection

A dissecting aortic aneurysm is not a free aneurysm of the aorta but rather a propagating hematoma extending initially within the media of the aorta to eventually rupture into intimately lined aortic lumen[17] (Fig. 13.6).

It is easily recognized on sonography with the classical appearance being a thin membrane fluttering in the lumen at different phases of cardiac cycle.[15] Color Doppler shows blood flow in both channel, although flow rates frequently differ between the channels.

Effort should be made to distinguish a true dissection from a pseudodissection which is caused by liquefaction of aneurysm thrombus.[18] The distinguishing features include no fluttering of the intravascular membrane, no flow in one lumen and a thick membrane in pseudolesion.[15]

Abdominal Aortic Pseudoaneurysm

Abdominal aortic pseudoaneurysms may occur as a complication of abdominal aortic aneurysm, abdominal interventional procedure or abdominal surgery. They may also result from vasculitis, mycotic aneurysms or abdominal surgery and may be associated with postprocedural hematoma particularly in patients receiving anticoagulant or antiplatelet medication.[19]

A pseudoaneurysm is an organized perivascular hematoma that has a lumen is continuity with the vascular lumen. Formation of a pseudoaneurysm generally involves an arterial injury, local hemorrhage and tamponade by surrounding tissues.[20] Pseudoaneurysm of the abdominal aorta is a rare finding accounting for only 1 percent of all abdominal aneurysms.[21]

On gray scale sonography pseudoaneurysms appears is as anechoic saccular collections in proximity to arteries (Figs. 13.7A and B). These collections are more easily perceived by color flow mapping. Pulsed Doppler studies show turbulent or arterial like flow (swirling or whirl wind flow) within the pseudoaneurysm lumen and systolic and diastolic continuous flow, the classic 'to and fro' spectral wave pattern, in the communicating channel. This pattern consists of high speed flow directed outward from the artery into the pseudoaneurysm during systole and slower flow out of the pseudoaneurysm during diastole.[22]

The 'to and fro' sign is helpful in identifying the exact point of communication between the pseudoaneurysms and aorta when planning a surgical approach.[3]

Hematoma or other fluid collections adjacent but not communicating with the aorta may move vigorously as the aorta pulsates. Such movement should not be mistaken for the concentric pulsations of a pseudoaneurysm.

The final diagnosis with Duplex Doppler sonography requires identification of the typical flow pattern within

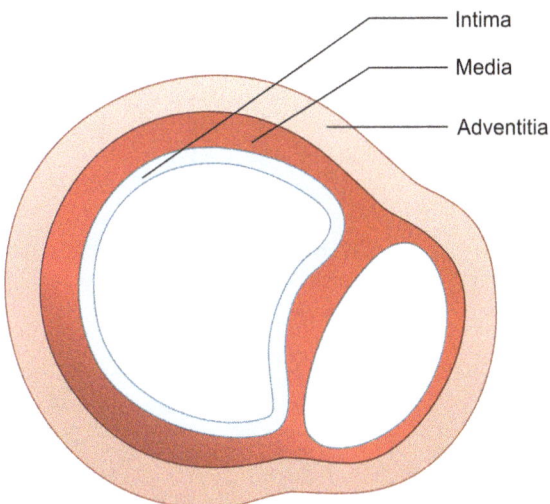

Fig. 13.6: Line diagram showing aortic dissection.

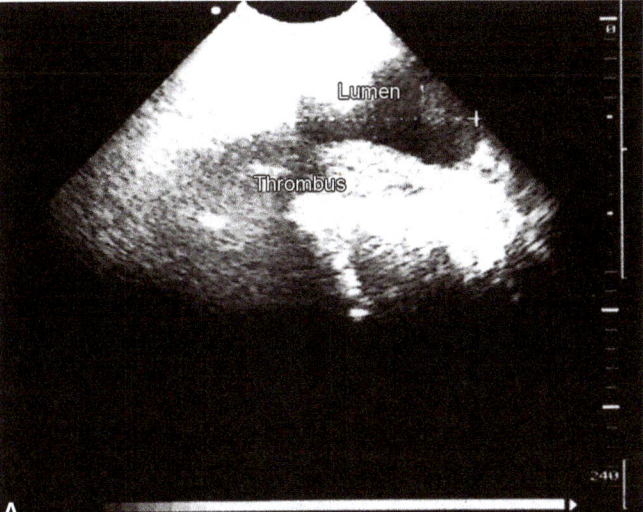
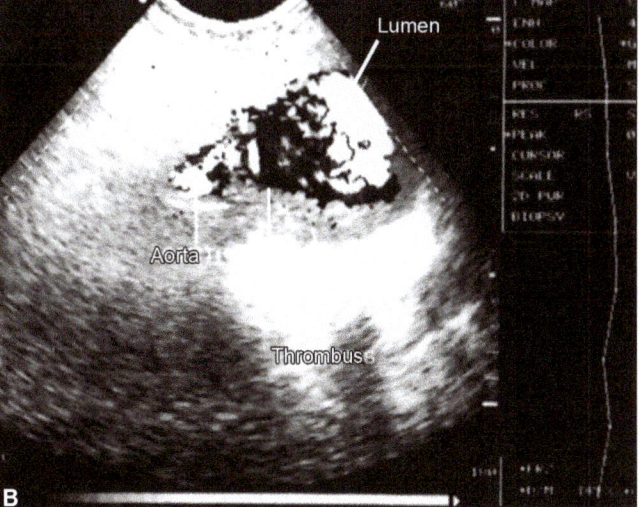

Figs. 13.7A and B: (A) Gray scale image in transverse plane at midaortic level showing well defined, anechoic saccular collection in continuity with the aorta. An echogenic thrombus is seen in the posterior wall of the pseudoaneurysm; (B) Color flow Doppler image of same patient showing luminal blood flow in the pseudoaneurysm.

the neck of the pseudoaneurysm. This finding usually demonstrated in post catheterization pseudoaneurysms' can be absent or less obvious in those that are due to a dehiscence of the anastomotic connection of synthetic bypass grafts, those due to involvement of peripancreatic arteries by chronic pancreatitis, or those complicating organ transplants.[22] The reason for this can be due to either the absence of or difficulty in locating a communicating channel or it can be due to the presence of a broad channel that shows a highly turbulent and disorganized atypical flow throughout the cardiac cycle. Combined Duplex and color flow sonography is the screening modality of choice to evaluate a pulsatile mass in the abdomen.

AORTIC GRAFTS

Distal Aortic Graft

The operative procedure for a patient with isolated infrarenal abdominal aortic aneurysms who has no evidence of peripheral vascular disease is a simple tube graft. This is appreciated sonographically by a rather sharp definition of parallel echogenic walls in the distal aorta.

Aortic aneurysms are repaired by incising the aneurysms, implanting the graft, then wrapping the aneurysmal sac around the implanted graft as a stabilizing force.

The relatively high incidence of complications following endovascular aneurysms surgery mandates rigorous postoperative surveillance program. Endo leaks have been described in all initial series of endovascular aneurysm repairs with an incidence ranging from 10-43%. Endoleak may be early or late and may arise from the proximal anastomosis, the distal anastomosis or as a result of retrograde filling from the lumbar, inferior mesenteric or common iliac vessels. Irrespective of the origin of the leak the consequences are potentially serious. Establishment of flow within the aneurysm sac may facilitate continued aneurysm expansion and rupture. Conventionally CT has been used to follow patients after endovascular aneurysm repair. Recent study has suggested than Duplex imaging may be useful in the setting.[23]

If bleeding occurs postoperatively hematoma tends to dissect between the graft and the encircling aneurysmal wall producing a characteristic ultrasonic appearance of a lumen within a lumen.

Duplex imaging demonstrates the presence of flow within the aneurysm as at the site of leak.[23]

Majority of patients with a proven endoleak have continued expansion of aneurysm sac.[23]

Studies have shown that successful exclusion of the aneurysm sac results in a reduction in aneurysm size.[23,24]

One theoretical problem associated with endovascular aneurysm repair concerns the fate of the proximal aortic neck. The proximal aortic neck may continue to dilate, which could cause migration and displacement of the proximal aortic stent.[23]

Duplex Doppler imaging may be used as the first line investigation to monitor patients following endovascular aneurysm repair. Cross-sectional imaging may then be reserved for patients with a demonstrable endoleak or increase in aneurysm diameter.[23]

KEY POINTS

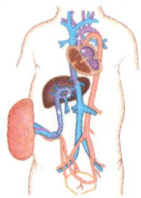

- **Aneurysm**
  - True aneurysm—localized dilatation > 3 cm diameter
  - Pseudoaneurysm—organized paravascular hematoma, lumen contiguous with aortic lumen
  - Doppler reveals swirling within pseudoaneurysm, continuous systolic and diastolic flow
  - To and fro move pattern at neck.
- **Aortic dissection**
  - Thin membrane fluttering in lumen—blood flow in both channels with different flow rates.
- **Aortic grafts—complications**
  - Duplex Doppler distinguishes pseudoaneurysms, (Pulsatile/turbulent flow) from perigraft fluid (transmitted pulsation).

Aortoiliac Graft

Often patients with extension of abdominal aortic aneurysm into iliac arteries have an aortoiliac prosthesis placed with an end to end proximal and distal anastomosis.

These grafts can be appreciated sonographically because of their very parallel echogenic walls.

Aortofemoral Graft

Aortofemoral grafts are placed in patients who have some vascular compromise below the distal aorta. These aortofemoral grafts have either end to end or end to side anastomosis. Sonographically the end to end grafts produce slight dilatation at the proximal anastomosis.

COMPLICATIONS OF GRAFT IMPLANTATION

Pseudoaneurysms

Pseudoaneurysms are by far the most common complication of vascular prosthetic surgery. Aortic anastomotic pseudoaneurysm is defined as a type of pseudoaneurysm due to extra-vasation of blood caused by a defect in the suture line at the junction of the prosthetic graft and the native aorta.[25]

A pseudoaneurysm is not surrounded by any layer of the wall of the native aorta. Usually partial thrombosis of the pseudoaneurysms occurs with blood flowing into nonthrombosed part.

False aneurysms can result from a number of causes, late failure of suture material, endarterectomy at the site of anastomosis, graft dilatation, hypertension and atherosclerotic degeneration of native vessel.[25]

Graft infection is another dreaded complication and leads to false aneurysm formation at the suture line as does the communicating hematoma from a leak of the suture line at the time of a fresh anastomosis.[17] With Duplex Doppler imaging pulsatile or turbulent flow within the pseudoaneurysm may be seen.[25]

Proximal anastomotic false aneurysms of the aorta have a serious prognosis and are associated with a high mortality.

Aneurysms when they occur in patients with vascular prosthetics are almost always anastomotic in location either proximally or distally, the only exception being those related to trauma or those secondary to an intrinsic defect is the prosthetic wall, a distinct rarely.[17]

Perigraft Fluid

Fluid around the graft either proximally, distally or along its length is a serious and important finding best seen with ultrasound or CT. Perigraft fluid produces a similar appearance sonographically whether it is secondary to hematoma, serum, lymph node, or abscess.

If the collection is large or echogenic or increasing in size or far away from the graft then infection must be considered[16] and fine needle aspiration is indicated. Lymphocele around the graft may be very hypoechoic and may simulate a dissection.[5]

Ordinarily ultrasound distinguishes between false aneurysm and perigraft fluid collections.

False aneurysms have definite discrete pulsations throughout other fluid collections may have some transmitted pulsation where the fluid abuts upon the pulsatile vessel but are never intrinsically pulsatile. Color spectral Doppler are very useful in there instances.

AORTIC BRANCHES

Celiac Trunk

Classically the celiac artery has a high resistive pattern at its origin with a small amount of reversed early diastolic flow.[5] As one goes distally it losses its early reversed diastolic flow. Distally the artery has continuous forward flow throughout the cardiac cycle of low resistance type.

With the cursor appropriately positioned waveforms can be sampled in the hepatic artery, splenic artery, and the left gastric artery.

The gastric artery demonstrated surprisingly high shifts and is easily seen ascending from the celiac trunk. The splenic artery shows low resistance flow and has a turbulent flow presumbambly associated with its common tortuousity.[1]

The hepatic artery rises solely from the celiac axis 72% of the time. The superior mesenteric artery given off the common hepatic artery in 4% of the cases the right hepatic artery in 11% of cases and the left hepatic artery in 10% of cases.[5]

The common hepatic artery can easily be sampled as well as its branch, the pancreatoduodenal artery lying on the superficial surface of the pancreas. Real time imaging allows the proper hepatic artery to be traced up to the portahepatis and the right hepatic artery can be sampled as it crosses anterior to the portal vein. The hepatic artery usually has a low resistance pattern (Fig. 13.8).

SUPERIOR MESENTERIC ARTERY (SME)

The normal SMA spectral pattern demonstrates organized flow throughout the cardiac cycle and in the fasting states. Characteristically has flow reversal in early diastole. This is similar to the higher resistance outflow vessels in the periphery. Normal celiac artery velocity waveform demonstrates organized flow in systolic and somewhat disorganized diastolic flow with continuous forward flow throughout diastole and no diastolic flow reversal. These waveforms are reminiscent of the low outflow resistance system seen in the internal carotid artery.[33]

Fasting peak systolic velocities of SMA and celiac artery have ranged from 103–196 cm/sec and 118–163 cm/sec respectively[33] (Figs. 13.8A to G).

Flow Responses to Physiology Stimulus

Jager et al.[9] have measured postprandial velocities in the SMA after 1,000 calories test meal: within 15 minutes after eating a significant increase in peak systolic velocity was observed. This reached a maximum of almost double the baseline flow velocity 45 minutes after eating and returned to normal by 90 minutes. During this time diastolic velocity increased to almost three times fasting levels. This dramatic postprandial increase in diastolic velocity appeared to be the most predictable spectral change in SMA velocity

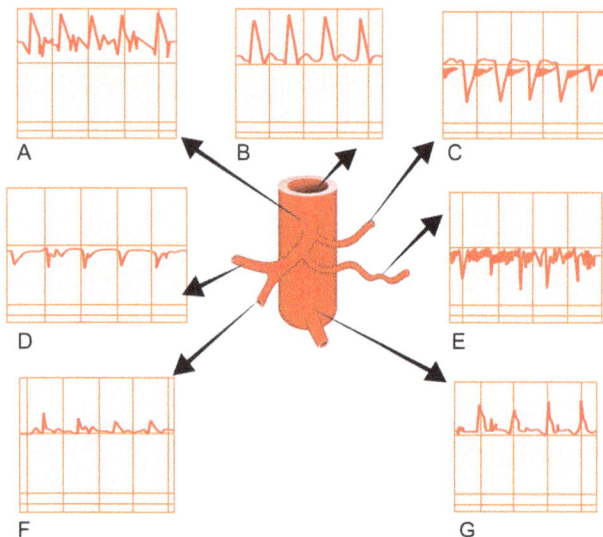

Figs. 13.8A to G: (A) Time velocity spectra in celiac trunk (B) proximal aorta, (C) left gastric artery, (D) common hepatic artery, (E) splenic artery, (F) gastroduodenal artery, and (G) superior mesenteric artery.

waveforms. There is also a complete disappearance of diastolic flow reversal in SMA after eating.

Moneta et al.[34] measured celiac and SMA flow velocities postprandially. There was 20–24% increase in iliac systolic and diastolic flow velocities after meals but the difference was not statistically significant. In contrast SMA flow velocities increased significantly after test meals.

Mesenteric Doppler

The arteries primarily responsible for mesenteric circulation include the SMA, IMA, and branches of celiac artery which provide anastomotic links in case of occlusive disease. The branches which provide collateral flow include common hepatic artery and gastroduodenal artery. Chronic mesenteric ischemia results due to atherosclerotic involvement of a least two of the three major vessels supplying the bowel. Abundant collateral exists in the mesenteric circulation hence it is possible at times that all three mesenteric vessels are occluded without bowel infarction or symptoms due to the rich collateral network. Mesenteric duplex scanning represents a noninvasive technique for anatomic and physiologic assessment of visceral vessels. It provides a rapid accurate method for the evaluation of patency of major splanchnic vessel. This aids in the selection of patients for arteriography and allow rational selection of alternative diagnostic studies.

Moneta et al.[35] found that a peak systolic velocity more than 275 cm/sec indicates a significant obstruction of SMA.

A peak systolic velocity more than 200 cm/sec for the celiac also correlated with a significant stenosis of the vessel.

When mesenteric ischemia requires surgical intervention bypass grafting from the aorta to the mesenteric arteries is frequently employed. Mesenteric duplex scanning may provide an improved, noninvasive technique for objective assessment of postoperative graft patency as well as a method for long-term follow-up of these arterial reconstruction procedures.[36]

Splanchnic Aneurysms

Splanchnic aneurysms may be congenital, atherosclerotic, post-traumatic, mycotic, or inflammatory. About 10% of patients with chronic pancreatitis develop these pseudo-aneurysms which occur in the hepatic artery, splenic artery, (Figs. 13.9A and B) SMA, gastroduodenal, and IMA. They may be saccular or fusiform and usually have no reverse within them. They may have layers of thrombus on the walls. They present a significant risk to the interventional radiologist as they may be mistaken for simple abscesses. It is prudent to evaluate with Doppler all collections prior to drainage.[15]

Real time identification of pulsation in the aneurysm is helpful in characterizing the vascular nature of mass. Pulsation may be absent or be diminished as a result of perianeurysmal fibrosis. Doppler ultrasound can make a precise diagnosis.[37]

RENAL ARTERIES

The renal arteries originate at or slightly below the origin of the superior mesenteric artery.

The normal right renal artery arises laterally or anterolaterally from the aorta and passes anterior to the right diaphragmatic crux and posterior to the inferior vena cava. The left renal artery arises lateral or posterolateral from aorta. Transverse scanning can usually visualize the renal arteries but coronal scan with the patient in the left lateral decubitus position may help identify the arteries in difficult case. The proximal renal artery waveform has a low pulsatility and a high continuous flow component (indicated by mean height from the zero line) and is dramatically different from that of the adjacent aortic signal. Similar waveforms are seen in the renal sinus the midregion of the kidney and the arcuate vessels at the corticomedullary junction (Figs. 13.10A to E).

Aneurysms

Renal artery aneurysms are rare. True aneurysms are usually secondary to arteriosclerosis, polyarteritis nodosa

The Retroperitoneum and Great Vessels | 125

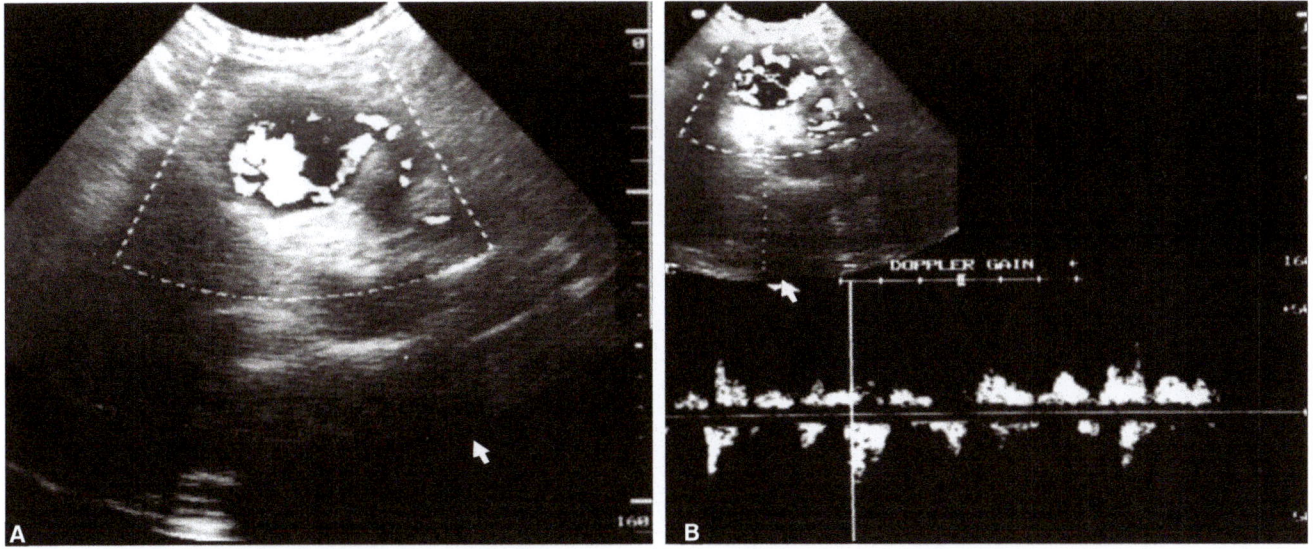

Figs. 13.9A and B: (A) Color and (B) Duplex Doppler images in a case of splenic artery aneurysm.

or fibromuscular dysplasia and false aneurysm are often the result of trauma. Pulsations in the aneurysms may be seen with real time imaging or arterial flow identified in them using Doppler ultrasound.[32]

Arteriovenous Malformations

Renal arteriovenous malformations may be congenital or acquired. Latter occur as a result of trauma, surgery, renal biopsy or neoplasms. Arteriovenous malformations may appear as a cluster of tortuous arteries and veins or more commonly a cystic structure representing either the aneurysmal artery or vein. A dilated renal vein or inferior vena cava above the renal vein suggests the presence of this lesion. Rim calcifications or mural thrombus may also be present and if a major component of the malformation is arterial pulsation may be identified. Doppler analysis may also be utilized.[32]

Stenosis and Occlusion

Doppler techniques have been applied to the renal artery with 83% sensitivity and 97% specificity in diagnosing stenosis greater than 60%.

A threshold velocity of 180 cm/sec of renal arteries is taken as normal with velocities greater than this suggestive of stenosis.

A ratio of peak systolic velocities in the aorta and stenotic renal artery segment of 3.5 of greater indicates 60% chance of RAS.[38]

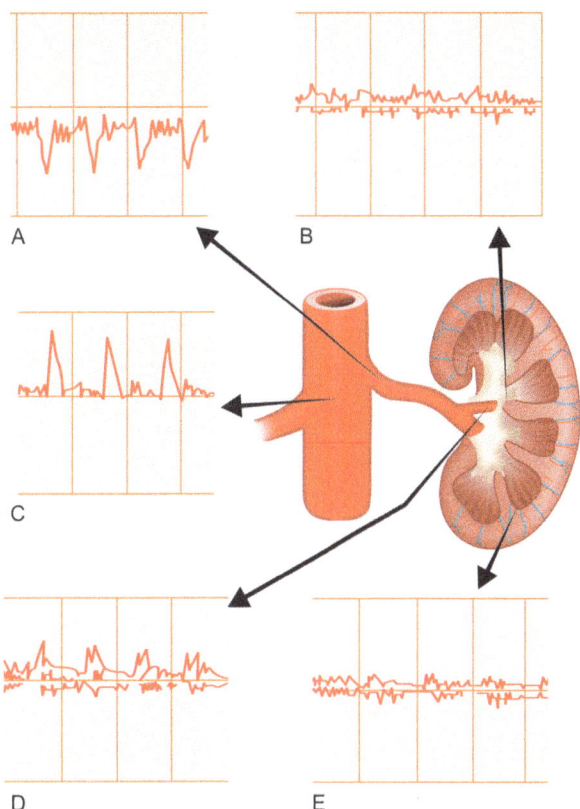

Figs. 13.10A to E: Time velocity spectra in: main renal artery at origin (A); mid zone of kidney (B); midaorta (C); renal sinus (D); arcuate artery (E).

Another technique evaluates spectral Doppler waveform intrarenally. The shape of systolic upstroke is evaluated and the acceleration time and index are calculation. An acceleration index of 3 m/sec^2 or greater is abnormal.[39] Lack of the normal early systolic peak in the renal artery tracing is also highly specific for diagnosing renal artery stenosis.[39]

INFERIOR VENA CAVA

Anatomy

The inferior vena cava is a large vein that returns blood from the lower limbs, pelvis, and abdomen to the right atrium. It is formed by the paired common iliac veins on the anterior surface of the L5 vertebral body and lies anteriorly and slightly to the right of the spine.[26] It traverses the diaphragm and enters the right atrium at the level of eight thoracic vertebra.

Its main branches are the hepatic veins, the renal veins, and the common iliac veins. The walls of inferior vena cava (IVC) are much thinner than those of aorta and the pressure of blood it deals is also much lower.

Sonography

The intrahepatic portion of the IVC is routinely viewed by using the liver as an acoustic window. The remainder of the vessel is inconsistently seen because it is intermittently flat and oval shaped and may be obscured by overlying bowel gas. Common iliac vein and external iliac veins are seen inconsistently with their arteries on the lateral aspect of the pelvic brim. The IVC lumen is anechoic although with slow flowing blood it becomes more echogenic and may show swirling. This is seen with right heart failure, fluid overload, and caudal to an IVC obstruction. The appearance varies with respiration. With deep inspiration, venous return decreases, and IVC dilates. With deep expiration, venous return improves and IVC diameter decreases. By doing a valsalva, venous return is blocked and flow temporarily reversed in the IVC: causing it to bulge. The IVC transmits both cardiac and respiratory pulsations, the transmission is more noticeably sonographically the closer one comes to heart. The classical tracing has a saw tooth pattern (Fig. 13.11). Most distally and in the common iliac veins there is a more phasic pattern similar to the pattern in proximal limbs.[5]

Pathology

The most commonly encountered intraluminal pathology of the IVC is thrombosis which usually spreads from another vein in the pelvis, lower limbs, liver, or kidney. IVC thrombosis is sonographically diagnosed as an intraluminal

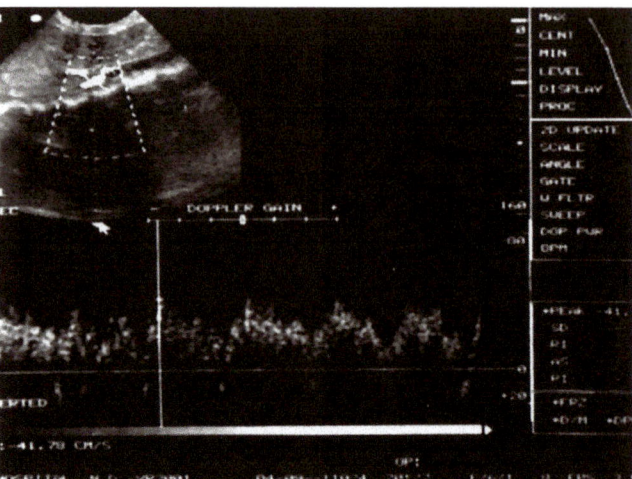

Fig. 13.11: Duplex Doppler of normal IVC showing wide variation in flow velocity and direction owing to effects of cardiac and respiratory cycles.

filling defect that usually expands the diameter of the vessel (Figs. 13.12A and B). The echogenicity of a thrombus depends on its age, chronic thrombi may calcify. If a thrombus is hypoechoic or isoechoic with the liver, color Doppler is very helpful in making the diagnosis as color frequently surrounds the thrombus.[5] Spectral Doppler analysis produces no signal from uncomplicated thrombus. Arterial type tracing may be seen within tumor thrombi. The presence of IVC tumor thrombus is usually diagnosed readily. The kidney is the most likely site of origin.

A variety of vena cava filters are now being used in the IVC to prevent distal venous thrombi from going onto pulmonary embolism. Ultrasound can sometimes see these as echogenic structures within the IVC and can monitor complications such as thrombosis that may occur at their site of insertion.[27] The Kimray Greenfield filter is one of the most common devices and consists of stainless steel wire cage that has a narrow apex with six diverging limb. Its optimal position is above iliac bifurcation but below the level of the renal veins (so as not interfere with blood flow from kidneys). Duplex Doppler demonstrates the patency of the inferior vena cava above and below the filter. Thrombus affecting the filter can be detected by Doppler ultrasound even when it is undetected by real time scanning.[32]

Mural Lesions

Mural based lesions include adherent thrombus and tumors. Primary tumors are rare but of them the leiomyosarcoma is the most common. It most frequently affects females in the fifth and sixth decade of life.[28] Typically this is a low grade

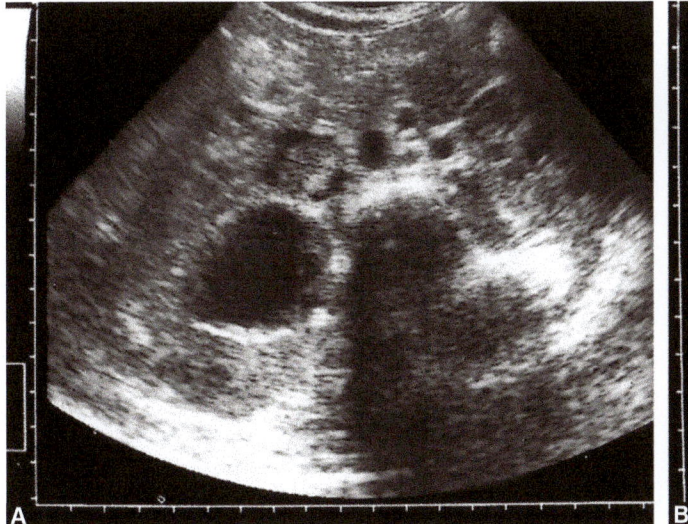 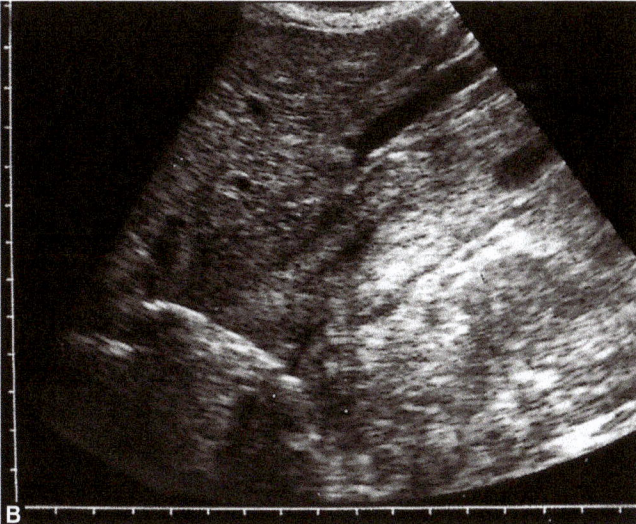

Figs. 13.12A and B: Gray scale image in transverse and longitudinal sections showing an echogenic thrombus obliterating the lumen of inferior vena cava and extending along its entire length.

malignancy with an early, relatively quiescent growth period of at least several months, during which collateral vessels may develop.[28] However, it is nearly always lethal because of its late stage at presentation. Frequent sites of metastases include liver and lung. Moreover, extension into right atrium usually precludes surgical resection.[29]

The typical gray scale ultrasound appearance of this tumor is a soft tissue mass which distends the IVC and may contain scattered foci of cystic necrosis. IVC thrombus may be bland due to extensive deep venous thrombosis or may represent malignant tissue. The diagnosis of a malignant thrombus is greatly aided by the detection of tumor neovascularity with Doppler ultrasound. Such vessels demonstrate opacity of smooth muscle in the intima and media, which causes arteriovenous shunting and low impedance high diastolic flow. Color Doppler demonstrates continually fluctuating color indicating pulsatile arterial flow. The detection of such arterial vascularity distinguishes this from the chief entity in the differential diagnosis, bland thrombus which is avascular.[29]

Although imaging studies may strongly suggest an IVC leiomyosarcoma biopsy is needed for definitive diagnosis.[29]

Metastatic lesions include direct spread from lymphoma, hepatocellular carcinoma, breast and renal cell carcinoma mural IVC lesions can exert mass effect and affect structures like the ureter (retrocaval ureter) or the lesions can spread into IVC branches such as renal hepatic veins.[5]

IVC rupture: Usually follows severe abdominal trauma or surgical or interventional therapy. It frequently results in large retroperitoneal bleed and it is associated with damage to other structures.

IVC BRANCHES AND TRIBUTARIES

Renal Veins

The right renal vein is very short while the left renal vein has a much longer course as it travels between the aorta and the SMA to reach the IVC. Both renal veins (especially the left) frequently collect blood from varies in portal hypertension patients. Circumaortic veins are rare. The left renal vein retroaortic variant which occurs in about 2% of patients is of great importance when contemplating surgery.

Renal vein thrombosis is associated with acute glomerulonephritis, lupus, amyloidosis, sepsis, trauma, and dehydration.[5] Of those who have undergone renal transplants 1% develop this problem. On sonography one may see dilatation of vein proximal to the occlusion. The kidney enlarges and there is decreased echogenicity secondary to edema in the kidney. Doppler study shows no renal vein flow and a high resistive arterial flow pattern.[5]

Hepatic Veins

Hepatic vein Doppler spectral tracings are usually triphasic and pulsatile reflecting transmitted cardiac pulsations. This pattern is abolished in about 20% of cases of cirrhosis and hypertension, and it is exaggerated in right heart failure.[30]

Iliac and Ovarian Veins

The common and external iliac veins with the adjacent arteries are predominantly medial and anterior at the inguinal ligament and they become posterior and lateral to the accompanying vessels close to the IVC. They have a respiratory phasicity and can be compressed by adjacent structures and pathology including lymphoceles, hematoma transplant kidney, abscess and aneurysm.

They collapse with a Valsalva maneuver because of their intra abdominal position but increase in diameter following augmentation by a squeezing of iliac or by elevation.

Ovarian vein thrombosis usually occurs postpartum and is associated with endometritis and surgery. Sonography frequently shows massive enlargement of all part of the ovarian vein often with an echogenic thrombus within it.[31] It usually occurs on the right side. Sonography detection should include evaluation of the expected entry of the vein directly into IVC.

INTRAOPERATIVE APPLICATIONS OF DOPPLER

Doppler ultrasound can be used in abdominal surgery to help assess intestinal viability.

Colonic ischemia may follow aortic reconstruction in 1.5–10% of patients. The ischemia is related to inadequate collateral flow following division of inferior mesenteric artery. After temporarily occluding the inferior mesenteric artery, a Doppler probe is applied to the colon. Marked diminution or loss of the arterial signal identifies those patients who need reimplantation of the inferior mesenteric artery. Doppler ultrasound can also assess colonic viability in colon esophageal bypasses and can delineate the borders of resection in surgery for small bowel ischemia.[40]

Intraoperative detection of abdominal and renal arteriovenous malformations is possible with Doppler.[41] It has also been employed in order to avoid damage to the major arteries of kidney during nephrostomy.

REFERENCES

1. Taylor KJW, Burns PN, Woodeock JP. Blood flow in deep abdominal and pelvic vessels: Ultrasonic pulsed Doppler analysis. Radiol. 1985;15:487-93.
2. Burns PN. Hemodynamics. In: Taylor KJW, Burns PN, Wills PNT (Eds). Clinical Applications of Doppler Ultrasound, 2nd edition. New York: Raven Press, 1995. p.3553.
3. Abu Yousef MM, Wirse JA, Shamma AR. Case report. The to and fro sign. Duplex Doppler evidence of femoral artery pseudoaneurysms. AJR. 1988;150:632-34.
4. Allison DJ. Arteriography. In: Grainger RG, Allison DJ (Eds). Diagnostic Radiology: An Anglo American Textbook of Imaging. Edinburgh: Churchill Livingstone. 1986;1.pp.2014-15.
5. Downey DB. The Retroperitoneum and great vessels. In: Rumack CM, WIlson SR, Charboneau JW (Eds). Diagnostic Ultrasound. Mosby Year Book. 1998;12:455-86.
6. Gooding EAW, Effeney DJ. Static and real time B mode sonography of arterial occlusion. AJR. 1982;139:4949-52.
7. Zwiebel WJ, Fracto D. Basics of abdominal and pelvis Doppler instrumentation, anatomy and vascular Doppler signatures. Semin Ultrasound CT MR. 1992;13:321.
8. Koher TR, Nance DR, Crames MM et al. Duplex scanning for diagnosis of aortoiliac and femoropopliteal disease: A prospective study. Circulation. 1987;76(5):1074-80.
9. Jager KA, Ricketls HJ, Strandness DE. Duplex scanning for the evaluation of lower limb arterial disease. In: Bernstein EF (Ed). Noninvasive Diagnostic Techniques in Vascular Disease. St Louis: The CV Mosby. 1985;10:619.
10. Pasch AR, Ricotta JJ, May AG. Abdominal aortic aneurysm: The case for elective resection. Circulation. 1984;70(Suppl 1):14.
11. Laroy LL, Cormier PJ, Matalon TAS, et al. Imaging of abdominal Aortic Aneurysms. AJR. 1989;152:785-92.
12. Carriero A, Jezzi NM, Filippone A, et al. Magnetic resonance angiography and color Doppler sonography in the evaluation of abdominal aortic aneurysm. Eur Radiol. 1997;7:495-500.
13. Schroeder WB, Holeg SW. The definition assessment of aneurysm by color flow Doppler. J Diagn Med Sonogr. 1991;7:20-109.
14. Giron J, Senae JP, Francois F et al. Place de la TDM Danspevaluation preoperative dis aneurisms de l' aorta abdominals. J Radiol. 1990;71:49-55.
15. Pennel RC, Hollier LH, Lui JT, et al. Clinical and therapeutics evaluation of inflammatory aortic aneurysms: A thirty year review: J Vase Surg. 1995;2:839.
16. Zwiebel WJ. Aortic and iliac aneurysm. Semin Ultrasound CT MRI. 1992;13:53-68.
17. Gooding GAW. Aneurysms of abdominal aorta, iliac and femoral arteries. Sem in Ultrasound. 1982;2:170-79.
18. King PS, Cooperberg PL, Madigan SM. The anechoic crescent in abdominal aortic aneurysms: Not a sign of dissection. AJR. 1986;146:345.
19. Erturk H, Erden A, Yusdakul M. Pseudoaneurysm of Abdominal Aorta diagnosed by color Duplex Doppler. Sonography. J Clin Ultrasound. 1999;27(4):202-05.
20. Bennet DE, Cherry JK. The natural history of traumatic aneurysm of the aorta. Surgery. 1967;61:516.
21. Richard GP, Patrich CA. Pseudoaneurysm of the abdominal aorta. A case report and review of literature. Am J Med Sci. 1991;301:25.
22. Llornte JG, Gallego MG, Arnaize AM. Chronic post traumatic pseudoaneurysm of the abdominal aorta diagnosed by duplex Doppler ultrasonography. Acta Radiol. 1997;38:121.
23. Thompson MM, Boyle JR, HaiIshorn T. Comparison of computed tomography and duplex imaging in assessing aorta morphology following endovascular aneurysm pair. Br J Surg. 1998;85:346-50.
24. May J, White GH, Yu W. A prospective study of changes in morphology and dimension of abdominal aorta aneurysm following endoluminal repair: a preliminary report. J Endov Surg. 1995;2:343-47.

25. Guinet C, Buy JN, Ghossain MA. Aorta anastomotic pseudoaneurysm: US, CT MR and angiography. J Comp Asst Tomography. 1992;26(2):182-88.
26. Gray G. Gray's Anatomy, 3rd edition. London: Longamans Green and Lo. 1954.pp.859-62.
27. McWissen MW, Erichson SJ, Foley WD. Thrombosis at venous insertion sites after inferior vena caval filter placement. Radiol. 1989;12:415-19.
28. Coughlen JH, Andrews S. Growth of a leiomyosarcoma is the inferior vena cava. Can Assoc Radiol J. 1992;43:221-4.
29. Paanghaal SS, Karenek TJ, Waehsberg RH. Inferior vena cava leiomyosarcoma: Diagnosis and biopsy with color Doppler sonography. J Clin Ultras. 1997;25:275-78.
30. Bolondi L, Gaiani S, Semincelli S. Changes in hepatic venous flow in liver disease assessed by Doppler US: Relationship with histology. J Hepatol. 1991;13(Suppl):98.
31. Adkin J, Wilson SR. Unusual course of the gonadal vein a case report of postpartum ovarian vein thrombosis mimicking acute appendicitis clinically and sonographically. JUM. 1996;15:409-12.
32. Needleman L, Rifken MD. Vascular ultrasonography: Abdominal applications. Radiol Clin North Am. 1986;24(3):461-84.
33. Flinn WR, Rizzo RJ, Park JS. Duplex scanning for assessment of mesenteric ischaemia. Surg Clin North Am. 1990;70(1):99-107.
34. Moneta EL, Taylor DC, Helton WS. Duplex ultrasound measurement of postprandial intestinal blood: Effect of meal composition. Gastroenterol. 1988;95:1294-301.
35. Moneta EL, Yeagu RA, Lea RW. Non invasive localization of arterial occlusive disease: A comparison of segmental pressures and arterial duplex mapping. J Vasc Surg. 1993;17:578-82.
36. Sandager E, Flinnn WR, McCarthy WJ et al. Assessment of visceral arterial reconstruction using duplex scan. J Vasc Technol. 1987;11:13-16.
37. Derchi LE, Biggi E, Cici GR. Aneurysms of the splenic artery non invasive diagnosis by pulsed Doppler sonography. J Ultrasound Med. 1984;3:41-44.
38. Olin JW, Piemonte MR, Young JR. The utility of duplex ultrasound scanning of diagnosing significant renal artery stenosis. Ann Intern Med. 1995;122:833-38.
39. Starros AT, Parker SH, Yakes WF. Segmental stenosis of the renal artery. Pattern recognition of tardus and parvus abnormality with duplex sonography. Radiol. 1992;184:487-92.
40. Hobson RW, Wright GB, O'Donnell JA: Determination of intestinal viability. Arch Surg. 1979;114:165-68.
41. Boyce WH. Ultrasonic velocimetry in resection of renal arteriovenous fistula and other intrarenal surgical procedures. J Urol. 1981;125:610-11.

Current Role of High Resolution Ultrasonography and Color Doppler in the Diagnosis of Scrotal Diseases

Advent of high resolution ultrasonography and high sensitivity of color Doppler imaging of scrotum has widened the diagnostic spectrum. Ultrasound probes using frequencies ranging from 7.5-10 MHz coupled with color Doppler equipment capable of picking up slow flows are essential modalities currently used for adequate diagnostic imaging of scrotal pathologies. Scrotal ultrasonography augments clinical examination and when interpreted with appropriate clinical background provides definitive diagnosis and prompt management often limiting the need for surgical intervention. The indications are:

- Palpable scrotal mass
  - Hydrocele, epididymal cyst, inguinal hernia, and varicocele
- Pain
  - Infection, torsion, and trauma
- Infertility
  - Hypogonadism, varicocele
- Cryptorchidism
  - Undescended testis
- Follow-up
  - Patients with previous disease, retroperitoneal mass, and undescended testis
- Search for unknown primary.

NORMAL ULTRASOUND ANATOMY

Scrotal wall: Its thickness ranges from 27 mm and is formed by various tissue layers, which cannot be separately imaged with present resolution of equipment.

Testes: They have ovoid shape, smooth contour and medium echogenicity. It measures 35 cm in length and 23 cm in transverse diameter. It consists of numerous convoluted tubules, split into various lobules by fibrous septa that radiate from mediastinum to the periphery.

Mediastinum testis: This seen as linear echogenic density in the posterior aspect of the testis and the site of attachment to the epididymis. Arteries and veins enter through this site.

Tunica vaginalis: It is a fibrous capsule of testis not visualized on imaging separate from the testis. It invaginates into the testis in the mediastinal area. It has the visceral and parietal layers with potential space that is filled with minimal fluid.

Epididymis: It is located posterolaterally to the testis. The triangular upper portionhead is larger than the rest and measures 8-12 mm and isoechoic with the testis. Body and tail are usually not well differentiated on ultrasound.

Vascular anatomy (Figs. 14.1 to 14.3): It can be easily studied with color Doppler mode. The arterial supply consists of peripheral capsular arteries, centripetal arteries and transmediastinal arteries.

Spectral waveforms of testicular flow typically show prominent diastolic component. Normal low flow in the testis is readily demonstrated on color Doppler study and it is also possible to diagnose hypo or hypervascular states in various disease processes.

Technique

It is generally helpful to explain the procedure to the patient and reassure them about the safety and simplicity of the procedure. Examination in a quiet dark room with minimal disturbance and in children, warm room temperature to avoid cremasteric reflex is extremely useful to derive utmost cooperation and diagnostic information. Patient is placed in supine position with thighs slightly separated and a towel placed under the scrotum to lift and support the contents. Examination in the erect position of the patient is preferred for diagnosis of varicocele and reducible hernia. Sedation is

Current Role of High Resolution Ultrasonography and Color Doppler in the Diagnosis of Scrotal Diseases | 131

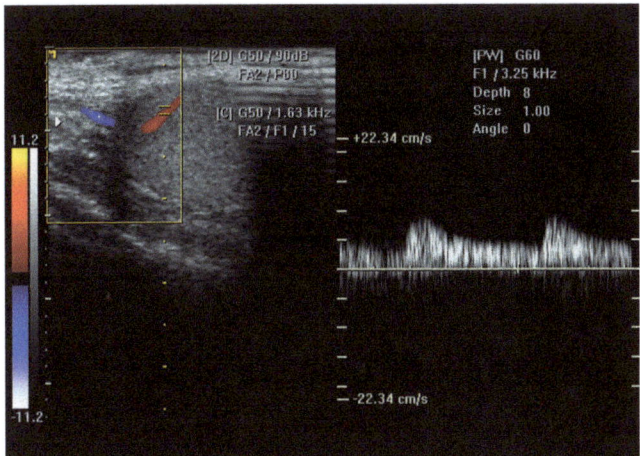

Fig. 14.1: Duplex Doppler shows low velocity and low resistance flow in the intratesticular artery.

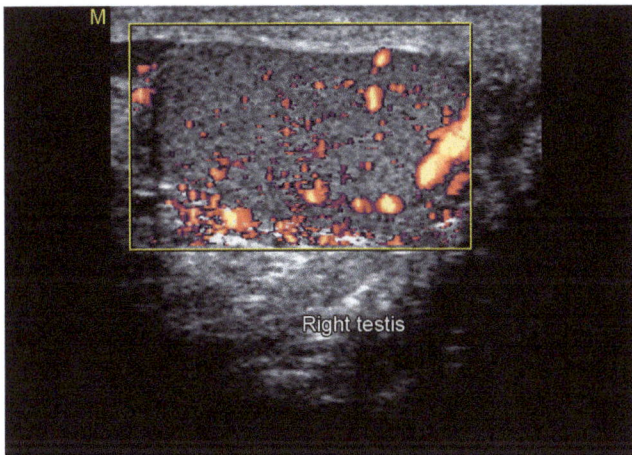

Fig. 14.2: Power Doppler shows normal testicular vascularity.

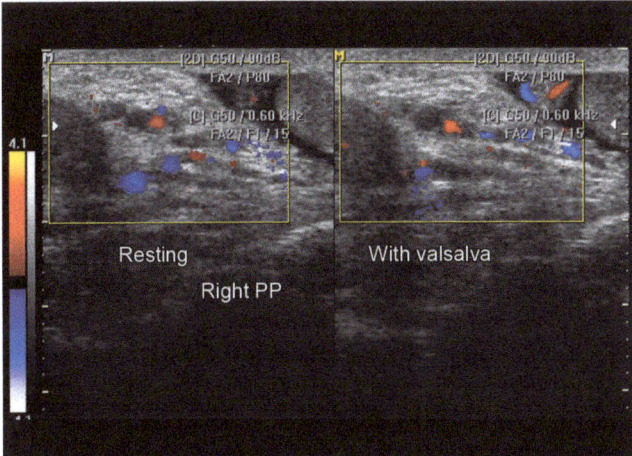

Fig. 14.3: Color Doppler shows normal pampiniform plexus in resting state and with valsalva maneuver.

seldom necessary in infants and young children if they are starved for an hour or two and feed is given during the examination while they rest in their mother's lap. High resolution linear probes in the range 7.5-10 MHz frequency should be used. It is recommended that color Duplex Doppler equipment be set to lowest possible PRF and wall filters to pickup low flows. Simultaneous visualization of both testicles for comparing the vascularity is extremely useful when one of the testis is normal.

TESTICULAR TORSION

Testicular torsion is a result of excessive mobility of testis. Most torsion is seen at puberty (intravaginal) with a peak during neonatal period (extravaginal at the cord) and is usually bilateral requiring bilateral orchiopexy.

Ultrasonography findings vary depending on the time elapsed between the onset of episode and the time of examination.

Acute phase (within 6 hours)
- Normal findings
- Scrotal wall thickening
- Small hematocele
- Enlarged hypoechoic testis and epididymis.

Early subacute phase (1-4 days)
- Acute findings are more obvious
- Echofree area of liquefactive necrosis
- Hypoechoic mass of hemorrhage.

Late subacute phase (5-10 days)
- Progressive decrease of early subacute phase findings.

Chronic phase (over 10 days)
- Normalisation of findings
- Testis small and echopoor
- Persistent epididymal enlargement and increased echogenicity.
  Color Doppler Findings

Acute phase (Fig. 14.4)
- Diminished or absent flow to the testis
- Normal peritesticular flow.

Late phase (3-8 days) (Figs. 14.5 and 14.6)
- Persistence of decreased flow to testis
- Increased peritesticular flow.

Although much has been written about the usefulness of color Doppler to detect torsion of testis, recent studies indicate that surgery need not be delayed by an ultrasound study if high degree of clinical suspicion persists. Color Doppler imaging is rendered less useful in following conditions:

1. Prepubertal testis which normally have low flow
2. Ectopic testis

3. Torsion detorsion state previously torsed testis is now reperfused and color flow may be normal or hypervascular
4. Severe epididymo-orchitis causing secondary ischemia. The recently reported most reliable sign is a "snail shell curl" of the epididymis and not the color flow abnormalities.

KEY POINTS

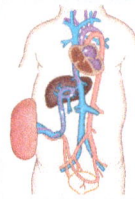

- Testicular vessels show low flow with prominent diastolic component.
- In testicular torsion, there is decreased or absent flow to testis with normal or increased peritesticular flow.
- Most reliable sign for testicular torsion is 'snail shell curl' of epididymis.
- Enlargement of epididymis and testis with increased vascularity is seen in acute inflammation.
- Epididymo-orchitis may mask underlying tumor.

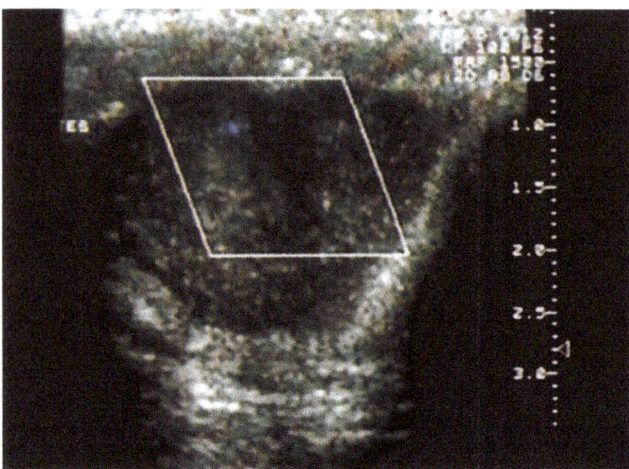

Fig. 14.4: Torsion of testis—Complete absence of color flow in the testis (lowest velocity settings used for Doppler study).

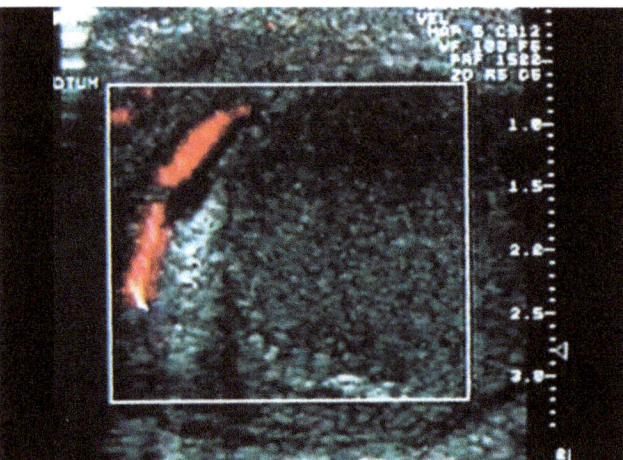

Fig. 14.5: Late phase of testicular torsion—No flow is seen in the testis. Peritesticular flow is present.

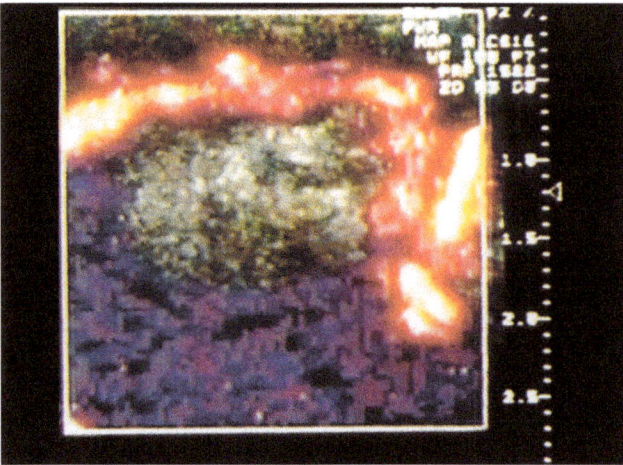

Fig. 14.6: Power Doppler highlights exuberant peritesticular flow and absence of flow in the testis.

INFLAMMATORY DISEASES

Acute inflammation: Most frequent cause of acute scrotum in adults is inflammation, particularly epididymitis in about 75% of cases. It is detected in about 44% cases by color Doppler. Isolated orchitis is commonly seen in viral disease like mumps. This condition exhibits clinical manifestations closely resembling those in acute testicular torsion and need to be differentiated clearly to select the correct management options.

Ultrasound findings (Figs. 14.7 to 14.9)
- Enlargement of epididymis and testis
- Focal or diffuse hypoechogenicity
- Scrotal wall thickening
- Fluid in tunica vaginalis
- Increased vascularity on Color Doppler.

An excellent general rule is that in acute painful enlargement of the scrotum, greater enlargement of epididymis and fewer changes in the testis, usually with increased free fluid, points to infective process viz. epididymitis or epididymo-orchitis.

Testicular tumors may be masked by a presenting epididymo-orchitis and hence, it is important to rescan patient after the therapy to detect the tumor.

Chronic inflammation: More frequently seen in underdeveloped countries and evolve with mild symptoms. This might result from inadequate treatment of an acute inflammation or from specific infection caused by *Mycobacterium tuberculosis* or *Treponema pallidum,* etc. Genitourinary tuberculosis is one of the most commonly encountered extrapulmonary sites of infections in our

country. Ultrasound features are not specific and the gamut of findings may overlap with those found in acute inflammation. The ultrasound features are (Figs. 14.10 and 14.11):
- Thickening and increased echogenicity of epididymis
- Confluent anechoic areas representing necrosis in testis
- Complex mass of epididymis-testicular complex
- Organized hydrocele
- Testicular calcification
- Scrotal wall calcification
- Color Doppler may reveal hypervascularity in the scrotal wall.

SCROTAL TRAUMA

Ultrasonography plays a profound role in defining the extent of injury in cases of blunt trauma. Early diagnosis

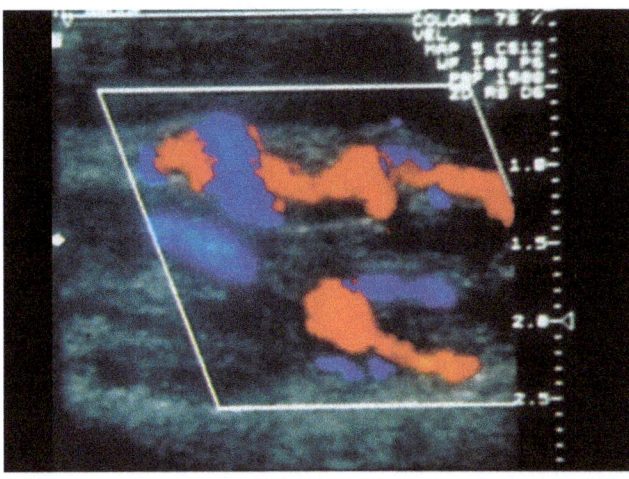

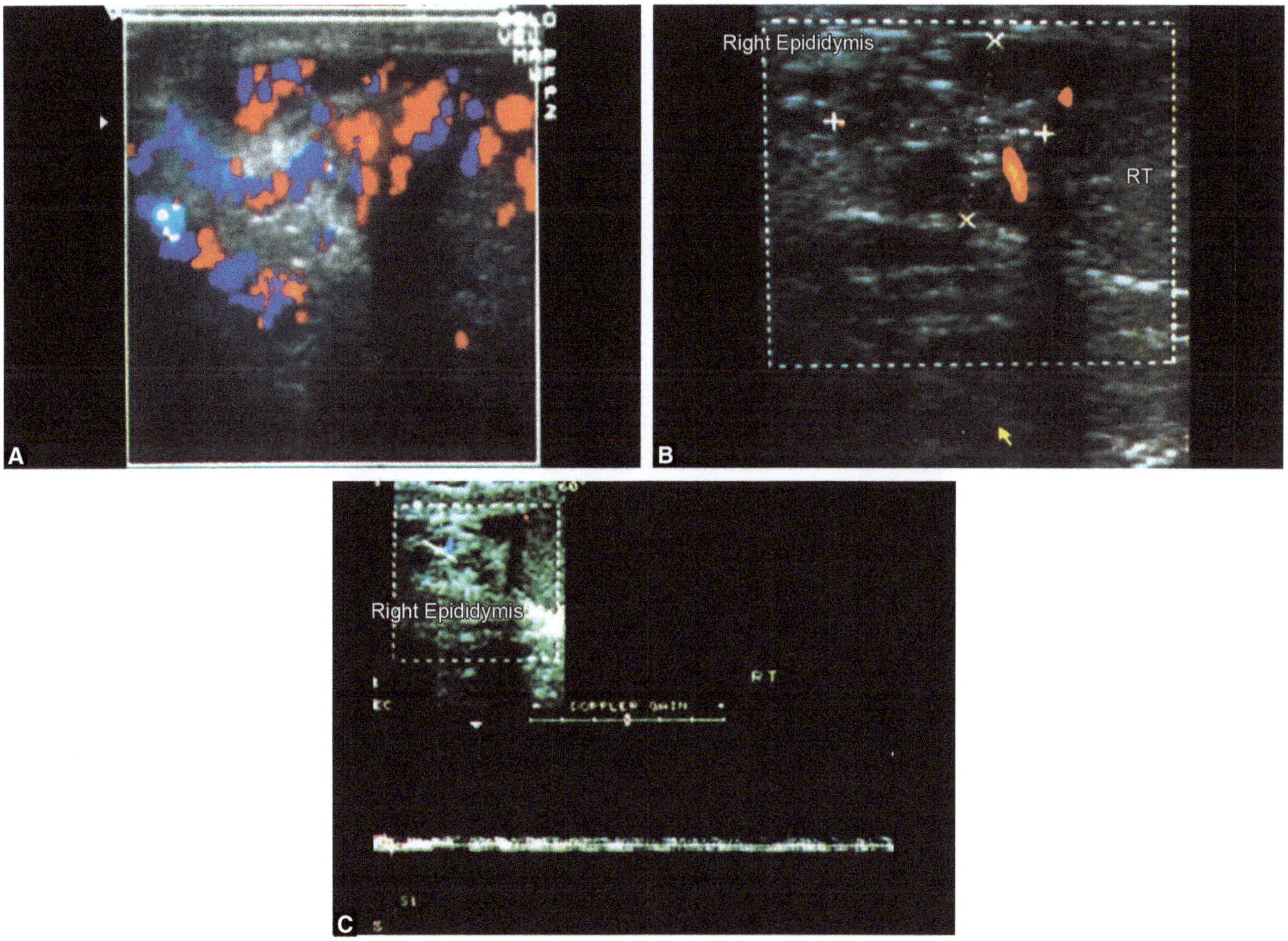

Fig. 14.7: Funiculitis-hypervascularity along the spermatic cord (postoperative infection).

Figs. 14.8A to C: (A) Acute epididymitis-Increased color flow in epididymis; (B) Color Doppler scan in another patient shows enlarged hypoechoic right epididymis with hypoechoic testis; (C) Velocity waveform from vein confirms venous flow in epididymis in this patient.

134 | Textbook of Color Doppler Imaging

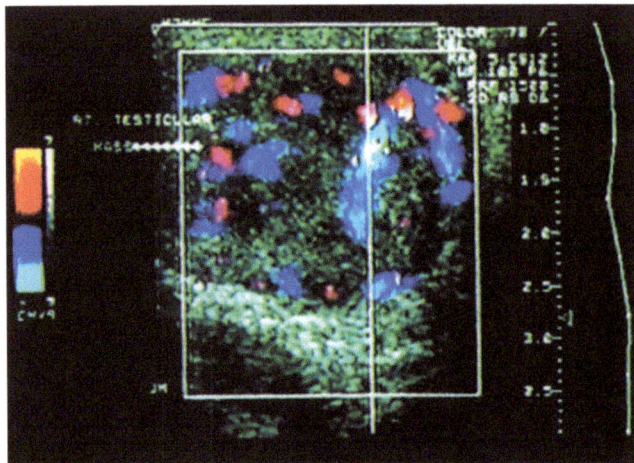

Fig. 14.9: Acute orchitis-increased color flow in the testis.

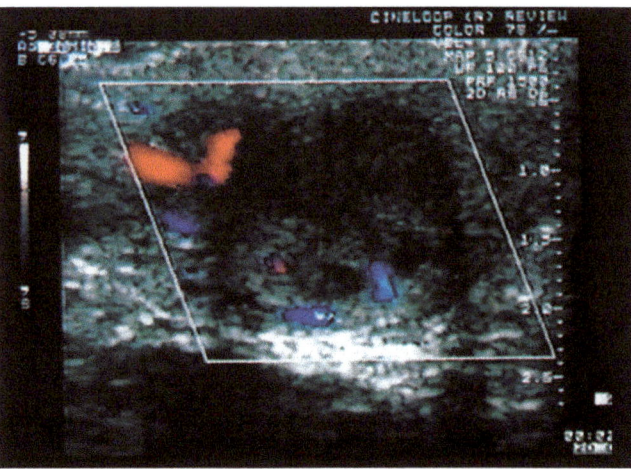

Fig. 14.10: Chronic epididymo-orchitis (Tuberculous).

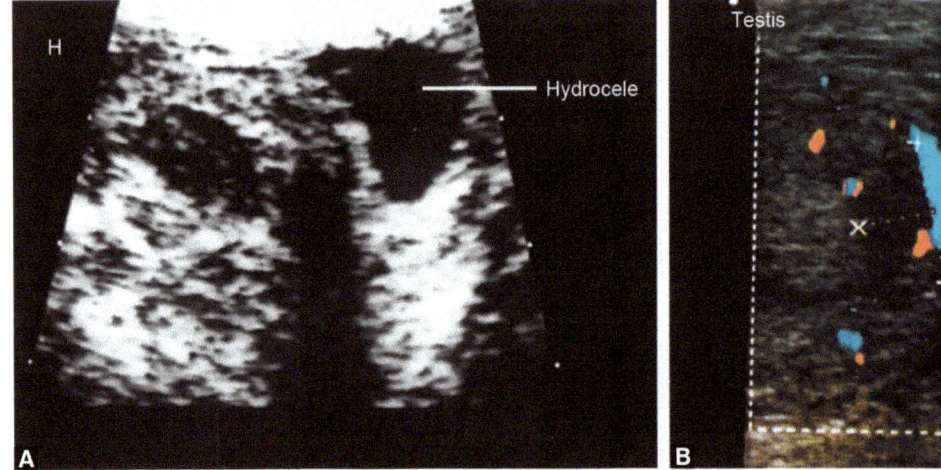

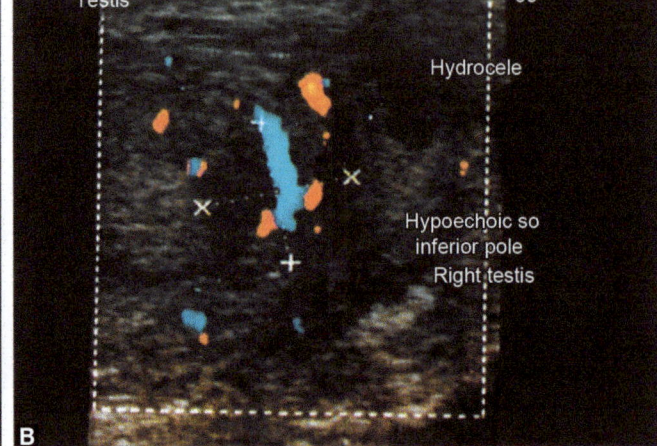

Figs. 14.11A and B: (A) Epididymo-orchitis with testicular abscess: Gray scale image in transverse plane shows enlarged testis within homogeneous texture and a hypoechoic mass at the inferior pole (abscess) associated with hydrocele; (B) Epididymo-orchitis with testicular abscess: Color Doppler image in same patient shows generalized increased vascularity in testis.

and surgical intervention within 72 hours after the injury significantly increases the salvage rate and prevents ischemic atrophy of the testis. Diagnosis of rupture, torsion and dislocation of testis are indicative of surgical exploration. About 50% of traumatic hematoceles are associated with rupture.

Ultrasonography findings are:
- Hematocele-echogenic or echopoor
- Testicular rupture presents as discontinuity in the normal smooth contour of the testis indicating break in the tunica albuginea
- Intratesticular hematoma may be echogenic or echo poor and may mimic tumors hence follow-up is recommended to avoid missing an undiagnosed tumor with superimposed hemorrhage secondary to trauma.

HYDROCELE

Hydrocele is the most common cause of scrotal swelling and is caused by collection of fluid in tunica vaginalis. It may be idiopathic or associated with trauma, infection, torsion, tumor, and infarction or due to obstructed lymphatic. Ultrasound reveals fluid surrounding the testis located posteriorly. Ultrasonography findings are (Figs. 14.12 to 14.14):

- Echo-free area representing clear fluid
- Echogenic debris in the fluid suggests presence of blood, pus, protein or cholesterol
- Septations
- Scrotal calculi

Current Role of High Resolution Ultrasonography and Color Doppler in the Diagnosis of Scrotal Diseases

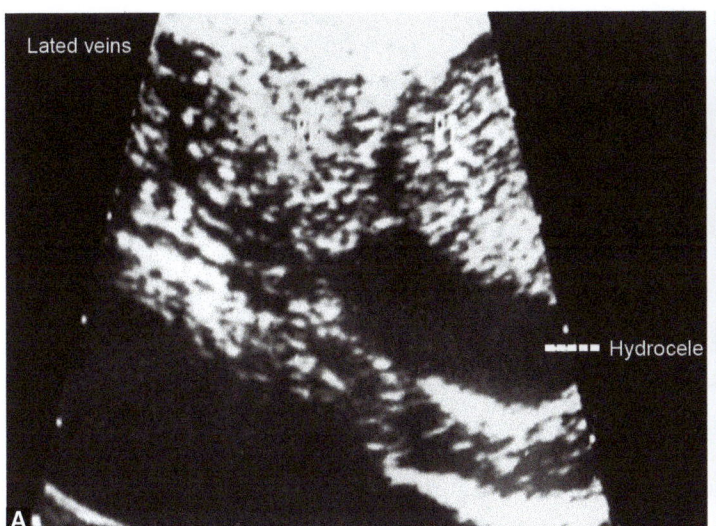
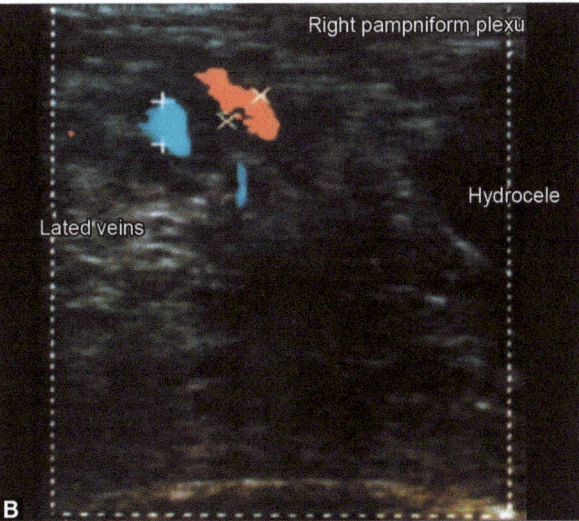

Figs. 14.12A and B: (A) Gray scale image in longitudinal plane shows echo free area adjacent to right testis in a case of hydrocele. Dilated veins are also seen superior to the epididymis, suggestive of associated varicocele; (B) Color Doppler flow image shows evidence of color flow in dilated veins.

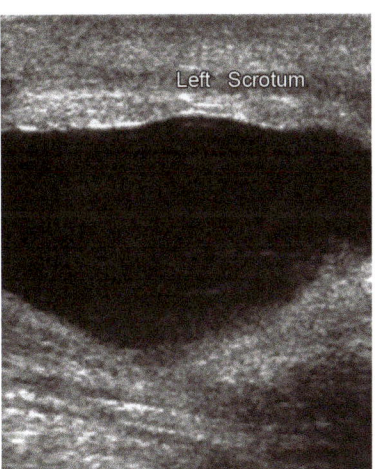

Fig. 14.13: Gray scale image shows a large hydrocele.

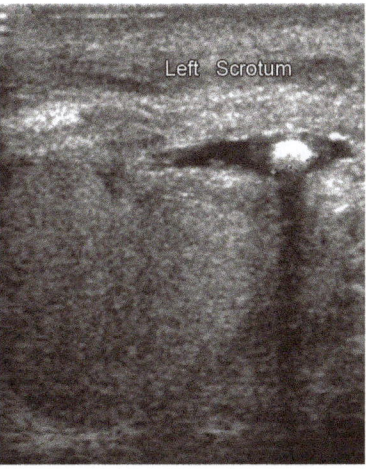

Fig. 14.14: Gray scale image shows scrotal calculus.

KEY POINTS

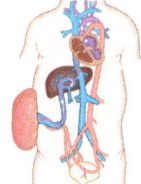

- Intratesticular hematoma may mimic a tumor.
- Undescended testis is usually located in superficial soft tissue or inguinal canal.
- In varicocele, veins are >2 mm in diameter with retrograde flow in internal spermatic veins.
- Majority of testicular tumors arise from germ cells.
- Testicular tumors have variable echogenecity and may show flow in the periphery of the lesion.

UNDESCENDED TESTIS

Undescended testis (Fig. 14.15) is the most common congenital abnormality found in about 1% of boys and men and it occurs due to pathological impairment of hypothalamo pituitary gonadal axis. The incidence of malignancies encountered in this testis is up to 45–48 times higher than the general population and are also more prone to rupture, torsion, and infertility. If repaired before 5 years of age, the risk for malignancy drops significantly. Fortunately, most of the undescended testis are located in superficial soft tissue or inguinal canal and are readily detected in about 97% of cases. The search usually begins from the scrotum upwards. The undescended testis is a small oval structures,

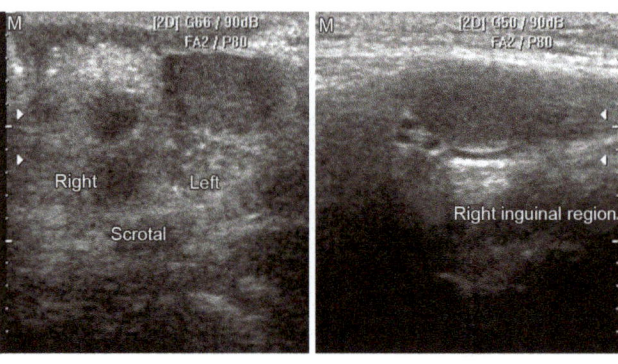

Fig. 14.15: Gray scale images show empty right scrotal sac and testis in right inguinal region s/o undescended testis.

may be slightly hypoechoic or isoechoic to the parenchyma of normal testis. The undescended testis cannot be imaged if located in the abdominal cavity. Confusion with an enlarged lymph node in the inguinal region may be avoided by noting following points:
- Enlarged inguinal nodes are uncommon in the age group
- Hilum of the lymph node is prominently echogenic as compared to faintly echoic mediastinum testis
- Enlarged node is hypervascular as compared to virtual vascular undescended testis
- Lymph nodes are fairly fixed in position as compared to mobile undescended testis.

SCROTAL CALCIFICATIONS

Isolated testicular calcifications are of no clinical significance and usually presents as spermatic granuloma, phleboliths or 'burned -out' tumors. It is seen in atrophic testis as evenly distributed, diffuse small calcifications. Irregular calcifications are seen in teratoma and embryonal cell carcinoma, chronic tuberculosis and as sequel to old trauma. Microlithiasis is seen in cryptorchidism, infertility, postorchiopexy, Klinefelter's syndrome and male pseudohermaphroditism and is considered benign but possible premalignant condition. Extratesticular calcifications are mainly benign in nature.

VARICOCELE

Varicocele is the most common correctable cause of male infertility. Ultrasonography and color Doppler play an important role in the diagnosis, particularly in subclinical cases (10%). The veins of the pampiniform plexus are dilated to exceed 2 mm in diameter. The veins are characterized by retrograde flow in the internal spermatic vein. The examination performed in standing posture and during valsalva the veins often dilate to 3 mm and more (Figs. 14.16 and 14.17).

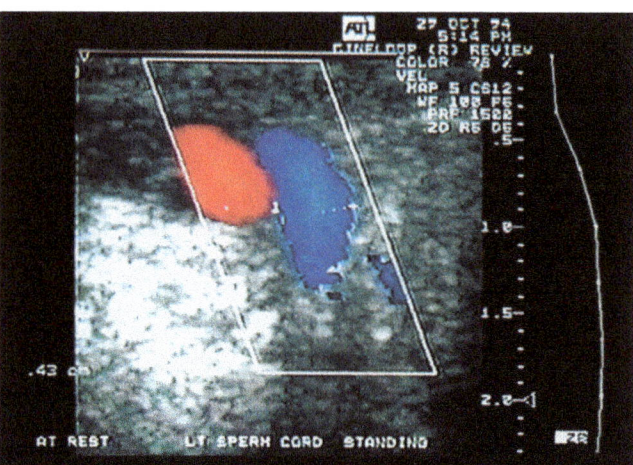

Fig. 14.16: Longitudinal color Doppler image of the left spermatic cord demonstrating dilated vascular channels suggestive of varicocele.

SCROTAL HERNIAS

Scrotal hernias are common paratesticular masses. Clinical history and physical examination are primary basis of diagnosis, however, sonography helps in atypical cases. The contents of the hernia sac may be small bowel, colon, and omentum. Presence of peristalsis and bowel mucosal pattern helps in distinguishing the nature of the contents. Highly echoic content within scrotal sac may be due to presence of omentum or fatty tissue. Sonography of the inguinal canal can establish the extension of the bowel/omentum from the scrotal sac. In the absence of peristalsis and signature bowel mucosal pattern, differentiation from other extra testicular masses may be difficult. Often a strangulated inguinoscrotal hernia may present as an "acute scrotum".

TESTICULAR TUMORS

Most neoplasms of testis are malignant and commonly present as a mass. The peak incidence occurs between the age group 25-35 years and majority of them arises from germ cells. There is a wide spectrum of ultrasonographic features ranging from hypoechoic, isoechoic, hyperechoic, and even complex echoic. Color Doppler sonography may reveal flow in the periphery of the mass lesion. Focal orchitis may mimic neoplasm and hence the importance of follow-up studies.

Seminoma is the most common occurring germ cell tumor (40-50%) which is radiosensitive with excellent prognosis. The only exception being an anaplastic seminoma which carries poorer prognosis. It shows

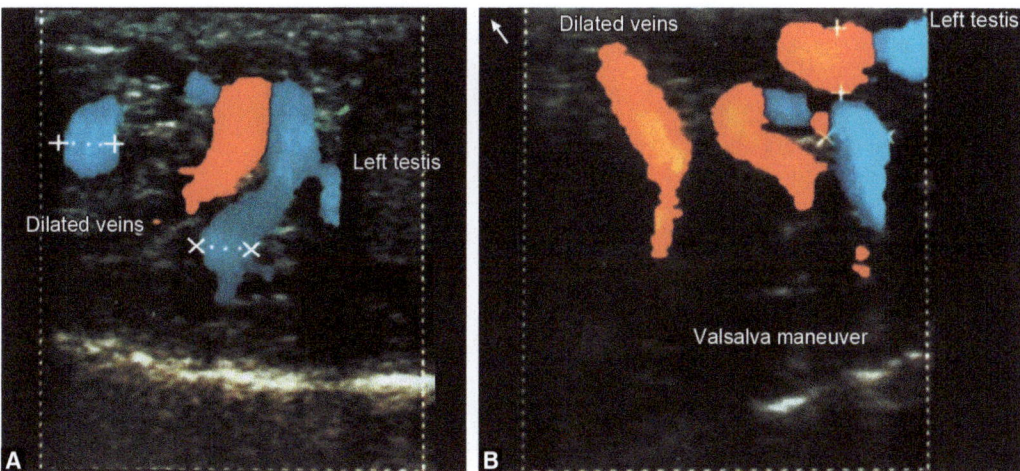

Figs. 14.17A and B: (A) Color Doppler in another patient shows dilated veins in standing position; (B) Color Doppler in another patient shows dilated veins during Valsalva maneuver.

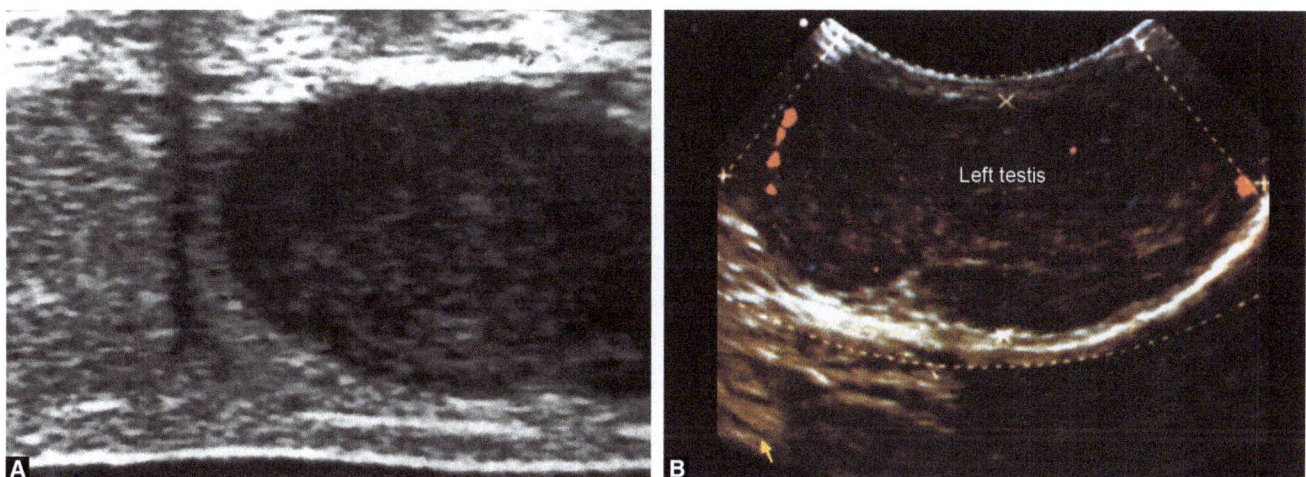

Figs. 14.18A and B: (A) Seminoma: gray scale image shows enlarged testis with uniform hypoechoic echotexture; (B) Seminoma: color Doppler image shows increased vascularity at the periphery of the lesion.

hypoechoic uniform echotexture with poor margins (Figs. 14.18A and B).

Embryonal cell carcinoma: It is the next common tumor (20–25%). It is aggressive causing early invasion of surrounding tissues, hemorrhage and cystic degeneration. The ultrasound shows a large tumor with distortion of testicular configuration and cystic-echoic areas. It carries poor prognosis.

Teratomas: They are less common (5–10%). In adults they are usually benign but in children they are also found to be malignant. Usually small, 2 mm size tumors composed of germ cell layers and may show calcifications, cyst, mixed echogenicity and whirled appearance (Figs. 14.19A and B).

Early preoperative diagnosis can often salvage the unaffected part of the testis (partial orchiectomy).

Teratocarcinoma: It is a combination of teratoma and embryonal cell carcinoma, which is the most frequent tumor after seminoma.

The other tumors occurring are yolk sac carcinoma, choriocarcinoma and 'burned-out' tumor. The nongerm cell tumors are Leydig cell and Sertoli cell type tumors.

Secondary tumors comprising of 5% of tumors are lymphoproliferative diseases, acute and chronic leukemia and non-Hodgkin's lymphoma. The ultrasound pattern is of diffusely hypoechoic, ill-defined lesion with normal or larger testis.

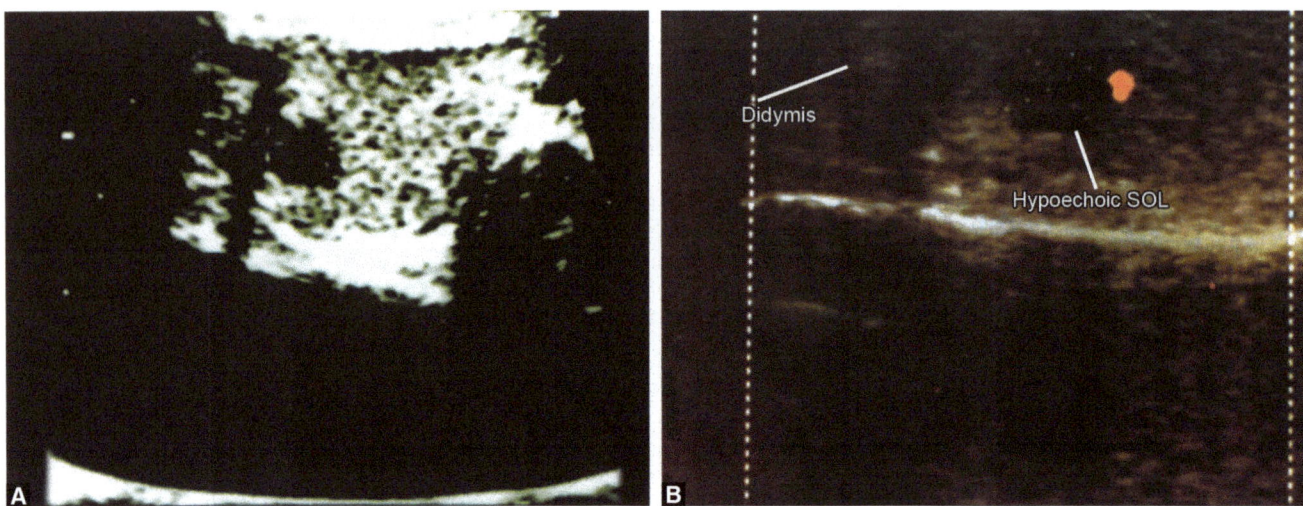

Figs. 14.19A and B: (A) Gray scale image in a patient with teratoma shows: hypoechoic mass with ill-defined margins at superior pole of left testis; (B) Gray scale image in a patient with teratoma shows: peripheral vascularity as evident on color Doppler image.

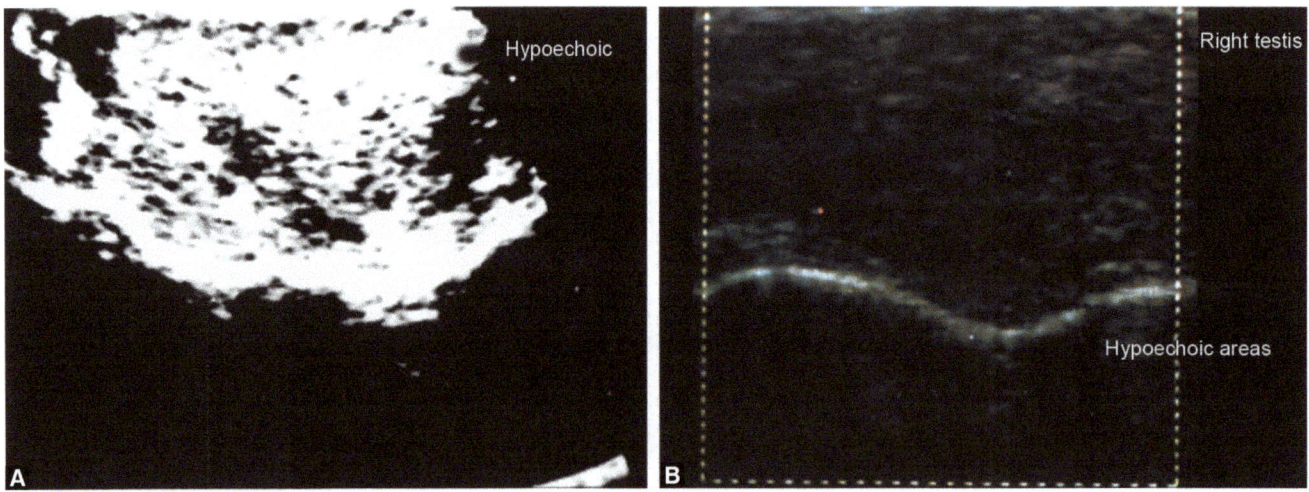

Figs. 14.20A and B: (A) Findings in a 62-year-old man with senile testicular atrophy: gray scale image reveals multiple hypoechoic areas within the testis; (B) Findings in a 62-year-old man with senile testicular atrophy: color Doppler flow image shows avascular nature of hypoechoic areas.

Secondary non-lymphoproliferative diseases are metastasis arising from primary tumors in kidney, prostate, stomach, melanoma, Wilms' tumor, neuroblastoma, histiocytosis, retinoblastoma and rhabdomyosarcoma. Ultrasound may show multiple lesions of variable echogenicity, usually hypoechoic.

The majority of extratesticular tumors are benign and originates from the spermatic cord. Lipomas are the most frequent benign while sarcomas are the most frequent malignant tumors seen.

Senile Atrophy of Testis

Age-related atrophy is evident ultrasonographically by multiple hypoechoic areas within the testis. On color Doppler imaging, hypoechoic areas appear avascular (Figs. 14.20A and B).

Duplex Ultrasonography of Erectile Dysfunction

Erectile dysfunction (ED) or impotence is defined as an inability to achieve rigidity of the penis, which is sufficient for penetration. It is broadly classified into two categories—organic and psychogenic. Vasculogenic impotence is the most common cause of organic impotence. Many patients with erectile dysfunction have combination of both organic and psychogenic components. Therefore, the term vasculogenic ED does not rule out the presence of underlying psychological factors. It merely means that vascular factors are predominant cause of ED. Vascular ED has two different possible mechanisms—obstruction in penile inflow tract, termed as arterial ED and the inability to trap the incoming blood at sufficient pressure in the cavernosa, termed as veno-occlusive ED.

ANATOMY AND PHYSIOLOGY OF PENILE ERECTION

Paired internal pudendal arteries give rise to common penile arteries on both sides. These divide into four arteries, one each to spongiosa, cavernosa, proximal urethra, and dorsum of the penis (deep dorsal artery). The cavernosal artery provides blood to cavernosa via multiple helicine arteries that open directly into the cavernosal sinusoids. Venules located within the subintimal space between the periphery of erectile tissue and the tunica albuginea provides venous outflow channel from corpora cavernosa via peripheral lacunae.

Penile erection is a neurovascular phenomena in which the neurological stimulus via parasympathetic nerves from sacral[2-4] leads to smooth muscle relaxation in helicine arteries leading to vasodilatation. There is also relaxation of trabecular smooth muscle relaxation in cavernosa, which coupled with increased blood flow leads to increase in size and length of the penis causing tumescence. In the next phase, subtunicalvenules are compressed against tunica albuginea due to dilatation of sinusoids and increase in intracavernosal pressure, leading to erectile response. If this veno-occlusive mechanism is competent, the arterial inflow leads to increase in intracavernosal pressure to the level of mean arterial pressure. Perineal muscles contractions generate to further increase in pressure and erectile response leads to the rigidity.

EVALUATION OF ERECTILE DYSFUNCTION

Various tests available for evaluation of vascular ED includes papaverine induced penile erection (PIPE) test, pharmacopenile Duplex ultrasonography (PPDU), cavernosometry with cavernosography, penile angiography and radionuclide imaging. PPDU is sufficient for majority of patients, other more invasive tests are reserved for patients actually considered for surgical treatment.

Traditionally, evaluation of ED begins with PIPE test in which the erectile response of the penis is studied after intracavernosal injection of papaverine or some other vasoactive agent. Normal erectile response is suggestive of normal vascular status and hence neurological or psychological factors are considered as a predominant cause. If only partial or short-lived erection is resulted, then the vascular ED is presumed.

Pharmacopenile Duplex Ultrasonography (PPDU)

The PPDU is fast becoming the first line investigation to define vascular ED and to differentiate between arterial insufficiency and incompetent veno-occlusive mechanism.

The different vasoactive agents used for PPDU are papaverine, prostaglandin (PGE_1) and combination of papaverine and phentolamine. Papaverine may lead to false negative erectile response in some patients or may lead to persistent painful erection (priapism) in others. Prostaglandin (PGE_1) has better erection rate and lesser incidence of priapism.[1] Genital self-stimulation, visual erotic stimulation or application of light tourniquet at penoscrotal junction may augment the erectile response to these agents.

TECHNIQUE

The examination must be carried out in an atmosphere of privacy. Anxiety and resultant sympathetic stimulation may interfere with the response to pharmacological stimulus, hence every effort should be made to relax the patient during the procedure. A rubber band is preferably placed at the root of the penis. The sonographic evaluation begins with scanning of the flaccid penis in transverse plane to measure the diameter of the cavernosal arteries. Then, under aseptic precautions, intracavernosal injection of 60 mg of papaverine is made with 26/27 G needle in either of the cavernosa. Injection on the contralateral side is not required as cross communications exist between both sides. Care must be taken not to inject in subcutaneous tissue, vessels or urethra. Erectile response is graded visually from E_0 to E_5 as described by Broderick.[2] E_0 refers to no response, E_1 to partial elongation of the shaft only, E_2 to moderate tumescence without any rigidity. E_3 erection achieves full tumescence but there is no rigidity and the penis is easily bendable. E_4 and E_5 grades show full erection with partial rigidity or full rigidity for at least 20 minutes respectively. After evaluating the erectile response, scanning is started from root of the penis to the distal part; both in transverse and longitudinal plane. Dorsal scanning in longitudinal plane is necessary to identify penile deformities and cavernosal collaterals. Post-injection diameters of both cavernosal arteries are measured in transverse plane. Angle corrected flow velocities are measured in cavernosal arteries as proximal as possible (Fig. 15.1). Initial flow velocities are taken five minutes after the injection. The measurements are repeated after short intervals till peak rigidity. Most accurate flowmetry values coincide with peak rigidity of the penis. If no rigidity is achieved initially, the flowmetry may be obtained at least till 15 minutes before termination of the examination, as some individuals may reach to that stage after some time.

Post-papaverine injection normal spectral waveform cavernosal artery normally has five reproducible phases[3] (Fig. 15.2). In phase 1, there is increase in both systolic and diastolic velocities. In phase 2, there is progressive

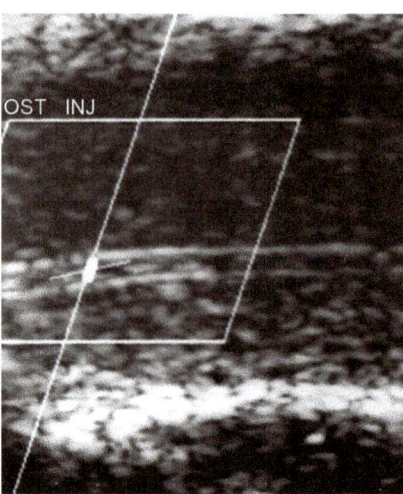

Fig. 15.1: PPDU examination shows technique for placement of sample volume in the cavernosal artery with angle correction.

decrease in end diastolic velocity and appearance of the dicrotic notch. Patients with severe venous leakage do not progress beyond phase 2. In phase 3, diastolic flow approximates zero and it is reversed in phase 4. Phase 5 is characterized by eventual loss of both systolic and diastolic flow signals. Various parameters and their accepted normal values studied on flowmetry are maximum recorded peak systolic velocity (PSV) of 30 cm/second or more, minimum end diastolic velocity (EDV) of 5 cm/second or less (zero or reversed diastolic flow included as normal), acceleration time (AT) of 0.11 second or less, and resistive index (RI) of 0.85 or more. Mild variations are seen in cut off values as described in various reported studies.

The studies that have been published regarding the normal Doppler flowmetry values have been on small number of healthy volunteers.[3,4] There has been no such study on Indian patients. At our institution, we could not conduct our study on normal healthy volunteers because of invasive nature of the procedure and feasibility and ethical considerations. Therefore, it was decided to study patients with psychogenic impotence with a normal erection elicited on pharmacological stimulus test since these patients can be presumed to have a normal vascular status.[5,6]

In our study comprising 30 men, the mean age was 24.8 years. This is significantly less than the mean age of patients in the earlier studies by Valji et al. and Quam et al. who reported the mean age of 51 and 56 years respectively in their studies.[7,8] This lower mean age of patients in our population is difficult to explain but probably it is related to observation of our clinical psychologist that elderly men are usually hesitant to seek medical advice for their sexual problems (personal communication). They also have a tendency to regard it as part of aging rather than a

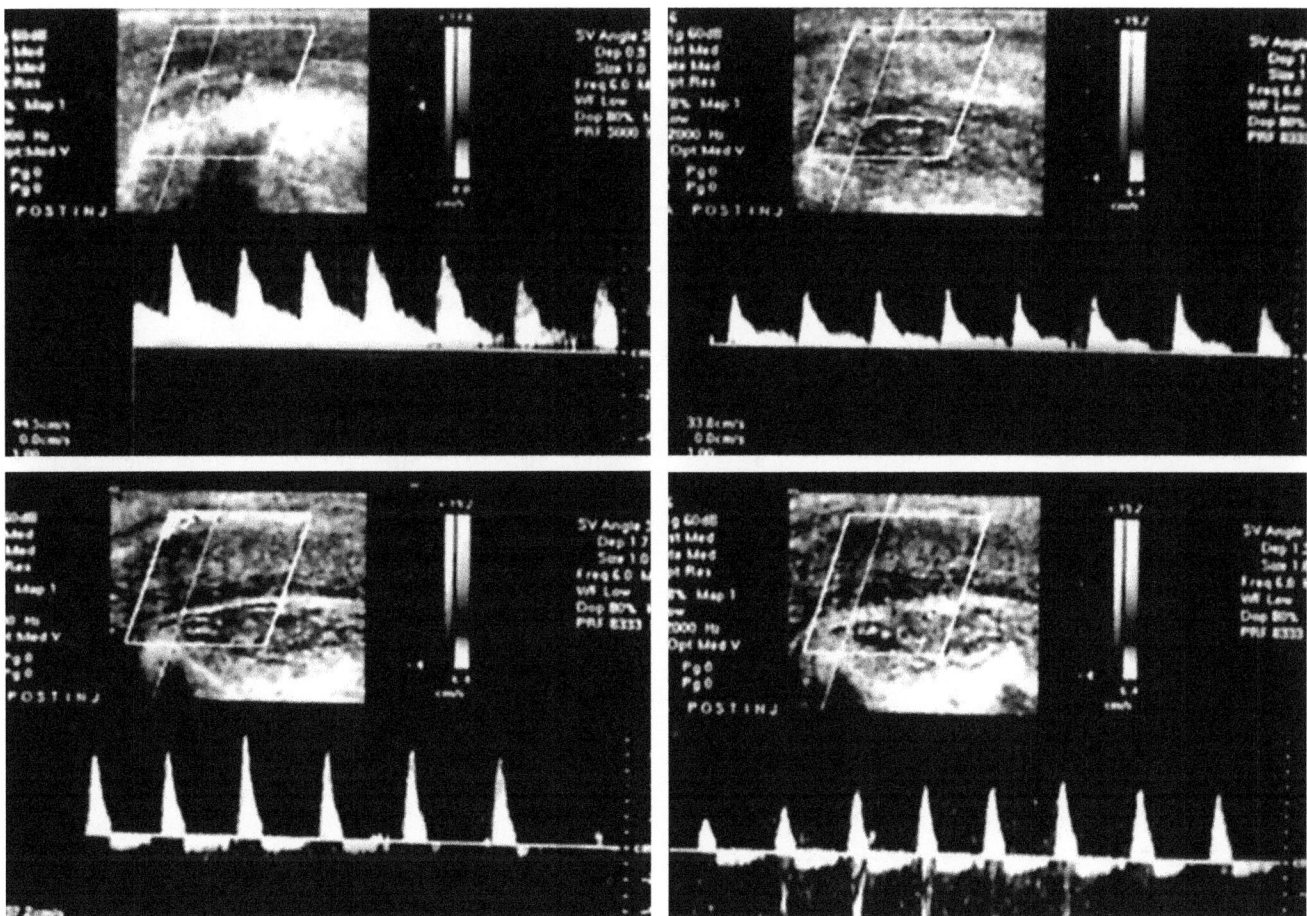

Fig. 15.2: Serial spectral tracings during PPDU shows various phases of flow pattern (refer text).

disease problem. All 30 men in our study were diagnosed to have nonvasculogenic ED. Their younger mean age emphasize the fact that the younger men have less incidence of organic impotence than older men as the later group are likely to suffer from atherosclerosis and a replacement of elastic collagen with non-distensible collagen leading to vasculogenic erectile dysfunction.[9] All the patients had peak systolic velocity above 35 cm/sec, which correlates well with that reported by Benson et al.[10] However, mean PSV was 61.3 cm/second which is significantly higher than all previously reported studies.[3,8] Analysis of PSV variation with age has shown that there is a negative correlation and thus a higher mean PSV in the present study can be attributed to younger age of the study population. Similar results have been reported by Chung WS et al.[11] The mean acceleration time, which is now considered the best discriminator of arterial impotence, was 0.06 sec and none of the patients had AT of more 0.1 sec which is in conformity with existing literature.

The mean end diastolic velocity was –1.2 cm/seconds (negative sign indicates flow reversal) and it also correlates well with the prevailing consensus in literature.[3] Mean RI was 0.93 in whom diastolic flow reversal was not achieved. Majority of the patients had either absent or reversed diastolic flow (20 patients) or EDV 5 cm/sec or less (six patients). Four patients had end diastolic velocity more than 5 cm/sec, however, these patients had a very high PSVs and normal resistive indices. They also showed normal rigid erection on pharmacological stimulation. Thus, it appears that EDV > 5 cm/sec alone may not be a specific indicator of veno-occlusive insufficiency and it should be correlated with resistive index for diagnosis of veno-occlusive insufficiency. Normal mean PSV is dependant upon the age of the individual and it decreases with advancing age.[12]

In summary, abnormal PSV and AT are suggestive of arterial cause while abnormal EDV and RI indicate venous leakage. RI is considered more accurate than EDV for assessment of venous competence as probe vessel angle, the most important variable associated with the process of sampling and velocity calculation is filtered out in calculation of RI. Any increase in cavernosal artery diameter by less than three-fourth of the baseline is also suggestive of arterial insufficiency. If arterial disease is present,

KEY POINTS

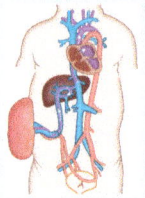

- Vasculogenic impotence is most common cause of organic impotence.
- PPDU differentiates arterial insufficiency and incompetent veno-occlusion.
- Abnormal peak systolic velocity and acceleration time suggest arterial cause.
- Abnormal end-diastolic volume and resistive index indicate venous leakage.
- Veno-occlusion cannot be assessed in presence of arterial insufficiency.

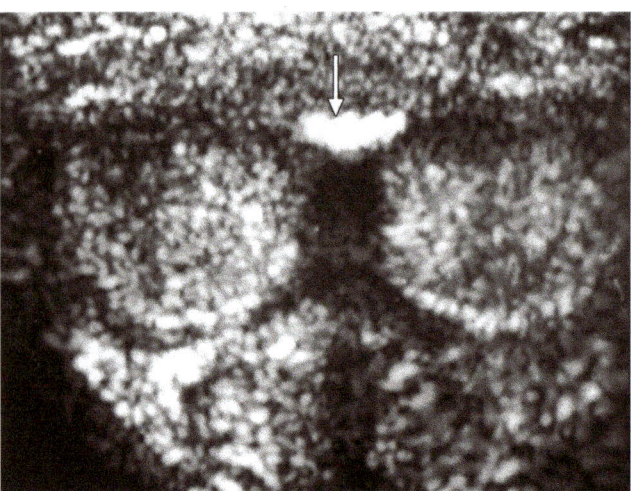

Fig. 15.3: Peyronie's disease: dense echogenic plaque of tunica with distal shadowing is seen on the dorsal surface of the penis.

intracavernosal pressure remains below systemic pressure and veno-occlusion cannot occur, even if this mechanism is intact, and diastolic flow will continue to persist. Therefore, veno-occlusive mechanism cannot be assessed in presence of arterial disease.

TREATMENT OF COMPLICATIONS

The most common complications during the diagnostic work-up and especially during the PPDU, is a papaverine induced prolonged, painful erection or priapism. Not all of them require specific treatment as penile detume-scence generally occurs within few hours. In case the duration of erection exceeds six hours, the corpora cavernosa are drained to decrease the pressure and 10 microgram of adrenaline is injected intracavernosally to induce cavernosal smooth muscle contraction, effective venous drainage and restriction of arterial flow. The adrenaline of 1 in 1000 strength can be diluted with appropriate amount of normal saline to produce adrenaline injection of the desired strength. Compression bandage is also applied for few minutes. In case the erection has recurred, the procedure can be repeated.

PEYRONIE'S DISEASE

This is a benign condition resulting from inelastic scar of tunica albuginea, which produce curvature deformities of penis and ED. On sonography, the penile plaques are seen as echogenic, avascular, focal thickening of tunica albuginea which may displace or encase cavernous vasculature. Dense plaques may contain calcification and produce acoustic shadowing (Fig. 15.3) however, calcification can be seen even without evidence of calcification on the plain radiographs. Most plaques are located on the dorsal surface of middle third of the shaft of the penis.

REFERENCES

1. Meuleman, Diemont WL. Investigation of erectile dysfunction. Urol Clin N Am. 1995;22:803-19.
2. Broderick GA, Arger P. Duplex Doppler ultrasonography: noninvasive assessment of penis anatomy and function. Seminroentgenology. 1993;28:43-56.
3. Shwartz AM, Lawe M, Berger RE, et al. Assessment of normal and abnormal erectile function–colour Doppler sonography versus conventional techniques. Radiology. 1991;180:105-09.
4. Shabsigh R, Fishman IR, Quesda ET, et al. Evaluation of vasculogenic erectile impotence using penile duplex sonography. J Urol. 1990;142:1469-74.
5. Lue TF, Tanagho EZ. Physiology of erection and pharmacological management of impotence. J Urol. 1987;137:829-35.
6. Merckx LA, DeBruyne RMG, Goes E, et al. The value of dynamic colour Doppler scanning in the diagnosis of venogenic impotence. J Urol. 1992;148:318-20.
7. Valji K, Bookstein JJ. Diagnosis of arteriogenic impotence: Efficacy of Duplex sonography as a screening tool. AJR Am J Roentgenology. 1993;160:65-69.
8. Quam JP, King BF, James EM, et al. Duplex and colour Doppler sonographic evaluation of vasculogenic impotence. AJR Am J Roentgenology. 1989;153:1141.
9. Padma Nathan H, Boyd SD, Chung D. The biochemical effect of ageing, diabetes and ischemia on corporal and tunical collagen. J Urol. 1991;145:342-518.
10. Benson CB, Aruny JE, Vickers MA. Correlation of Duplex sonography with angiography in-patients with erectile dysfunction. AJR Am J Roentgenology. 1993;160:71-73.
11. Chung WS, Park YY, Kwon SW. The impact of aging on penile hemodynamics in normal responders to pharmacological injection: Doppler sonographic study. J Urol. 1989;157:2129-31.
12. Bhargava R, Srivastava DN, Thulkar S, et al. Colour Duplex Doppler ultrasonography evaluation of non-vasculogenic male erectile dysfunction: an Indian perspective. Australian Radiology. 2002;46:170-3.

Chapter 16: Color Doppler of Small Parts

MUSCULOSKELETAL SYSTEM

Ultrasound is often the first step in the assessment of musculoskeletal soft tissue masses. It can confirm the presence of a lesion, and provide information regarding its size, location, margin, and internal structures. It can easily differentiate solid from fluid masses. Further characterization of the solid masses is not very specific. Sonography is usually not able to distinguish benign from malignant mass lesions. Newly formed tumor vessels in a malignant neoplasm shows some distinct features like abnormal branching pattern, irregular size, wide sinusoids, and arteriovenous shunts. Such features and resulting blood flow abnormalities can be detected by color Doppler and pulsed Doppler sonography.

Instrumentation and Technique

An adequate frequency probe should be chosen depending upon the size and depth of the lesion. Frequency varies from 3.5-7.5 MHz. Color Doppler parameters should be optimized for low blood flow velocities. For spectral analysis low value of PRF and low wall filters should be used. The values can be adjusted upwards if medium to high velocities are encountered. Sample values should be adjusted to the vessel size. For each lesions, a minimum of three values should be taken. Absolute velocities should be obtained after angle correction. When different peak systolic values are found within a lesion, highest value should be considered for evaluation.

Color Doppler evaluation should be preceded by thorough gray scale examination. The lesion should be examined for growth pattern, margins, echogenicity and internal texture. On gray scale imaging, feature which are suggestive of a malignant lesion are: infiltrating or mixed pattern of tumor growth, blurred or irregular margins, hypoechoic pattern and heterogeneous texture.

On color Doppler flow imaging extent and configuration of tumor vascularity should be assessed on the basis of following features:
a. Flow signals: present or absent
b. Number of vessels
c. Vessel arrangement within the lesion—regularly distributed or randomly dispersed
d. Vessel course—linear or tortuous
e. Presence or absence of abrupt variation in calibre.

On pulsed Doppler evaluation, systolic and diastolic velocities, and pulsatility index should be measured.

Color and pulsed wave Doppler data are more helpful in categorizing a lesion as benign or malignant compared to gray scale sonography alone. Absence of flow is a characteristic feature of the benign lesion. Presence of flow however, can be found in both benign and malignant lesions. The number of vessels in the lesion is also not of much help in distinction. It correlates more with the tumor size and not with benign or malignant nature. Arrangement of the vessels within the lesion is more useful. A regular arrangement with a linear course is usually suggestive of a benign mass.

KEY POINTS

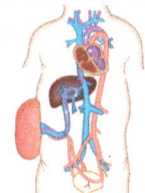

Doppler in musculoskeletal mass lesions
- Regular arrangement of vessels with linear course suggests presence of a benign mass.
- Malignant lesions have randomly distributed vessels with abrupt variations in size as well as flow signals.
- Peak systolic velocity more than 50 cm/sec is highly suggestive of a malignant lesion.

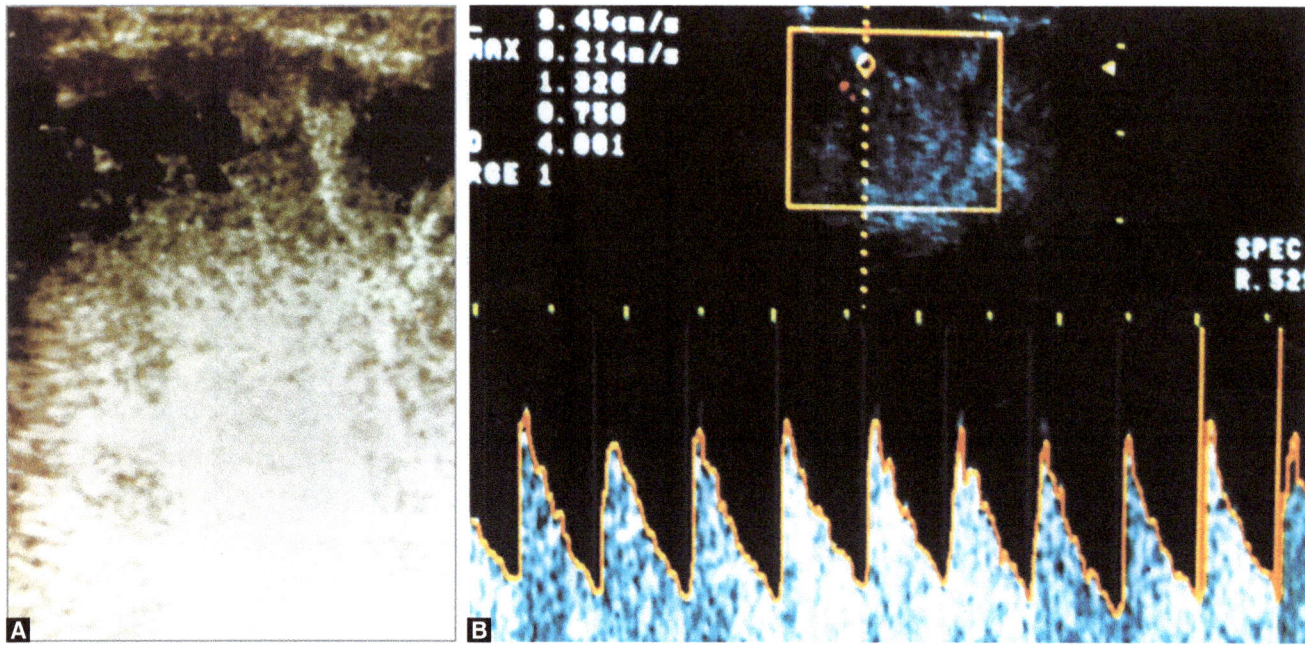

Figs. 16.1A and B: Rhabdomyosarcoma—(A) Gray scale image reveals a large heterogeneous mass in the neck; (B) Color and pulse Doppler image shows central, high velocity flow signal in the lesion.

Randomly distributed vessels with abrupt variation in size as well as spot flow signals are seen in malignant lesions. On spectral evaluation peak systolic velocity is the single most reliable parameter for discriminating benign and malignant lesions (Figs. 16.1A and B). A threshold of 50 cm/sec is the best criterion. Diagnostic accuracy is enhanced by composite analysis of sonographic, color, and pulsed Doppler findings.

SKIN AND SUBCUTANEOUS TISSUES

Evaluation of the skin and subcutaneous tissue is one of the most recent achievements of sonography. Availability of very high resolution probe (10-20 MHz) enables acquisition of excellent image with great anatomic details, including an accurate definition of various layers of the skin. Lesions of the skin are a frequent and possibly serious dermatological problems, as some of the most aggressive neoplasms arise from the skin and are clinically indistinguishable from benign ones. High frequency sonography alone is now specific in evaluation of these lesions. Color Doppler sonography increases the specificity of the sonography by providing real time evaluation of the vascularity, which is an important clue in distinguishing benign from the malignant lesions. Malignant tumors are expected to show increased vascularity compared to their benign counterparts.

The sonographic examination should be carried by a high resolution linear transducer. Doppler parameters should be adjusted to detect low velocity or low volume flow. Power Doppler can be used to increase vessel conspicuity and demonstrate vessel continuity.

The lesion should be scanned slowly with minimum probe pressure, as even slight compression with transducer can obliterate thin vessel pedicles supplying the nodules. Nodules are classified as:

Type I : Avascular
Type II : Hypovascular with a single vascular pole in the hilum
Type III : Hypervascular with multiple peripheral poles, and
Type IV : Hypervascular with internal vessels.

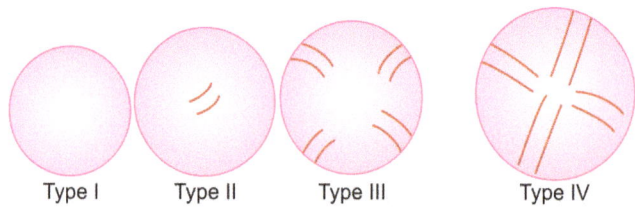

Majority of the malignant nodules show both peripheral (Type III) and intralesional vascularity (Type IV), where as hypovascularity is seen mainly in the benign lesions. Malignant tumors of the skin produce angiogenic factors that promote the development of multiple small arterial vessels, which enter the tumor peripherally at right angles and give rise to multiple intralesional vessels which contain stagnant blood. The subsequent central necrosis progressively obstructs and destroys the intralesional vessels and eventually progresses to stop blood flow in the peripheral arteries, because of high resistance of the intralesional blood vessels. Thus, Type IV pattern is more likely to be present in a malignant tumor without necrosis (Fig. 16.2A), whereas Type III pattern would be found in tumor with central necrosis. Type I (avascular nodule) [Figs. 16.2B (i, ii)] is the least specific, because it can be found in totally necrotic malignant, as well as benign tumors. Type II pattern is probably a variant of Type I and can be observed when the main artery of a benign tumor is large enough to be detected, possibly because the benign lesion is larger than usual. Pulse Doppler may also sometimes help in distinguishing benign and malignant lesions. Benign lesions show low systolic and diastolic velocities while high velocities are seen in malignant lesions [Figs. 16.2C (i, ii) and Table 16.1].

Color Doppler sonography has still not found acceptance as a primary diagnostic modality, because the superficial nodule can be effectively evaluated by physical examination and biopsy alone. So, dermatologists are reluctant to perform further investigations. Differentiation of local relapse of malignant tumors from scar may be potential application of color Doppler imaging.

VASCULAR LESIONS

Hemangioma

Hemangiomas are among one of common soft tissue masses in infants. Clinically they appear as slightly raised bluish

KEY POINTS

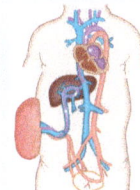

Doppler in skin and subcutaneous tissue lesions
- Very high frequency probe (10–20 MHz) is needed for evaluation.
- Malignant nodules show peripheral and intralesional vessels with high velocities.
- Benign nodules are usually hypovascular with low systolic and diastolic velocities.

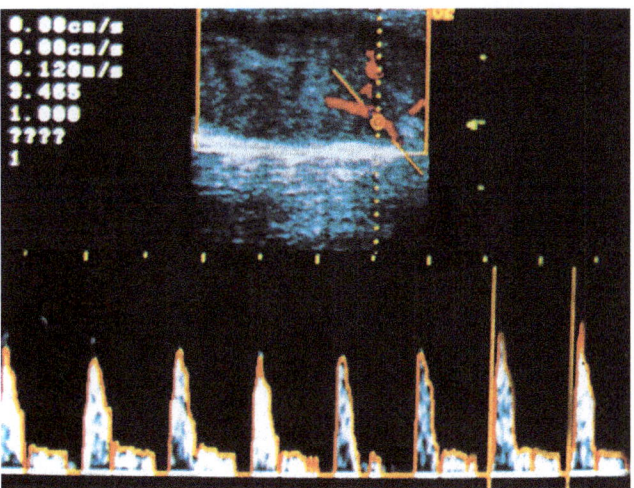

Fig. 16.2A: Color Doppler of right arm shows a subcutaneous metastasis with intralesional vascularity and central high velocity flow signal.

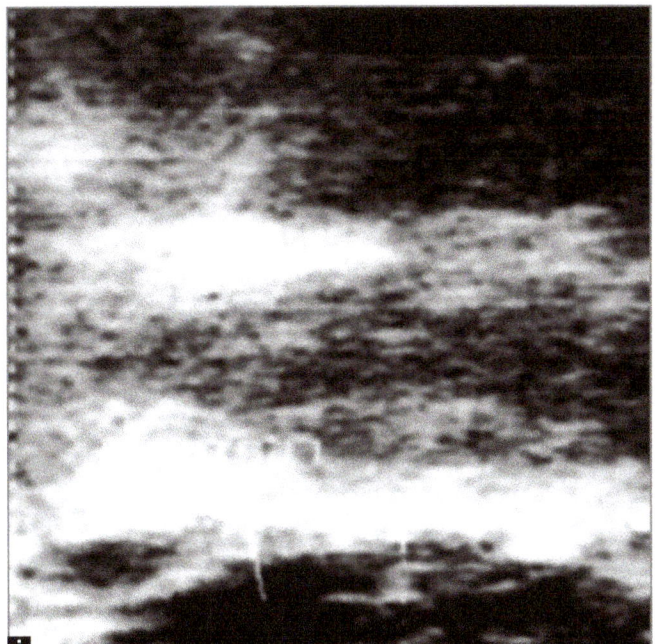

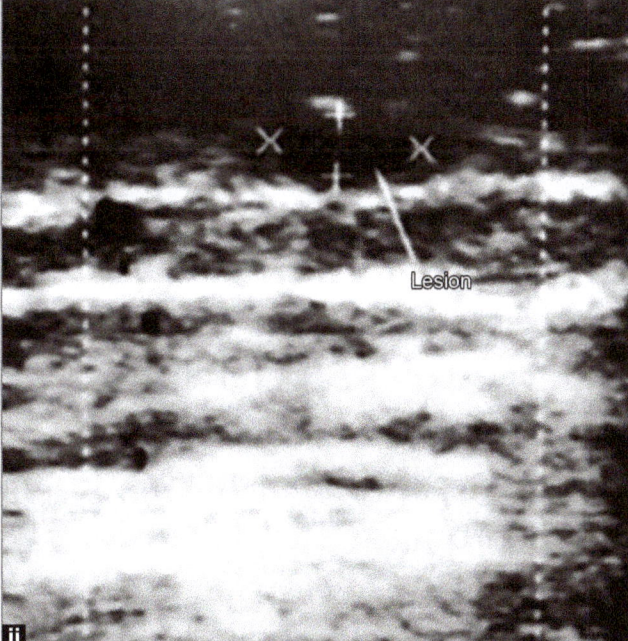

Figs. 16.2B(i, ii): Basal cell carcinoma: A well-defined hypo to anechoic skin lesion showing no color flow in color Doppler analysis.

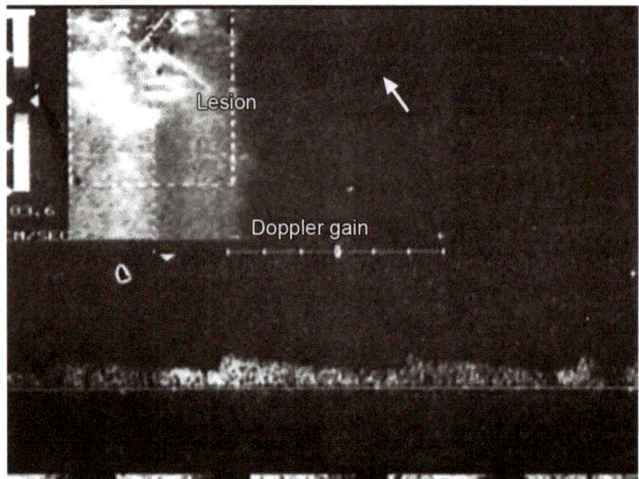

Fig. 16.2C(i): Pyogenic granuloma: a well-defined hypoechoic skin lesion seen with Doppler analysis showing low systolic and end diastolic velocity suggestive of a benign lesion.

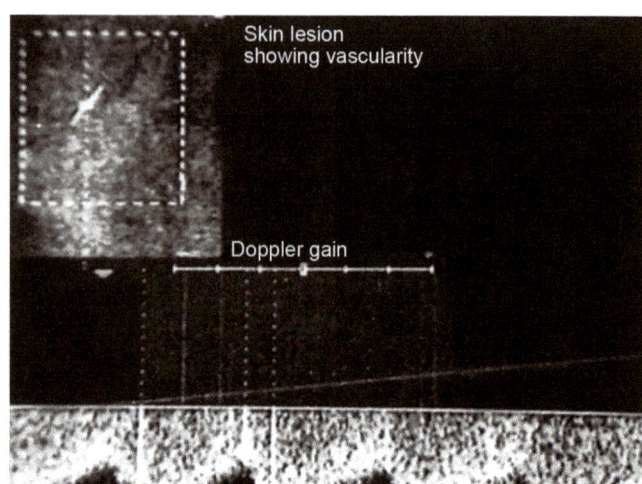

Fig. 16.2C(ii): Metastasis: A large well-defined hypoechoic skin lesion is seen in the scalp from carcinoma thyroid showing a high systolic and end-diastolic velocity suggestive of a malignant lesion.

TABLE 16.1: Color flow Doppler findings in skin lesions.

Lesion	Vascularity	Max-systolic (cm/sec)	End-diastolic (cm/sec)	RI
Pyogenic granuloma	+	6	3	0.50
Pyogenic granuloma	+	5	3	0.40
Pyogenic granuloma	+	6	3	0.50
Pyogenic granuloma	+	6	3	0.50
Squamous cell Ca	+	36.20	16.00	0.50
Squamous cell Ca	+	36.00	14.00	0.60
Metastasis	+	34.00	17.00	0.50

red subcutaneous masses. They regress as the child grows older. Some hemangiomas however, do not have this typical experience because part of or the entire lesion is deep in the soft tissue and the overlying skin appears normal. These lesions are difficult to distinguish clinically from more suspicious soft tissue masses such as soft tissue tumors and infantile myofibrosis.

Gray scale imaging shows a heterogeneous density soft tissue density mass. Some times vessels may also be visualized within the lesion, calcification may also be present (Fig. 16.3A).

On CDFI hemangiomas show presence of large number of intralesional vessels. Presence of more than five vessels per square centimeter has been seen. On spectral imaging a high frequency shift measuring more than 2 kHz is seen (Figs. 16.3B and C).

Cavernous hemangioma may show dilated and compressible venous channels that may show color flow only on PDI or on release of pressure. Some of the venous channels may show thrombosis or phleboliths.

Arteriovenous malformations may also show similar features on CDFI and pulse Doppler imaging, viz number of vessels more than five per square centimeter and Doppler shift greater than 2 kHz. However, distinction can some times be made on gray scale imaging in these cases, because of multiple sites of arteriovenous shunting large number of prominent vessels may be seen (Figs. 16.4A and B). Doppler evaluation may show arterialization of the waveform. Associated increase in blood flow and caliber is noted in the feeding arteries and draining veins.

Breast

Incidence of carcinoma of the breast has been rising steadily, and this along with the carcinoma of cervix is the leading cause of cancer in India. Early detection of this lesion is therefore extremely important as it offers chance of getting cured. X-ray mammography is the most frequent imaging modality used for evaluation of the breast abnormalities. Ultrasound was first used in the diagnostic work up of breast lesions in 1954. Since then many ultrasonic modalities dedicated to the examination of the breast have been developed. Advent of high resolution real time sonography has enabled excellent visualization and characterization of breast nodules. In addition, it provides an accurate guidance for aspiration and biopsy of these lesions. Though sonography is not better than

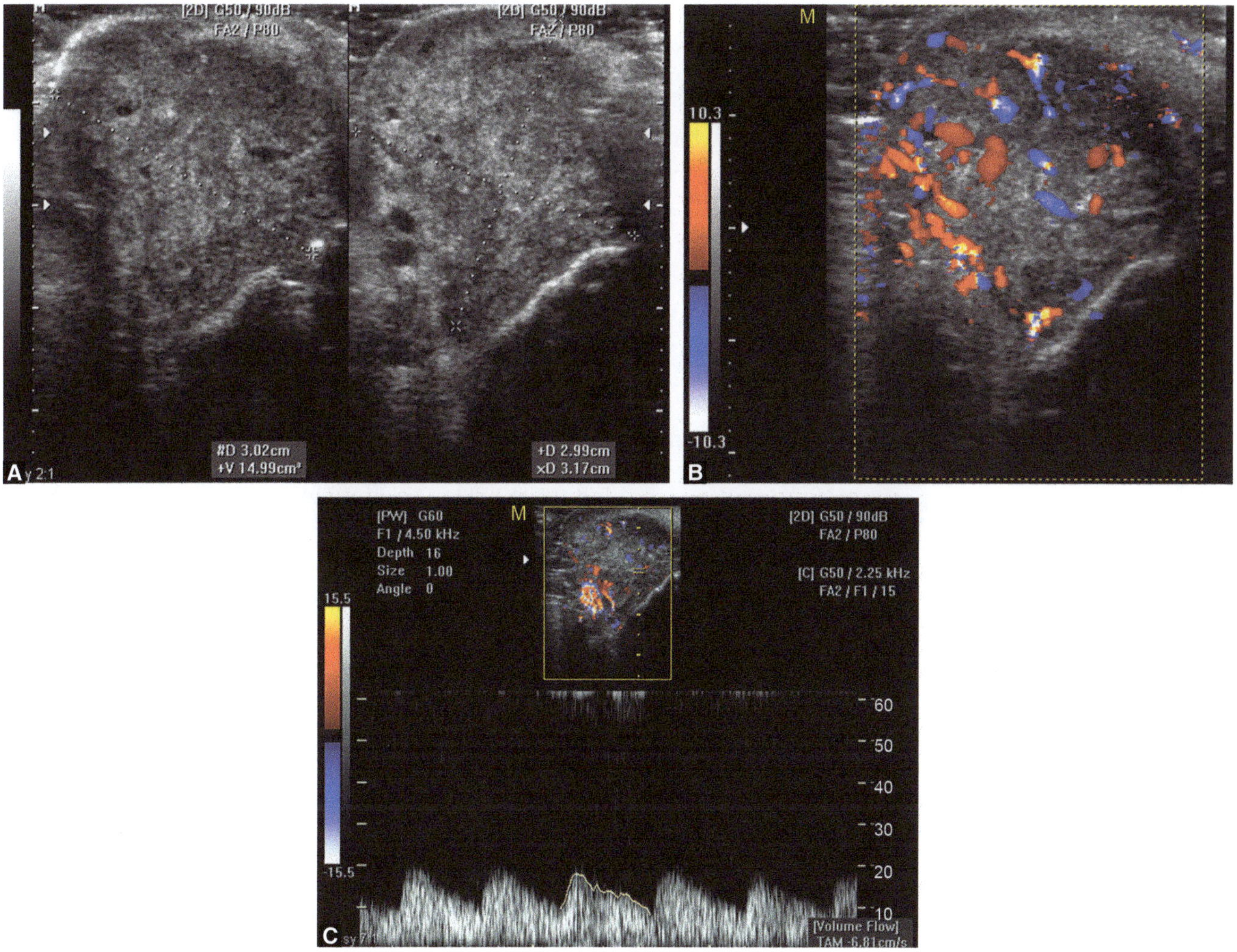

Color Doppler of Small Parts | 147

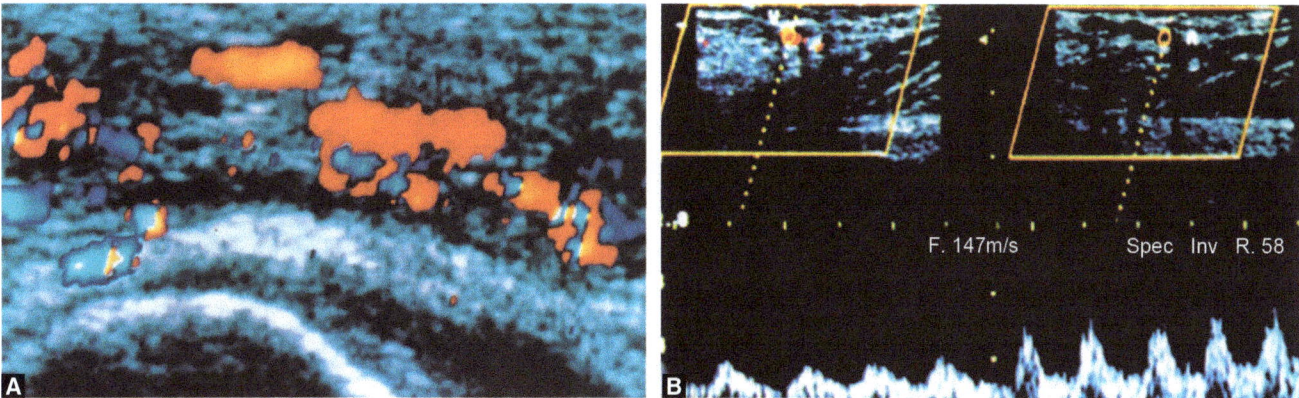

Figs. 16.3A to C: Hemangioma superficial (A) On Gray scale sonogram of wrist a mixed echogenic mass lesion is seen with multiple tortuousity suggestive of a vascular lesion; (B) Spectral Doppler shows evidence of flow with frequency shift of 3.1 kHz, suggestive of hemangioma Color Doppler shows numerous vessels within the hemangioma; (C) Spectral flow shows low velocity and low resistance arterial flow within hemangioma.

Figs. 16.4A and B: Arteriovenous malformation in the leg—(A) Color Doppler image shows multiple vascular spaces in a swelling of knee; (B) Spectral tracing shows arterialization of venous flow.

conventional mammography for screening of breast cancer, it is the most beneficial aid to the mammography. Certain features observed on sonography raise a high suspicion of malignancy, but none of them appears to be specific for malignancy. Combinations of features are more reliable than presence of a single finding. Various findings which may arouse suspicion of a malignant lesion on B-mode imaging include:
- Irregularity of borders
- Round shape, long axis perpendicular to skin
- Hypoechoic relative to surrounding breast parenchyma
- Presence of heterogeneity and posterior acoustic shadowing
- Echogenic rim of variable thickness.

Other investigative modalities have also been used in the evaluation of suspected breast disease for achieving the hitherto elusive goal of obtaining non-invasive diagnosis of breast carcinoma. These modalities include spectral and color Doppler flow imaging, MRI, CT, radionuclide studies with ^{99m}Tcsestamibi and ^{99}Tc sulfur colloid and digital mammography. Application of Doppler studies in differentiation of benign and malignant lesions is based on premise that the malignant lesions are likely to be more vascular.

For the sonographic and Doppler examination of the breast 7.5 MHz linear transducer is usually required. For the Doppler, gain settings are adjusted so that the clutter noise disappears. Velocity range is adjusted to avoid aliasing. Minimal transducer pressure is applied so that the slow blood flow is not obscured. The tumor vessels are visualized with the help of CDFI and power Doppler imaging and the vessels with the largest diameters are interrogated with pulsed Doppler for spectral analysis.

Blood vessels are more clearly seen with the power Doppler imaging than with color Doppler. Vascular continuity is also better demonstrated by power Doppler imaging. Blood flow signals are more numerous in breast cancers than in benign lesions. This is consistent with the fact that malignant lesions are more vascular (Figs. 16.5A and B) than their benign counterparts. Due to increased sensitivity of flow detection with PDI, some benign lesion may also appear hypervascular. These include benign phyllod tumors, intraductalpapillomatosis, inflammatory lesions, fibroadenoma and fibrocystic disease. Absence of vascularity differentiates inspissated ductal secretions from intraductal papilloma/carcinoma.

Various Doppler parameters have been evaluated for their use in differentiating between benign and malignant lesions (Tables 16.2 to 16.4). These include peak systolic velocity, pulsatility index and resistive index. In malignant neoplasm peak systolic velocity is increased but there is no universal agreement in the cut off velocity beyond which lesion can be classified as malignant. A PI value of >1.4 and RI value of >0.8 have been suggested as clinically useful cut off points. With these threshold values CDFI has 80% specificity with higher sensitivity and positive predictive value. Use of intravenous contrast agents such as microphilized albumin in increasing the specificity and sensitivity of color Doppler flow imaging and power Doppler imaging in tumor detection and differentiation between benign and malignant lesion glands is being studied at present.

Thyroid and Parathyroid Glands

Ultrasound has been successfully used as an adjunct to nuclear scintigraphy in evaluating the thyroid gland. Development of color Doppler flow imaging has permitted the assessment of blood supply in addition to morphology. Thyroid gland is one of the most vascular organs in the body. So Doppler may be useful in providing information in some thyroid diseases.

High frequency transducers (7-12 MHz) are used for thyroid and parathyroid imaging. Gray scale longitudinal and transverse images of the thyroid gland are obtained from the level of mandibular angle to the sternal notch. The patient is examined in supine position with neck extended. A pad may be placed under the shoulder to provide better exposure of the neck. Doppler parameters are optimized for low flow sensitivity in the case of suspected parathyroid adenoma. With presently available Doppler systems, rich vascularization of thyroid gland can be easily seen, which is most pronounced at the upper and lower pole. Superior thyroid vessels are found at the upper pole of each lobe. Inferior thyroid artery is present posterior to lower third of the lobe. Mean diameter of the arteries is 1-2 mm, the veins may be up to 8 mm in diameter. Peak systolic velocities are 20-40 cm/sec in major thyroid arteries and 15-30 cm/sec in intraparen-chymal arteries.

Graves' disease: It is characterized by generalized enlargement of the thyroid gland with biochemical hyperfunction. Color Doppler is useful in evaluation of this disease. Markedly increased vascularity is seen on CDFI and power Doppler imaging. This appearance has been referred to as "Thyroid inferno" (Fig. 16.6). Spectral Doppler shows increased peak systolic velocity, which may exceed 70 cm/sec. None of the other thyroid diseases show such high velocities. Doppler examination can also be used to monitor the response to therapy in these patients. Following treatment significant decrease in vascularity and the velocities of thyroid vessels is seen (Fig. 16.7).

Thyroid nodules: Hyperplastic thyroid nodules are less vascular than the normal thyroid parenchyma.

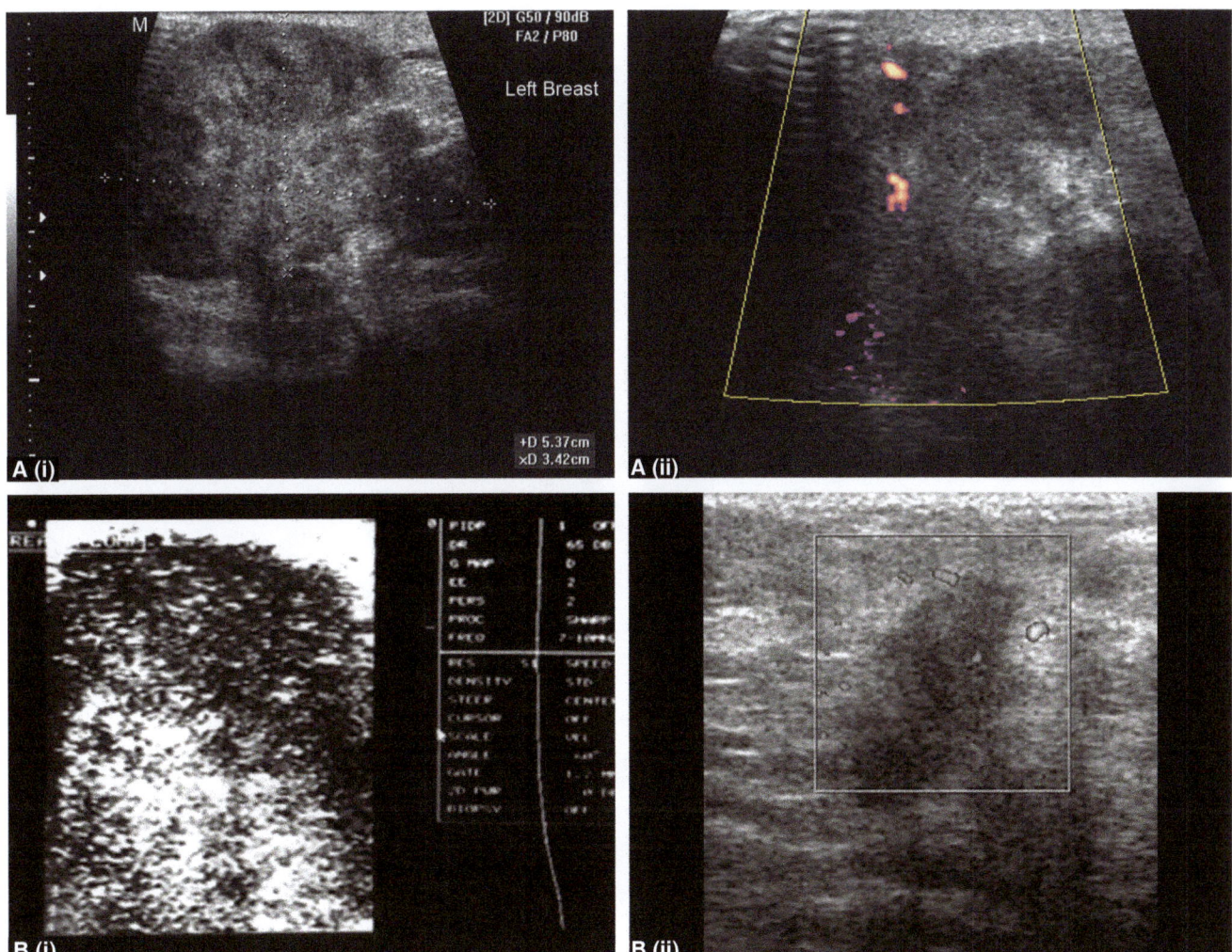

Figs. 16.5A(i) to B(ii): Carcinoma of breast—(A-i) Gray scale sonogram shows a large irregular mass lesion in the right breast; (A-ii) On CDFI blood vessels are seen in the center of the lesion, consistent with malignancy; (B-i) Gray scale US shows a large well-defined mass with homogeneous internal echotexture and no significant change in through; transmission; (B-ii) Color Doppler scan shows color signals located within the mass lesion.

TABLE 16.2: Doppler flow studies in benign vs malignant breast lumps.

	Malignant lumps		Benign breast		p value
	Mean ± SD	Range	Mean ± SD	Range	
1. Doppler signal	+++		±		
2. Peak systolic flow (Hz)	2429.75 ± 521.65	1267–3233	1584.69–726.80	867–2900	< 0.0001
3. Minimum diastolic flow 885 (Hz)	78 ± 862.28	233–1800	574.30 ± 314.97	133–1000	< 0.0001
4. DFT (mm^3) Max. frequency envelop	104.07 ± 32.04	42–1520	66.07 ± 28.91	31.133	< 0.0001
5. Pulsatility index	0.4810 ± 0.1276	0.239–0.689	0.4868 ± 0.1536	0.233–0.790	NS

TABLE 16.3: Doppler flow signals vs various clinical parameters in malignant lumps.

Histopathology	Maximum systolic freq. (Hz)	Minimum diagnostic (Hz)	DFT (mm³)
Fibroadenoma	1256	492	62
Fibroadenosis	1067	767	46
Cystosarcoma phylloides	2744	978	121
Infiltrating duct carcinoma	2367	686	99
Lobular carcinoma	2514	707	124
Squamous cell carcinoma	2867	767	109

TABLE 16.4: Doppler flow signals vs various clinical parameters in malignant lumps.

	Maximum diastolic Frequency (Mean) Hz	Minimum diagnostic Frequency (Mean) Hz	DFT (mm³)
Tumor size			
<2 cm	1643	517	57
2–5 cm	1794	588	72
5–10 cm	2612	1009	118
>10 cm	3000	1167	121
Tumor area			
0–10 cm²	1948	678	73
11–20 cm²	2006	745	86
21–30 cm²	2095	814	90
31–40 cm²	2192	814	94
41–50 cm²	2192	814	94
> 50 cm²	2793	1280	122
Stage of disease			
Stage II	1294	412	50
Stage III	2013	756	91
Stage IV	2754	1067	86
Grade of tumor			
Well differentiated	1467	707	68
Mod. differentiated	1866	686	83
Poor differentiated	1967	767	75

Well differentiated carcinomas are relatively hypervascular and show tortuous vessels with arteriovenous shunting. Poorly differentiating and anaplastic carcinomas are rapidly growing tumors with propensity to undergo necrosis and thus are most often hypovascular.

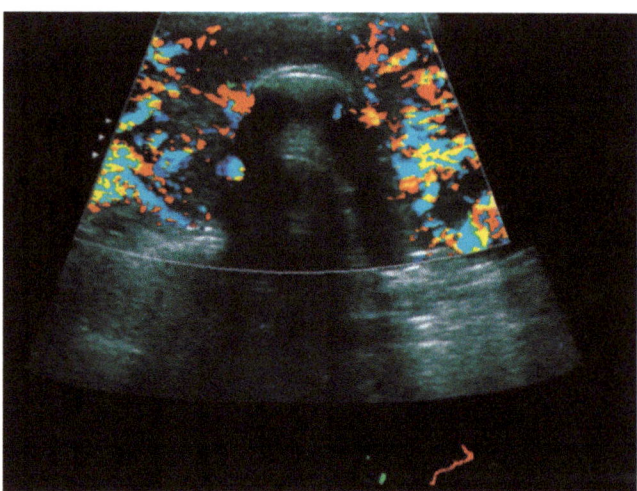

Fig. 16.6: Color Doppler image in a case of thyrotoxicosis. Both lobes of thyroid display marked increase in vascularity, also known as the 'Thyroid inferno' sign.

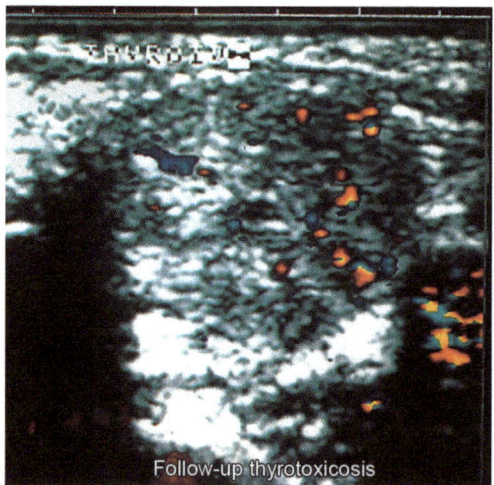

Fig. 16.7: Follow-up case of thyrotoxicosis on therapy, color Doppler image shows decreased flow in the thyroid gland, suggesting response to therapy.

KEY POINTS

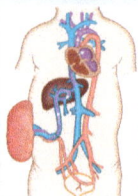

- Doppler in thyroid and parathyroid gland lesions
- "Thyroid inferno" sign on the CDFI with peak systolic velocities greater than 70 cm/sec is virtually pathognomonic of thyrotoxicosis.
- Majority of the benign thyroid nodules show peripheral vascularity.
- Vessels inside the lesion with or without peripheral vessels suggest malignant nodules in the thyroid gland.
- An extrathyroidal feeding artery is a useful guide for localizing a parathyroid adenoma on the CDFI.

Quantitative analysis of flow velocities is not accurate in differentiating benign from malignant nodules. Doppler finding that may be useful in differentiation, is the distribution of the vessels. With presently available high definition color Doppler systems, some degree of vascularity is demonstrated in all nodules. Two types of vascular distribution may be seen:
- Nodule with peripheral vascularity (Figs. 16.8A and B)
- Nodule with internal vessels, which may or may not be associated with peripheral vessels (Figs. 16.9A and B).

Large majority of hyperplastic, adenomatous, and goitrous nodules show peripheral distribution of the blood vessels (Figs. 16.8A and B), while majority of the thyroid malignancies show internal vessels with or without peripheral components (Figs. 16.9A and B). Role of color Doppler in evaluation of thyroid nodule is however controversial, and there is no universal agreement regarding its use in evaluation of a suspected thyroid nodule.

PARATHYROID ADENOMA

Primary hyperparathyroidism is caused by an adenoma in 80-90% of the cases. Other causes include enlargement of multiple glands (10-20%) and carcinoma (<1%). Value of preoperative localizing studies in patient with primary hyperparathyroidism is controversial. Many surgeons prefer routine bilateral neck exploration as the initial treatment for this condition. Some surgeons advocate unilateral neck exploration, because of following factors:
- Decreased operating room time

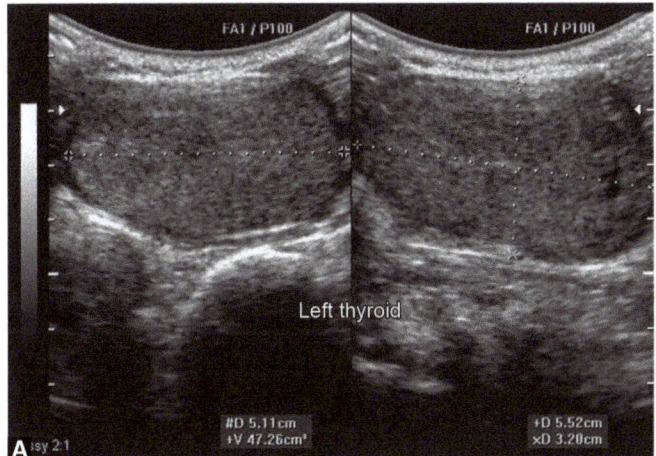 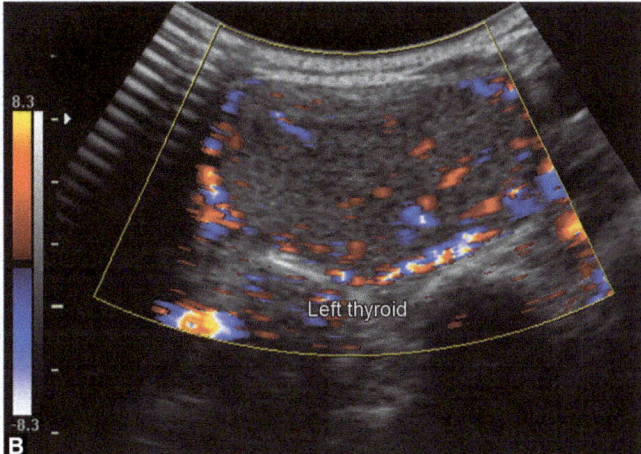

Figs. 16.8A and B: Benign lesion of thyroid—(A) Gray scale sonogram shows a solitary nodule in thyroid. Hypoechoic halo is visible around the nodule; (B) Doppler image of same lesion reveals mild vascularity in the mass. Color flow corresponding to the halo is seen.

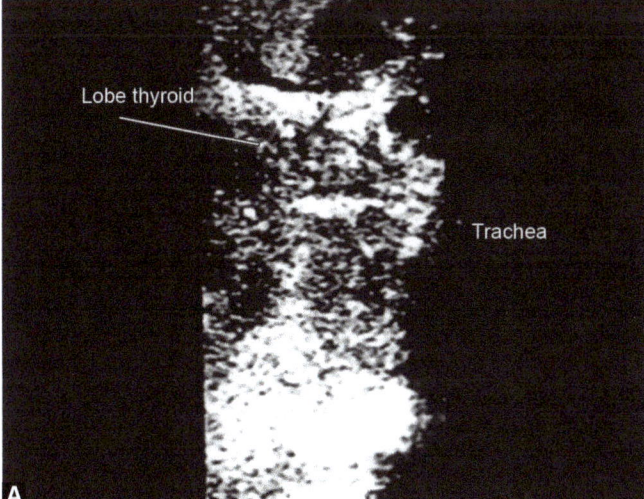 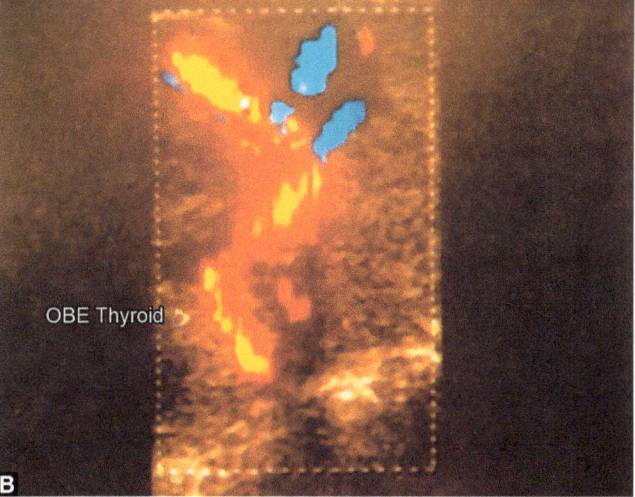

Figs. 16.9A and B: (A) Heterogeneous parenchymatous pattern seen in thyroid gland. There is obscuration of anatomical planes; (B) Color Doppler image in a thyroid nodule shows evidence of increased peripheral and central vascularity consistent with malignancy.

- Decreased risk of injury to the recurrent laryngeal nerve and normal parathyroid gland.

When unilateral surgery is being contemplated, accurate preoperative localization of the adenoma is critical. Sonography has sensitivity of 70-80% for localization of an abnormal parathyroid gland. Typical sonographic appearance of parathyroid adenoma on gray scale imaging is a hypoechoic ovoid or lobulated mass posterior or lateral to the thyroid gland. Approximately 95% of the adenoma occur in neck and usually obtain their blood supply from the branches of inferior thyroid artery. Parathyroid adenomas are hypervascular (Fig. 16.10). They are suspended by a vascular pedicle consisting of an extrathyroidal artery enveloped in fat. This extrathyroidal feeding artery can be visualised with color or power Doppler sonography. Identification of this feeding artery can lead to an abnormal parathyroid gland, which may be inconspicuous on gray scale imaging. Thus, CDFI increases the sensitivity and specificity of sonographic examination, in localizing an adenoma.

Salivary Glands

Real time sonography is a well-established modality for evaluating the head and neck region and its value in diagnosing abnormalities of the salivary gland is well-documented. Sonography helps to clarify clinically equivocal swellings of the salivary glands, and has a high accuracy rate for detection of salivary stone as well as differentiation of inflammation from tumors. In cases of salivary tumors, their location, size, extent in the superficial part of the gland and presence of cystic/necrotic areas can be reliably diagnosed with ultrasound. There is classical ultrasound description of the pleomorphic salivary gland adenoma (PSGA) and Warthin's tumor and it is possible to demonstrate these pathologies on real time ultrasound. The ultrasound features of pleomorphic salivary gland adenoma are those of a mass which is round or lobulated, hyperechoic, well-defined and demonstrates through transmission. Warthin's' tumors occur in the older age group and appear similar to PSGA, but are more likely to be multiple and show intralesional cystic areas or septations. Differentiation of benign from malignant salivary gland tumor may be difficult with gray scale sonography alone. Up to 20% of the malignant lesions can have sharp margins, making it difficult to use this criterion alone to differentiate benign from malignant lesions. Incidence of malignant salivary gland lesions is only 5-10% of the cases, but it is helpful for the surgeon to be aware of any neoplastic lesion, as the treatment options may vary from local to wide excision, with or without adjuvant therapy.

Increased vascularity in salivary gland tumors can be recognized on color Doppler flow imaging, a characteristic peripheral pattern for pleomorphic salivary gland adenoma has been described. The lesion may show fine centripetal branches. The RI value ranges from 0.6-1.1 and peak systolic velocity is less than 50 cm per sec. Warthin's tumor shows evenly scattered flow throughout the tumor. RI value is 0.55-0.8 and peak systolic velocity is always less than 60 cm/sec. The peak systolic velocity in malignant tumors is more than 60 cm/sec. A study by Bradly et al. found no correlation between the color pattern, peak systolic velocity and presence of malignancy. In their study, malignant lesions showed an increased vascular pattern. The Doppler indices (PI, RI) were at the higher end of the spectrum. Most of the malignant lesions had PI > 1.8 and RI > 0.8. PI < 1.8 and RI < 0.8 virtually excludes malignancy (Fig. 16.11). The authors concluded that risk of malignancy rises by a third in those with high PI and RI factors. They suggested that this information should be correlated with ultrasound morphology and clinical history.

Vascular malformation in the salivary gland have similar feature as in other superficial organ. Multiple tortuous vascular channels with color flow are seen (Fig. 16.12).

COLOR DOPPLER IMAGING IN ORBIT

Doppler imaging has been used as an adjunct to routine A and B scanning of orbit since 1960. With the advent of color Doppler imaging it is now possible to obtain information on the perfusion of the orbital structures in real time. It is possible to carry out a vessel specific analysis in a fast and easy manner.

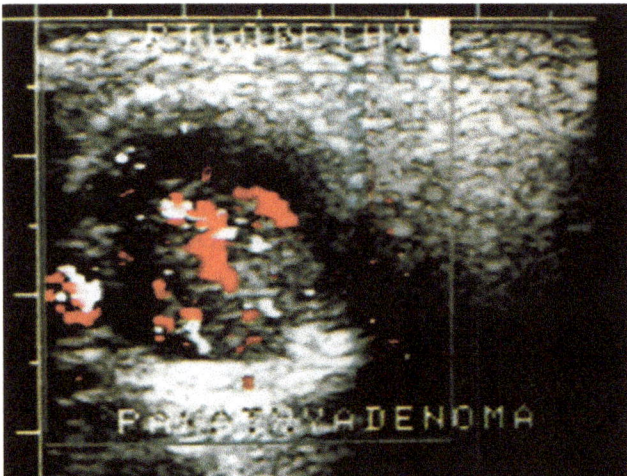

Fig. 16.10: Parathyroid adenoma—color Doppler of neck in a patient with clinical and biochemical evidence of hyperparathyroidism. A rounded mass lesion is seen posterior to the thyroid gland with increased vascularity. On surgery an adenoma was resected.

Color Doppler of Small Parts | 153

Normal Orbital Vessels

Central retinal artery (CRA) and central retinal vein (CRV) can be visualized at the level of the optic nerve. These vessels are seen within 2-12 mm of the optic nerve shadow. As the flow in CRA is towards the transducer, it is displayed in red color. CRV is displayed in blue. Absence of detectable CRA may indicate CRA occlusion in cases of acute loss of vision. Ciliary vessels can be identified on the side of the optic nerves. Ophthalmic artery enters the orbit temporal to the optic nerve. In the middle orbit the ophthalmic artery crosses over the optic nerve to occupy the nasal position relative to the optic nerve. Vortex veins may also be visualized entering into the superior and inferior ophthalmic veins.

Applications

Ocular Tumors

Recruitment of vessels is required for tumor growth. These vessels include the existing and newly proliferating vessels. Most of the tumors can be diagnosed clinically. Imaging techniques are more often used to confirm and document the diagnosis (Fig. 16.13A). Diagnostic accuracy of A and B scan for characterisation of the tumors is well-established. Color Doppler is being increasingly used to enhance the efficacy of these techniques. Intraocular mass lesions show evidence of Doppler signals. Choroidal melanomas show abnormal Doppler signals within the lesions (Fig. 16.13B). The flow spectrum pattern in these lesions is a medium to high systolic Doppler shift with high diastolic flow velocity. The flow decreases after brachy therapy in these patients. This is thought to be due to damage and sclerosis of tumor supplying vessels. Post therapy a decrease in peak systolic and an end diastolic velocity is seen. In choroidal hemangiomas, a high maximum systolic Doppler shift is seen along with high diastolic shifts. This is compatible with the pathologic features of this tumor which consist of a network of vascular channels. Evidence of increased flow is also seen in uveal metastases and retinoblastoma (Figs. 16.14A and B). Some intraocular lesions like age-related macular degeneration, with subretinal hemorrhage and dense vitreous hemorrhage may simulate the appearance of tumor on B-mode imaging. CDFI can help in differentiating these lesions by demonstrating these lesions by demonstrating lack of abnormal blood flow.

Orbital Tumors and Vascular Lesions

Most orbital neoplasms show presence of intratumoral and Doppler signals. In cavernous hemangiomas flow may be

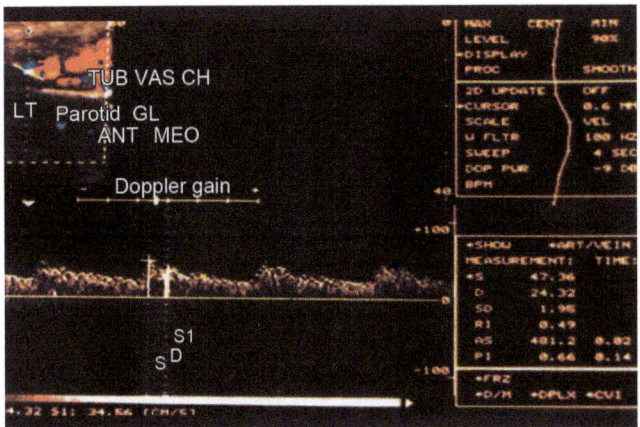

Fig. 16.11: Color Doppler sonography in a benign parotid lesion shows a mass lesion with vascular channels. Few vascular channels show continuous venous flow, arterial waveform shows peak velocity 47.36 and mean RI 0.49.

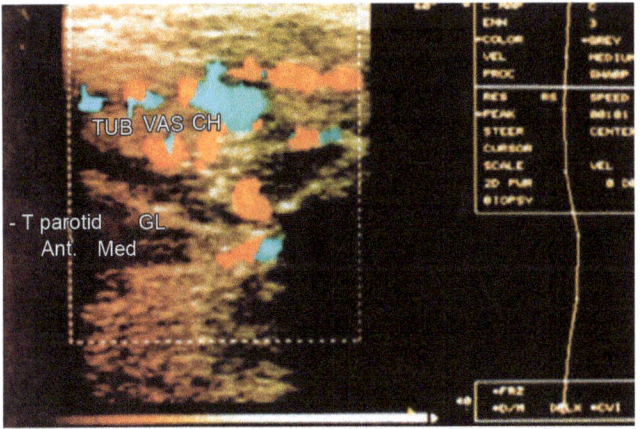

Fig. 16.12: Parotid hemangioma—Color Doppler sonography shows mass lesion with multiple vascular color flow signals.

The color Doppler examination can be performed with 7.5 MHz linear transducer. The transducer is applied to the close eyelid using a coupling gel. Patient is scanned in the supine position. Pressure should not be applied, as artifact can occur due to raised intraocular pressure. Horizontal and vertical scan through the eyes and orbit are obtained. The flow is assigned red or blue color. Flow towards the transducer is coded red and flow away from the transducer coded blue. Spectral analysis can be performed at selected sites. It is possible to distinguish between arteries and veins. Arteries show evidence of pulsatile flow on color images and spectral tracing, while the veins show continuous or minimally pulsatile flow. All examinations are performed in a low or medium flow setting. High flow setting may be applied for ophthalmic artery as this vessel has high flow velocity. The gain settings are adjusted, so as to minimize artifacts by lid and involuntary eye movement.

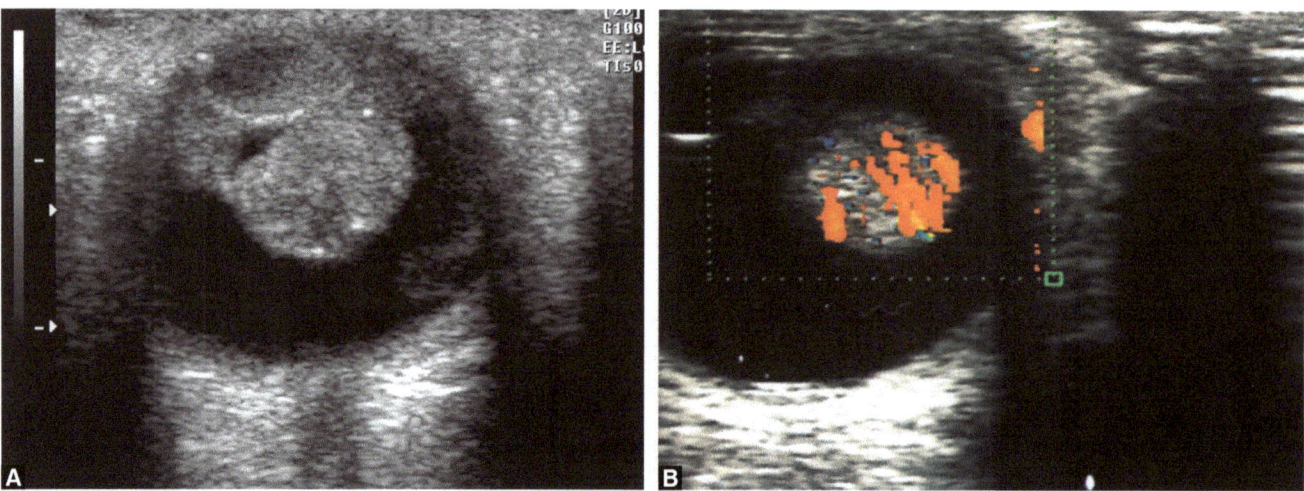

Figs. 16.13A and B: (A) Gray scale image showing choroidal melanoma; (B) Ocular melanoma: color Doppler flow images reveal evidence of increased vascularity in an intraocular mass. Melanoma was found at histopathologic examination.

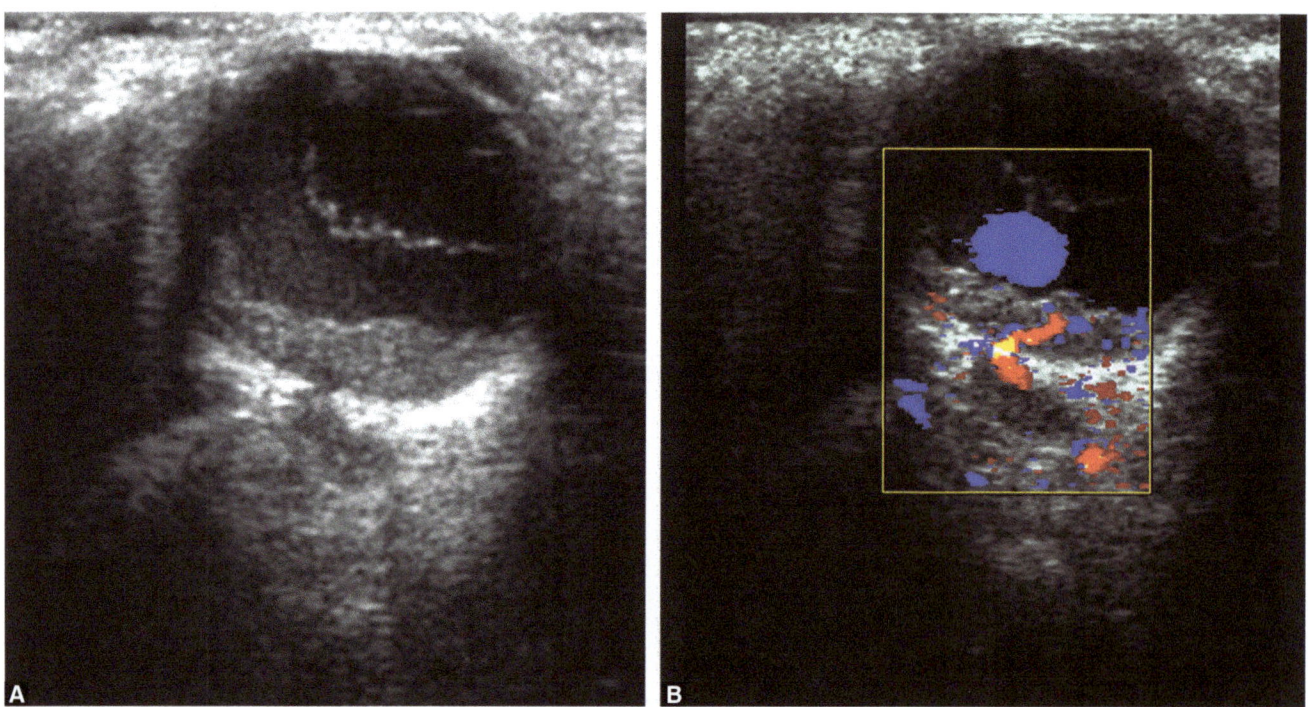

Figs. 16.14A and B: (A) Gray scale image of the globe in a child shows a mass lesion in the region of retina. Calcification is also seen within the lesion along with retinal detachment; (B) CDFI shows a hypervascular lesion, suggesting malignant nature. On surgery, retinoblastoma was found.

KEY POINTS

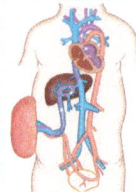

Orbital Doppler
- Orbital varices show respiratory variations in caliber with continuous nonpulsatile venous flow on the Doppler examination.
- Dilatation of the superior ophthalmic vein with arterialized high velocity flow in the posteroanterior direction is a characteristic feature of the carotid cavernous fistula.

seen on decreased gain settings (Fig. 16.15). Significantly increased vascularity is usually seen in malignant tumors. Sometimes benign tumor can cause blindness by pressing upon the optic nerve and its blood supply and this compression can be easily demonstrated by CDFI. Orbital varices have a characteristic pattern on Doppler imaging. They show dynamic changes throughout inspiration and expiration. During inspiration active filling and distension of the lesion is seen, flow is seen towards the transducer. On expiration the size of the lesion slowly decreases with flow away from the transducer. On pulsed Doppler evaluation the flow is continuous and nonpulsatile during both phases. This is characteristic of venous flow seen in this lesion.

Carotid Cavernous Sinus Fistulas

A carotid cavernous sinus fistula (CCSF) is an abnormal communication between a branch of the carotid arteries and the cavernous sinus. CDFI clearly demonstrates the dilated arterialized superior ophthalmic vein with high velocity blood flow towards the transducer (posterior to anterior). This finding, well seen on CDFI is highly suggestive of CCSF. High preseptal vascularity and thickening of extraocular muscles can also be seen. Doppler interrogation of vessels shows high systolic and diastolic velocities. CDFI can also be used to document reduced flow after balloon embolization.

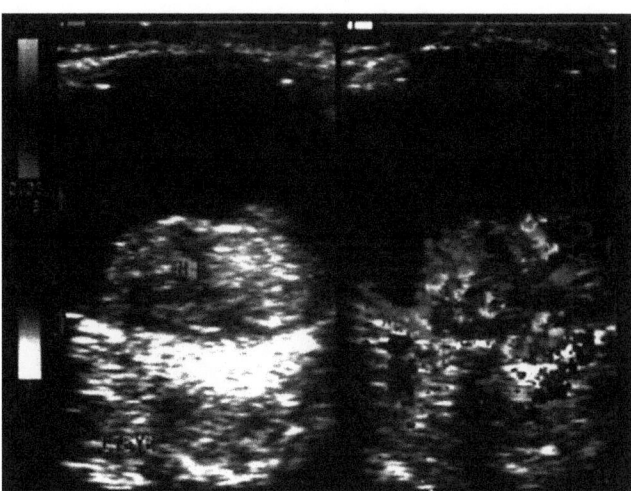

Fig. 16.15: Intraocular hemangioma: Color Doppler image shows a mass lesion in the posterior compartment of globe with increased vascularity.

Retinal Vessels Abnormalities

In occlusion of central retinal artery absence or marked reduction in flow can be seen on CDFI. Systolic and diastolic velocities are also reduced. Occlusion of central retinal veins shows a characteristic Doppler pattern. Central retinal artery show reduced flow in systole. Peak systolic waveform is blunted. Markedly decreased or absent flow is seen during diastole indicating high resistance caused by the blockage.

Chapter 17

Doppler Imaging of Peripheral Arteries

The diagnosis of diseases involving peripheral arteries can usually be made on the basis of a thorough history and physical examination. Some form of additional testing is usually required for further characterization and/or quantification of the pathologic process. Easy accessibility of the limb arteries to sonography enables it to play a decisive role in the evaluation of disease. With the advent of high resolution ultrasound, it is possible to image the peripheral arteries without the limitations encountered in abdominal and thoracic vessels. Gray scale imaging has a limited role in evaluation. It can detect presence of an atherosclerotic plaque, aneurysm and juxtavascular masses which may appear to be of arterial origin on clinical evaluation. Duplex scanning plays an important role in vascular evaluation. Hemodynamic changes in a vessel can be studied by obtaining spectral waveform. Thus, obstructive arterial lesions can be quantified, arterial stenosis can be differentiated from occlusion and the nature of perivascular masses can be determined. The addition of color Doppler flow imaging (CDFI) has transformed peripheral arterial imaging from a time consuming tedious task to an efficient practical examination. It has also improved the diagnostic accuracy of the examination. A rapid survey by CDFI can identify the zone of abnormal flow in a diseased vessel which can be evaluated by pulsed Doppler. CDFI enables accurate gate placement in the area of maximum flow disturbance. Power mode imaging or Doppler angiography displays the peak amplitude of the flowing blood. The color obtained is uniform, aliasing is not a problem, as with pulsed and CDFI mode and slow flow is better detected, a disadvantage is the lack of information about the flow direction.

INSTRUMENTATION

Peripheral arteries are small in size, so high resolution transducers are required for imaging the vascular wall and the lumen. Frequencies in the range of 5 to 10 MHz are preferred. For larger region like thigh 5 to 7.5 MHz is usually adequate. Examination of small superficial vessels is usually done by 7.5 to 10 MHz transducers. A linear transducer design with electronic steering capability is ideal, as it permits rapid coverage of long arterial segments. For examining iliac arteries and abdominal aorta, a frequency range of 2.5 to 5 MHz is needed depending upon the body habitus of the patient. Doppler frequencies vary between 3-10 MHz, they should be lower than the frequency used for acquiring gray scale image. Color flow imaging rapidly identifies the area of flow disturbance, which can be evaluated by pulsed Doppler. Lower frequencies than gray scale imaging are used, this partially over comes the early aliasing of the color flow image.

NORMAL ANATOMY AND DOPPLER WAVEFORM

Lower Limb

Common femoral artery is the continuation of the external iliac artery at the level of the inguinal ligament. After a distance of about 4-7 cm, it divides into superficial and deep femoral (profunda) artery. The profundafemoris artery branches just beyond the origin to supply the femoral head and deep muscles of the thigh. Superficial femoral artery continues its downward course along the medial thigh till it reaches the adductor canal. At the lower limit of adductor canal it comes out through the adductor hiatus and continues as popliteal artery in the popliteal fossa. Popliteal artery lies along the posterior aspect of the knee, after giving off geniculate branches it divides into the anterior tibia artery and the tibioperoneal trunk at the lower edge of the popliteal fossa. Anterior tibial artery travels through the interosseous membrane to reach the anterior compartment of the leg. In the leg it is lateral to the anterior border of tibia. It crosses the ankle joint to be known as the dorsalispedis artery. Tibioperoneal trunk lies posteriorly and divides into the posterior tibial and peroneal artery. Posterior tibial artery lies in the posterior compartment and in its distal course can be easily localized behind medial malleolus.

Doppler Waveform (Fig. 17.1)

Triphasic flow pattern is seen in all the arteries. There is a phase of early systolic acceleration. This is followed by a period of small flow reversal before antegrade low velocity diastolic flow is seen. This triphasic waveform is characteristic of arteries supplying muscular bed, which has high peripheral resistance. During exercise or transient ischemia, there is loss of triphasic pattern. A monophasic pattern characterized by persistent antegrade diastolic flow is observed. Peak systolic velocities of arteries vary with location. It is approximately 100 cm/sec at the level of common femoral artery and 40-50 cm/sec in the leg arteries.

Technique

Arterial occlusive disease is the main indication of the lower limb arterial Doppler study. Atherosclerosis is the major cause and as it also involves proximal vessels including aorta and iliac arteries, evaluation of aortoiliac arteries should be integral part of Doppler study of lower limb arterial occlusive disease.

With the advent of CDFI, the aorta and iliac arteries can be visualized easily. Thus, preparation of the patient to reduce the bowel gas is not usually required. The study begins with the patient supine and transducer placed below the xiphoid process. A 2.5-3.5 MHz transducer is usually required. 5 MHz probe may be needed in thin individuals. Aorta is imaged in the sagittal section. Celiac axis and the superior mesenteric arteries can be seen arising anteriorly. Renal arteries arise from posterolateral aspect of the aorta just below the superior mesenteric artery. Aorta is followed to the iliac bifurcation and common and external iliac arteries are examined till the groin. Evaluation of vessels at and below the groin requires high frequency transducers. For evaluation of femoral arteries the hip is abducted and leg is flexed at the knees. Common femoral artery is evaluated till its bifurcation. Proximal segment of

KEY POINTS

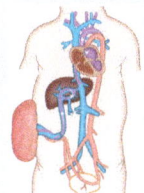

Lower limb arterial Doppler technique
- Complete examination mandates evaluation from the aortoiliac level to the dorsalispedis artery using gray scale, CDFI and pulsed Doppler.
- Aortoiliac vessels are examined with 2.5–3.5 MHz transducer with patient in the supine position.
- For femoral artery evaluation the patient is placed in supine position with abduction at hip and flexion at the knee joint.
- Popliteal segment should be examined with patient in the prone position with slight flexion at the knee joint.
- Anterior tibial artery is localized lateral to the anterior tibial cortex below the knee joint and followed distally till ankle.
- Posterior tibial artery should be looked for behind the medial malleolus and then followed proximally, till it joins the peroneal artery.

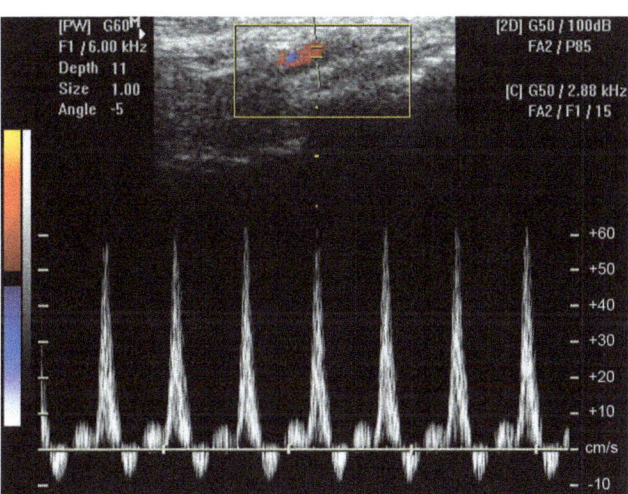

Fig. 17.1: Duplex Doppler tracing from right femoral artery shows triphasic waveform characteristic of a peripheral artery.

the profundafemoris is examined. The superficial femoral artery is followed distally. The transducer may have to be placed posteromedially in the lower thigh for examining the adductor canal region. A lower frequency transducer may be used if there is any difficulty in visualization. Popliteal artery is examined with the patient in prone position with knees slightly flexed. It is followed till its bifurcation. At this point, the anterior tibial artery goes deep to transducer, as it perforates the interosseous membrane to enter the anterior compartment of the leg. Posterior tibial artery is best evaluated by first looking for it behind the medial malleolus with the patient in prone position. Alternatively the patient may be in supine position with leg abducted and flexed at knee. Once localized the artery is followed proximally till it meets the peroneal artery. Peroneal artery is difficult to evaluate as compared to posterior tibial artery. It is seen posterior to fibula with the patient in prone position. Anterior tibial artery is seen below the knee, lateral to the anterior border of the tibia, as it emerges through the interosseous membrane. It can be easily followed along its course till the ankle joint where it becomes the dorsalispedis artery.

Arterial waveforms are obtained from following locations:
- Aorta
- Common and external iliac arteries
- Proximal, middle, and distal superficial femoral arteries
- Popliteal artery
- Anterior and posterior tibial arteries
- Dorsalis pedis artery.

Any sites of increased flow disturbance are noted. Entire length of each vessel must be scanned to avoid missing sites of localized stenosis. Color mapping provides only a single velocity parameter, which is a mean frequency estimate. Color imaging is also subject to aliasing, which may be seen as apparent change in direction. Dependence on angle of insonation may result in color changes caused by change in direction of flow rather than change in velocity. Finally relatively slow frame rate of image acquisition for color scanning results in spatial and temporal distortion, one portion of the vessel may be imaged in systole and another during diastole, resulting in appearance of a velocity change along the length of the vessel. Thus, it is important to confirm the findings by taking the spectral tracing in the region of abnormality seen on CDFI. Spectral waveforms should be obtained from the center of the vessel to avoid spectral broadening caused by the steep velocity gradient at the wall.

Upper Limb

Subclavian artery continues as axillary artery lateral to the first rib. It course medially over the proximal humerus to become the brachial artery. Brachial artery divides into radial, ulnar and interosseous artery in the interosseous fossa. Doppler flow pattern of the upper limb arteries is similar to that seen in the lower limb arteries.

Technique

Proximal subclavian arteries can be imaged above the sternoclavicular joint. Caudal angulation of transducer is usually required for optimal visualization. It can also be seen by placing the transducer in the supraclavicular fossa. Axillary artery can be imaged through the axilla, along the medial aspect of the proximal humerus. Brachial artery can be easily identified in the arm and traced distally. Another alternative approach to image the vessel at the elbow is where it is superficial and then follow it proximally. Radial artery can similarly be localized at the wrist and followed proximally.

Clinical Aspect of Peripheral Arterial Disease

The most common cause of peripheral arterial occlusive disease is atherosclerosis. Predisposing factors for this includes hypertension, diabetes and smoking. Aortoarteritis is a common cause in India, which usually affects proximal vessels in young females. This disease causes marked thickening of the arterial walls with luminal narrowing. Thromboangiitis obliterans or Buerger's disease is seen in males with history of smoking.

Clinical features of the peripheral arterial disease include intermittent claudication, rest pain, non-healing ulcer in the leg and gangrene. Extremities may be numb or cold. Patient may have one or more of the features mentioned above. On examination affected limb may be cold on palpation. Skin may show trophic changes. Arterial pulses can be weak or absent. On auscultation a bruit may be heard in the region of stenosis.

Other noninvasive tests are also used for evaluation of peripheral arterial disease. These include pressure studies, segmental pressure measurements, ankle/brachial indices, etc. These tests help in establishing the presence of arterial disease, its possible site and severity.

Ankle/brachial index is one of most frequently used test. Blood pressure is taken at the level of ankle joint and in the brachial artery. Normal value of this index is more than one. Value less than 0.9 suggests that an arterial problem is present in lower extremity. Ankle-brachial index corelates well with clinical symptoms of the disease (Table 17.1).

Once the suspicion of the peripheral arterial disease is aroused on ankle brachial index measurement, segmental pressure measurements are taken in the thigh and the leg for approximate localization of the diseased segment. A drop of more than 20 mm Hg pressure indicates likely presence

TABLE 17.1: Relation between symptoms and ankle/brachial index.

Ankle/brachial index	Presentation
> 1.0	Normal
0.9–1.0	Asymptomatic or minimal disease
0.5–0.9	Intermittent claudication
< 0.5	Rest pain, severe disease

of disease in that particular segment. However, precise localization of site of disease is usually difficult and they are of limited value in disease involving multiple segments.

Diagnosis on Doppler Imaging

The waveform of a normal peripheral artery is triphasic (Fig. 17.1). This waveform is altered in presence of arterial stenosis or occlusion. Analysis of the velocity pattern provides the most useful information regarding the hemodynamic significance of atherosclerotic lesion. Loss of triphasic pattern, variable loss of spectral window and widening of spectra with fairly-preserved color flow and PSV are signs of atherosclerosis signifying loss of pliability of vessel wall. As already described initial survey carried out by CDFI enables rapid identification of site of flow abnormality, which is then interrogated by pulsed Doppler to obtain the spectral wave forms. Waveforms are also obtained proximal and distal to stenosis. Ratio of peak systolic velocity in the stenosed segment to that in proximal segment is calculated to determine hemodynamically significant stenosis.

Proximal to the stenosis the waveform is usually normal. The findings in the stenotic region depend upon the severity of lesion and help in determining the degree of stenosis (Table 17.2).

In mild to moderate stenosis, the early diastolic reversal decreases and disappears with increasing severity of the lesion. Along with this increase in the diastolic flow is seen. With increasing severity of the lesion, forward flow through the artery increases and the diastolic velocity may approach near the systolic velocity. This increasing diastolic velocity is probably due to decreased peripheral resistance caused by dilatation of arterioles in the muscular bed in response to release of metabolites caused by local ischemia. Opening up of many small collateral pathways also contribute to decrease in peripheral resistance. Peak systolic velocity is less affected by vasodilatation. Therefore, this parameter is used to quantify the degree of stenosis. Artery distal to a high grade stenosis or occlusion show a slow rise, low amplitude (Tardus-Parvus) waveform (Figs. 17.2 to 17.4).

Accuracy

Many studies have compared sensitivity, specificity and diagnostic accuracy of Doppler with angiography as gold standard. Result of these studies are summarized in Table 17.3. Detection of calcification and thrombus is better with CDFI as compared to angiography. Detection of collateral vessel is poor.

Therapeutic Approaches

Once a hemodynamically significant stenosis or occlusion has been confirmed, some sort of therapeutic intervention is required to stop the progression of disease and to provide symptomatic relief to the patient. The therapeutic approach depends upon site, extent and severity of the lesion. Various options available are listed in Table 17.4.

TABLE 17.2: Findings and stenotic region depend on severity of lesion.

Stenosis	Findings
1. Normal	• Normal triphasic waveform
2. 1–19%	• Normal waveform outline • Normal peak systolic velocity • Slight spectral broadening
3. 20–49%	• At least 30% increase in peak systolic velocity compared to normal proximal segment • Prominent spectral broadening • Normal proximal and distal waveform
4. 50–99%	• More than 100% increase in peak systolic velocity compared to proximal segment • Loss of reverse flow (monophasic signal) • Extensive spectral broadening • Distal waveform monophasic with reduced systolic velocity
5. Complete occlusion (Fig. 17.2)	• No color on CDFI no flow on pulsed Doppler • Echogenic thrombus in artery • Damped waveform proximal to occlusion • Distal waveforms monophasic with decreased velocities (tardus-parvus waveform)

Evaluation of Bypass Graft by Doppler

The CDFI and Duplex Doppler ultrasound are the technique of choice for the postoperative monitoring of the bypass graft patency and to detect focal stenosis or any other cause of graft dysfunction.

In the immediate postoperative period, gray scale imaging is useful to evaluate the surgical bed of the graft, to locate perigraft collection which may be due to infection or pseudoaneurysm (discussed later in the chapter).

Synthetic Bypass Grafts

Complications affecting the synthetic graft depend upon the type of graft and time since surgery. In the early period (1-2 years since surgery) graft stenosis and occlusion may be due to technical reasons or development of fibrointimal

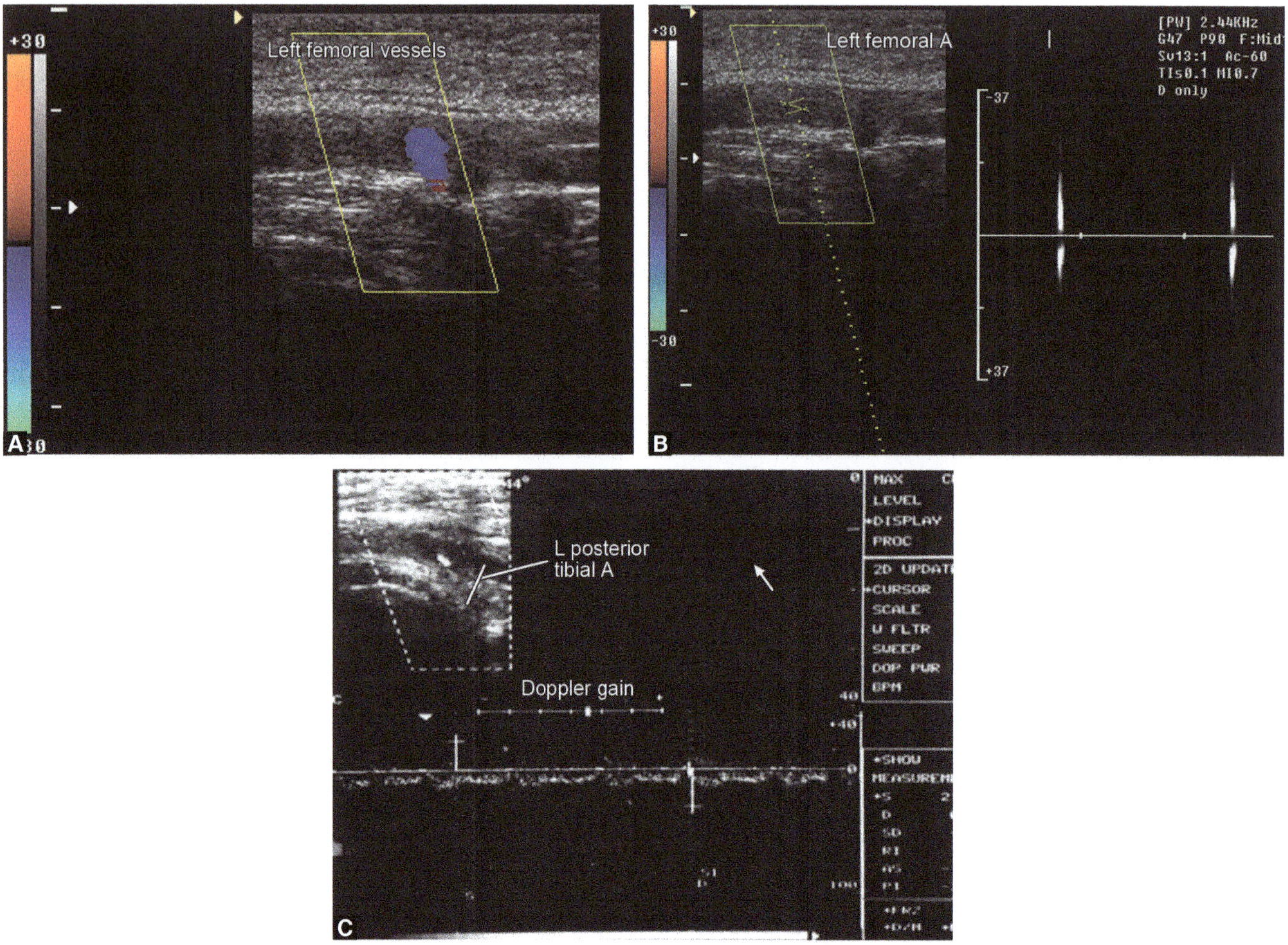

Figs. 17.2A to C: Thrombosis of superficial femoral artery—(A) Color Doppler image shows absence of flow in the distal superficial femoral artery; (B) Pulse Doppler shows attenuated waveform proximal to the point of occlusion; (C) Spectral tracing from posterior tibial artery in the same patient shows delayed peak with low amplitude (Tardus-Parvus) waveform.

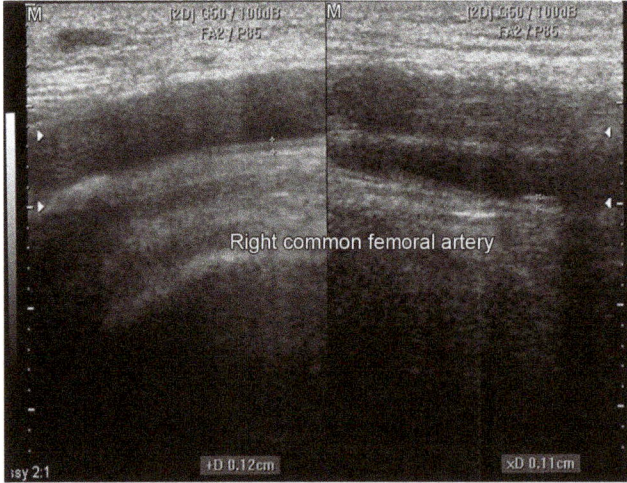

Fig. 17.3: Gray scale image showing thickening of the intima media complex s/o arteriosclerosis.

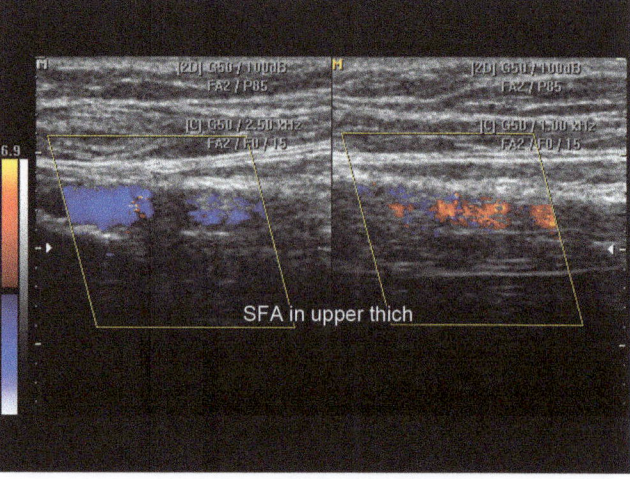

Fig. 17.4: Color Doppler shows fragmented color pattern in the superficial femoral artery s/o chronic partially recanalized thrombus.

TABLE 17.3: Efficacy of Doppler examination in the evaluation of lower limb arterio-occlusive disease.

	Jager et al. (1986)	Moneta et al. (1987)	Kohler et al. (1987)	Cossman et al. (1989)	Polak et al. (1990)	Whalen et al. (1992)	Sharma et al. (1996)
Sensitivity	96	77	82	83	88	92	65.6
Specificity	81	98	92	96	95	97	96.2
Positive predictive value	92	94	80	91	—	90	88.5
Negative predictive value	91	92	93	91	—	98	86.3
Accuracy	76.3	—	—	90	93	96	86.8

TABLE 17.4: Therapeutic options in peripheral arterio-occlusive disease.

Lesion	Preferred mode of therapy*
1. Diffuse aorto-femoral or aortoiliac disease	Dacron graft

2. Popliteal artery above the knee joint (occlusion or long segment narrowing)	• Polytetrafluoroethylene graft (PTFE)
	• Venous graft
	  – Reversed superficial vein
	  – *In situ* superficial vein

3. Popliteal artery below the knee and other leg vessels (occlusion, long segment of narrowing)	• Venous graft

4. Short segment narrowing in limb vessels	• Percutaneous interventions
	  – angioplasty
	  – atherectomy
	  – stent

*Extensive lesions may also be recanalized with the help of thrombolytic agents.

lesions at the anastomotic site. In the later stage graft failure is usually due to development of stenotic/occluding lesion in the native vessel proximal or distal to the graft. Late anastomotic pseudoaneurysm may occur in femoral anastomosis of aortofemoral graft.

Development of an anastomotic stenosis will cause significant increase in the velocity signals but increase in velocity, or turbulence of flow may be normal depending upon the nature of connection. This normal increase may be up to 100% without being pathologic. If such finding is noted, serial monitoring is indicated. If there is progressive increase in the velocity at the site of turbulence, it indicates development of stenotic lesion. Absence of signal in a graft is diagnostic of occlusion.

Autologous Vein Graft

Two types of venous grafts are used in bypass surgery reverse vein and *in situ* vein. In the reverse vein type of graft a native superficial vein is harvested and reversed. It is then anastomosed to the native artery, proximal and distal to the diseased segment. In the *in situ* technique the superficial vein is left in its bed (greater or lesser saphenous vein). The valves in the veins are lysed. Perforating branches are ligated. Proximal and distal segments of the veins are mobilized and anastomosed with the arterial segments.

Early cause of graft malfunction differs depending upon the time since the surgery. In early failure seen within one month, technical factors are the main causes. These include poor vein selection, poor suture line placement, poor selection of the anastomotic site, unsuspected arteriovenous fistula and poorly lysed venous valves. In second period lasting from one month to 2 years following surgery, graft malfunction may occur secondary to fibrointimal hyperplasia at the site of anastomosis or at the site of venous valves. Late failures beyond 2 years period are secondary to progression of atherosclerotic disease in the arteries proximal and distal to anastomosis.

Monitoring of venous bypass grafts has traditionally been performed by serial measurements of the lower extremity pressures, but Doppler sonography is superior to pressure measurements for monitoring and evaluation of suspected graft dysfunction. Measurement of the velocity can be used to identify the graft with high possibility of failure. Previously this approach consisted of measuring the peak systolic velocity in the narrowest segment of graft,

KEY POINTS

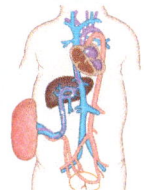

Peripheral arterial aneurysm
➠ Arteriosclerosis is the most common cause with involvement of the Popliteal arteries being the commonest.
➠ Focal enlargement of the artery with diameter more than 20% of the normal is highly specific for the diagnosis.
➠ CDFI is most helpful in diagnosis of completely thrombosed aneurysm.
➠ Other peripheral arteries and the aorta must always be examined for presence of associated aneurysm(s), which are present in many of these patients.

with velocity less than 45 cm/sec indicating presence of graft malfunction. But this criterion identifies only the severely diseased graft. Present approach aims at identifying the areas of stenosis in the graft which are likely to progress, causing restriction and finally occlusion of the flow. The graft is surveyed with CDFI. Site of stenosis is identified and spectral analysis is performed. Severity of stenosis can be determined by obtaining ratio of peak systolic velocities in the diseased segment with the velocity obtained in segment 2-4 cm proximal to it. Ratios greater than two correspond to 50% diameter stenosis, ratio greater than three indicates 75% stenosis. Presence of tandem lesions limits the usefulness of this technique. It has been shown that early lesions can develop within three months after surgery and can be detected by Doppler evaluation even before the patient develops symptoms. Intervention in the form of surgical revision of stenosis is indicated. Stenosis with systolic ratio above three or four usually requires this form of intervention.

Aneurysms

Peripheral arterial aneurysms are usually due to arteriosclerosis which causes weakening of the vessel walls. Popliteal artery is the most common site of aneurysm in the lower limb followed by the superficial femoral artery.

Ultrasound is now universally accepted as imaging modality of choice for diagnosis of a suspected aneurysm. A bulge or focal enlargement of 20% of the expected vessel diameter is consistent with diagnosis of aneurysm. Ultrasound can visualize the presence of intraluminal thrombus. With color Doppler patent lumen can be visualized and complete thrombosis can be diagnosed with more certainty, compared to ultrasound alone (Fig. 17.5A). Ultrasound is the ideal modality for follow-up of these cases. There are no strict criteria to determine the suitability of the patient for surgery. An aneurysm more than 2 cm in size usually requires surgical repair. Presence of distal embolization is an absolute indication for surgery, irrespective of its size. Since arteriosclerosis is a generalized diffuse process involving all parts of the arterial system, one might expect that aneurysmal degeneration would occur at multiple locations. In fact, the 40% of peripheral arterial aneurysms are multiple. Thus, detection of any aneurysm in the peripheral artery mandates a thorough search for detection of aneurysm in the other limbs and aortoiliac vessels (Fig. 17.5B).

Pseudoaneurysm

Pseudoaneurysm is defined as a contained rupture of the arterial wall. It develops sometimes as a complication of penetrating trauma or arterial catheterization. Common femoral artery is the most frequent site, because most of these lesions develop following arterial catheterization. Risk of development depends upon the size of catheter and anticoagulant therapy. On ultrasound a cystic mass is seen in relation to parent vessel. Communicating channel may be visualized on gray scale sonography. Appearances on CDFI are characteristic. A swirling motion of color 'ying-yang' sign (Fig. 17.6A) is seen within the cystic mass. The communicating channel or the 'neck' of the pseudoaneurysm is exceeding well seen with color Doppler on Duplex sonography, "to and fro" (Fig. 17.6B) sign is

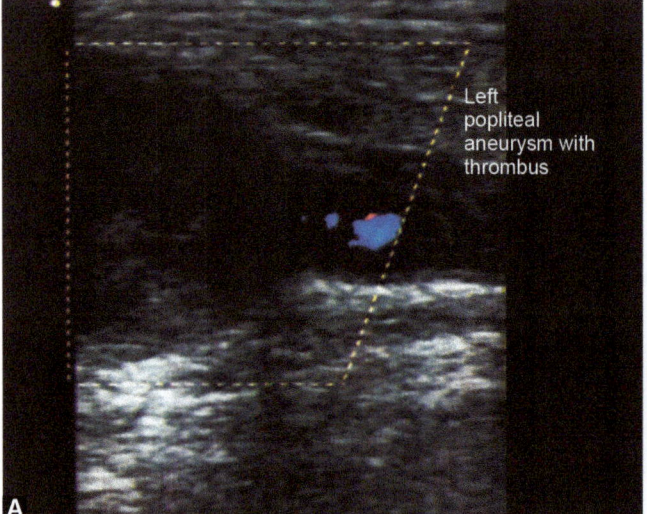
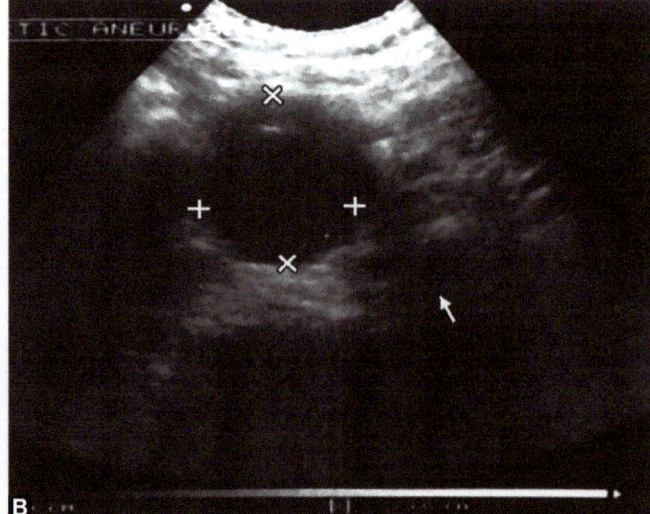

Figs. 17.5A and B: (A) Color Doppler flow image at the level of popliteal artery. Fusiform enlargement of popliteal artery is seen suggesting presence of an aneurysm. No color flow is demonstrable; (B) Gray scale image in the same patient shows associated aneurysm, with mural thrombus, in aorta below the level of renal hilum.

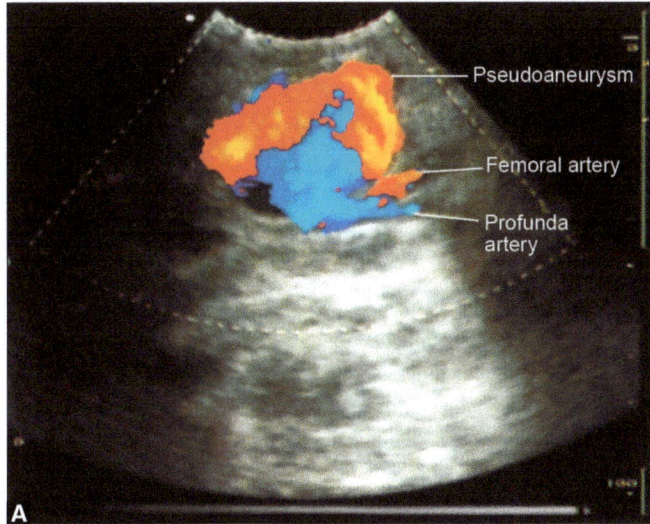 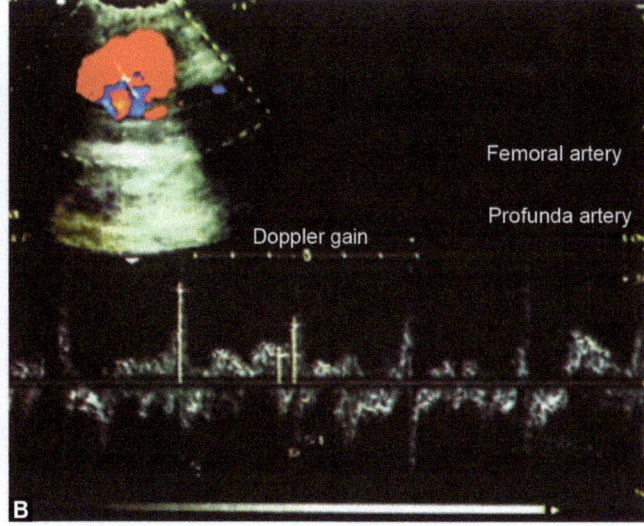

Figs. 17.6A and B: (A) Color Doppler shows swirling motion of color with the cystic mass; (B) The communicating channel is also well seen on color Doppler as "to and fro" sign.

KEY POINTS

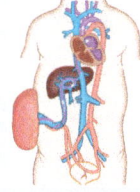

Pseudoaneurysms
- These are most commonly due to penetrating trauma or arterial catheterization.
- "Color swirl" on CDFI and "to and fro" sign on pulsed Doppler examination are diagnostic.
- Transcutaneous compression therapy with the ultrasound probe can obliterate many of these lesion.

typically seen in the neck or the communicating channel. The 'to' component is seen due to blood entering through the communicating channel into the pseudoaneurysm. High velocity settings may be needed for detection. During diastole, the blood present in the cavity returns to main arterial lumen causing the 'fro' component. Pseudoaneurysms can have multiple compartments.

Left to themselves pseudoaneurysms may undergo spontaneous thrombosis and closure on bed rest. There are two therapeutic approaches to this problem. If the surgeon decides to do surgery, the site of communication can be marked on skin and preoperative angiogram is not required. Direct "transcutaneous compression therapy" can also be used for obliterating these lesions with CDFI as guide. This intervention is successful if applied to pseudoaneurysm developing within a week of acute event. Later than this, endothelialization of communicating channel occurs, which hamper its occlusion. Direct pressure is applied with ultrasound probe over the neck of pseudoaneurysm. Probe is positioned in the long axis of the artery and flow in pseudoaneurysm cavity is obliterated by firm compression applied till twenty minutes. If initial compression is not successful the procedure can be repeated up to three times. Many reports have documented high success rate of this procedure. Pseudoaneurysm in upper limb arteries can also be treated by this therapy. Arterial or venous thrombosis, may occur rarely. Pseudoaneurysms may also occur following bypass graft. These postsurgical pseudoaneurysms are usually seen with synthetic vascular graft, at the site of distal anastomosis. This is probably due to weakening of the arterial wall at the anastomotic site, causing dehiscence. The communicating channel is not seen and the pseudoaneurysm is contiguous with the anastomosis. Thus, the doppler 'to and fro' sign is not seen. 'Ying yang' appearance is seen on CDFI. A patulous anastomosis should be distinguished from the anastomotic pseudoaneurysm. Surgical anastomosis is made wider to compensate for diameter differences between the graft and artery and subsequent fibrointimal hyperplasia. This causes appearance of vessel dilatation at the site of anastomosis. Patulous anastomosis shows continuation of wall of the artery and the graft, while pseudoaneurysm is seen as an eccentric mass lying in the soft tissues. Thrombus may be seen in the wall of pseudoaneurysm.

Arteriovenous Fistula

Arteriovenous fistula may be:
- Congenital
- Traumatic which may be due to penetrating injury or following angiography
- Created as part of dialysis shunt.

Congenital arteriovenous fistulas are communications between artery and large distended veins. These lesions are clinically obvious, as they cause discoloration of skin and trophic changes. Multiple venous channels with arterial branches feeding them can be seen on the skin. Diagnostic utility of ultrasound is limited. It can help in selecting the area for injection of sclerosing compounds and monitor the lesion following sclerotherapy.

Traumatic fistula may develop following penetrating trauma or following catheterization of the artery or vein. These lesions can be readily diagnosed with CDFI (Fig. 17.7A). The affected vein shows turbulence and is enlarged in size compared to its counterpart in the opposite limb. The fistulous communication is more easily seen with CDFI than with the Duplex scanning. On Duplex scanning the affected vein shows turbulence and arterialized waveform (Fig. 17.7B). Turbulent waveform in the vein can also be seen if there is extrinsic compression of the vein due to hematoma, another complication which can occur due to catheterization. CDFI is extremely helpful in such cases, as it can demonstrate the arteriovenous connection with ease. Arterial waveform proximal to the communication will show increase in the diastolic flow due to reduced resistance in the vein (Fig. 17.7C). Distal artery will show a normal waveform. The arteriovenous fistula should also be evaluated for venous flow during Valsalva maneuver. In lesion with small communicating channel the venous velocity will decrease. If there is complete cessation of flow, it indicates that the lesion in all probability will undergo spontaneous closure over a period of time. These lesions can be followed with CDFI and active intervention is not needed. Transcutaneous compression therapy under ultrasound guidance has been tried in larger lesions. Success rate for this form of therapy is 30% or lower.

Arteriovenous fistula may be created for hemodialysis. In the present day, clinical practice bypass grafts are most frequently used. They are inserted in the forearm and are made of either synthetic material (polytetrafluoroethylene or PTFE) or autologous vein. Complications which may occur in these access channels include development of small or large aneurysm, pseudoaneurysm or graft stenosis. These complications can be evaluated readily by color

KEY POINTS

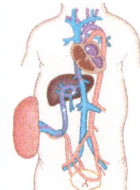

Arteriovenous fistula
- Causes: congenital, traumatic, as part of the dialysis shunt.
- Increased diastolic flow is seen in the feeding artery.
- Venous waveform shows turbulence and arterialization.

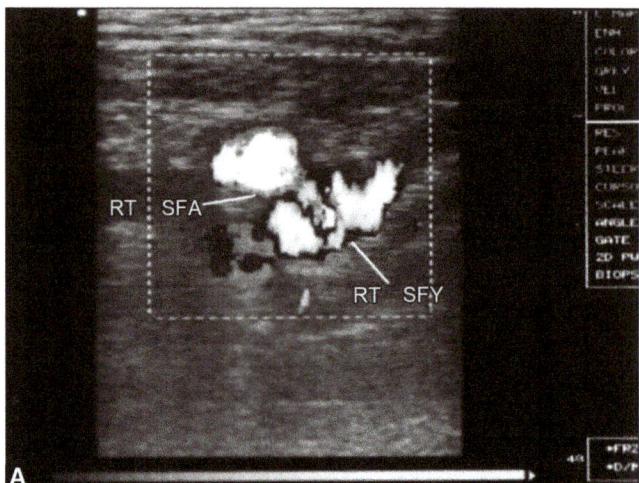

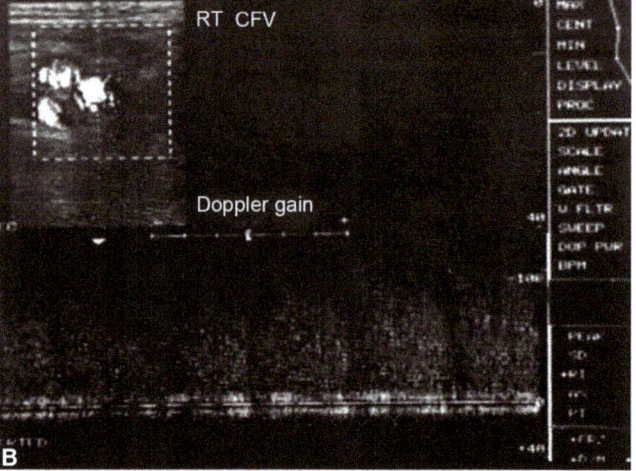

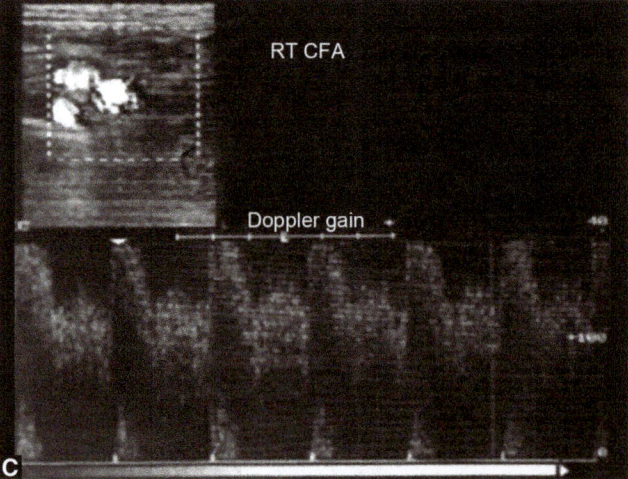

Figs. 17.7A to C: (A) Color Doppler image at the level of upper thigh shows a communication between superficial femoral vessels; (B) Pulse Doppler in common femoral vein shows turbulent high velocity waveform; (C) Pulse Doppler in common femoral artery proximal to fistula shows persistent antegrade flow in diastole.

Doppler flow imaging. Pseudoaneurysms can be diagnosed with accuracy greater than 90%. The detection of stenosis accuracy depends upon the type of graft. In straight segment graft the sensitivity and specificity have been reported to be 95% and 97% respectively. In graft having a tortuous path sensitivity and specificity are reportedly less (92% and 84% respectively). Overall accuracy is 86%.

In a normal graft peak systolic velocities range between 100 and 200 cm/sec. Waveform shows turbulence, this is seen as irregular waveform contour and filling of the spectral window. A significant stenosis is diagnosed in presence of a focal area within the graft showing peak systolic velocity ratio greater than two when compared with the velocity of the feeding artery. Presence of velocities less than or equal to 50 cm/sec also indicate presence of high grade stenosis.

Evaluation of dialysis shunts should also include examination of subclavian vein. Stenosis occurs at the site of proximal subclavian vein in 20-50% of the cases. They are seen in individuals, who had temporary hemodialysis access with placement of large diameter catheters.

Chapter 18

Venous System

Sonography is the preferred modality for the evaluation of the venous system. Veins are easily visualized on the gray scale sonography. Addition of Duplex and more recently color Doppler flow imaging has enabled quick visualization of normal and abnormal venous dynamics. With the advent of CDFI, role of venography has become limited. Additional benefits of CDFI include:
- Short examination time
- Elegant real time visual demonstration of physiological and pathological states
- Evaluation of deep seated veins like subclavian veins.

LOWER LIMB VEINS

These consist of superficial veins, deep veins and perforating veins.

Superficial veins: Greater and lesser (small) saphenous veins form the superficial venous system. Greater saphenous vein begins near the medial malleolus and terminates in the common femoral vein below the inguinal ligament. It is the longest vein in the body. It may be duplicated. Lesser saphenous vein begins adjacent to the medical malleolus and terminates in the popliteal vein in the calf.

Perforating veins: These are the channels between the superficial and deep venous system, which allow the flow to occur from superficial to the deep venous system. They communicate with the saphenous veins through the arch branches of the saphenous veins.

Deep veins of the limbs comprise of three paired veins in the calf namely posterior tibial veins, anterior tibial veins and peroneal veins. They join to form the popliteal vein in the popliteal fossa. Popliteal vein continues as the superficial femoral vein at the level of the adductor canal. This vein is joined by the profundafemoris vein in the thigh to form the common femoral vein. Above the inguinal ligament, this vein is known as external iliac vein. The external iliac vein joins the internal iliac vein to form the common iliac vein. The common iliac veins from two sides join together to form the inferior vena cava. Deep veins contain numerous valves to prevent backflow of the blood. The veins are accompanied by the arteries which bear the same name. The veins are usually larger than the arteries in caliber.

UPPER LIMB VEINS

Superficial venous system of the upper limb consists of cephalic and basilic veins. Cephalic veins run laterally. The basilic vein runs along the medial aspect of the forearm.

Deep venous system comprises of radial and ulnar veins, which join to form brachial vein in the proximal forearm. This vein continues as the axillary vein at the lower border of the teres major. Axillary vein becomes the subclavian vein at the outer border of the first rib. This vein joins the internal jugular vein to form the brachiocephalic vein. The brachiocephalic veins from two sides unite to form the superior vena cava.

INSTRUMENTATION AND TECHNIQUE

The ultrasound equipment for evaluation for venous system of the extremities should have a high resolution imaging capability with additional facility of Duplex and color flow imaging capable of picking up slow flow.

In most patients 5–7.5 MHz linear array transducer is adequate for the gray scale evaluation. In obese patients lower frequency transducer may be required. Evaluation of the pelvic veins and the inferior vena cava is done with

Venous System

KEY POINTS

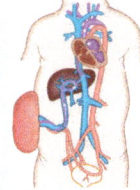

Technique for lower extremity venous Doppler
- 5–7.5 MHz linear array transducer is required for the limb veins; 3.5–5.0 MHz curvilinear array transducer for pelvic veins and the inferior vena cava.
- Patient position supine with elevation of the head. Hip is kept in flexion and external rotation.
- Identify the common femoral vein in the transverse plane, continue examination distally; oblique orientation is needed for adequate visualization of the saphenofemoral junction.
- CDFI and pulsed Doppler is performed intermittently to evaluate phasicity, compressibility, response to Valsalva maneuver and augmentation.
- In adductor canal region CDFI and pulsed Doppler examination is a must as compression may not obliterate the vein completely.
- Popliteal vein is evaluated in the prone position.
- Posterior tibial vein is localized posterior to the medial malleolus and followed proximally, anterior tibial vein is examined from below knee in supine position lateral to the anterior tibial cortex and then followed distally.

3.5 MHz transducer. Doppler evaluation can be performed with same transducer frequency. Additional capability of beam steering is desirable as it allows use of shallower Doppler angles. The Doppler parameters should be adjusted to pick up slow flow. Larger sample volume should be used to cover the entire diameter of the vein.

Lower Limb Veins

Optimum positioning, patient comfort, and cooperation are essential prerequisite for a high quality Doppler examination of the lower extremity venous system. The patient should be in supine position with elevation at the head end. This position increases venous filling and makes them prominent, thus enabling adequate evaluation of small veins. For the evaluation of the femoral veins the leg should be partially flexed at the hip and the hip should be in external rotation. Ultrasound gel is applied from the groin to the knee to facilitate continuous examination. The evaluation, which includes gray scale, Duplex and color flow imaging, should begin from just above the inguinal ligament in the transverse plane. Longitudinal sections are helpful for pulsed Doppler evaluation. Common femoral vein is identified adjacent to the common femoral artery. Vein can be distinguished from the artery because of following features:
- Medial location
- Larger size
- Lack of pulsations
- Compressibility on applying pressure.

The examination continues distally in the transverse plane, with compression of vein at regular intervals. Saphenofemoral junction is identified and examined for competence. Inferiorly bifurcation into the superficial femoral vein and the profundafemoris vein can be seen. Superficial vein is then followed distally till the lower third of the thigh, where it moves away from the transducer to enter the adductor canal. A lower frequency transducer is required for evaluation. The vein is less amenable to compression in this region, thus careful Duplex and color Doppler evaluation is needed to determine the normal hemodynamics.

Popliteal vein is examined in the prone or the lateral decubitus position. The examination begins from the upper popliteal fossa and continues inferiorly till the bifurcation. Posterior tibial vein evaluation usually starts posterior to the medial malleolus of tibia, where it is visualized as paired structure along side the artery of the same name. The examination is then continued upward till the tibioperoneal trunk. Peroneal veins can be visualized lateral to the posterior tibial vessels; they most often lie in relation to the posterior surface of the fibula. Anterior tibial veins are scanned in the supine position of the leg between the anterior surface of the tibia and fibula. They are difficult to evaluate in the superior part as they may be obscured by bony outlines of the tibia and fibula.

In cases of thrombosis of common femoral vein, external iliac and common iliac veins up to the formation of inferior vena cava must be examined to determine the extent of disease.

Saphenofemoral junction: It is identified just below the groin. Examination in oblique plane may be required for proper visualization. A valve may be identified at this level. The great saphenous vein is followed into the upper thigh. *Small saphenous vein* may be seen in the popliteal fossa. It is followed upwards till its entry in the popliteal vein. Gastrocnemius vein may cause confusion, but the small saphenous vein can be followed from the popliteal vein into the subcutaneous plane, while the gastrocnemius vein is limited to the muscle plane. The perforating veins are not seen in the normal patients.

Gray scale examination should include assessment of compressibility, presence of thrombus and presence of valves. Evaluation of flow dynamics like phasicity, augmentation, competence of valves can be done by color Doppler (Figs. 18.1A and B). Spectral analysis is performed to confirm and document the findings visualized on CDFI.

Upper Limb

Upper limb veins are examined in the supine position with head tilted away from the side being examined. The subclavian vein is seen above the sternoclavicular joint at the root of neck, its junction with the internal jugular vein may be seen in some patients. CDFI and Duplex evaluation is done in this medial portion, as the vein is not amenable to compression by the transducer. A phasic flow should be seen in the normal vein. Middle portion is not directly accessible due to overlying clavicle; patency of this segment can be ascertained by presence of normal flow in the proximal and distal segments. Lateral portion of the subclavian vein continues as the axillary vein. Junction of the cephalic and axillary vein is seen at the outer end of the first rib. Axillary vein is examined by raising the arm and resting it on the examination table with palm facing upwards. Distally the examination continues till the brachial venous bifurcation. Examination of the radial and ulnar veins should be started at the wrist and the veins should be followed proximally along their accompanying arteries.

Examination of the neck veins is also performed along with proximal veins of the upper limbs, as the pathology may involve both of them simultaneously. Internal jugular vein is traced from the root of neck to the angle of mandible. The vein is located anterolateral to the common carotid artery. Doppler evaluation shows prominent bidirectional flow due to transmitted cardiac pulsation. External jugular vein is smaller in size than the internal jugular vein. It lies lateral to the internal jugular vein along the posterior border of the sternocleidomastoid muscle.

CHARACTERISTICS OF A NORMAL VEIN

On gray scale imaging a normal vein has echo free lumen. Walls are thin and may be slightly echogenic. Venous valvular leaflets may be seen as thin echogenic structures in the lumen. On pulsed Doppler, monophasic, and low velocity blood flow is seen. Mild fluctuation in velocity is seen with phase of respiratory cycle, slow flow is seen during inspiration and faster flow during expiration (phasicity) (Fig. 18.2). In normal upper limb veins, spontaneous phasic flow is seen with bidirectional pattern. The retrograde component is due to contraction of the heart. Various maneuvers are employed to demonstrate patency and normal hemodynamics.

Compression (Figs. 18.3A and B): Gentle pressure over the vein by the transducer causes apposition of the wall and obliteration of the lumen in a normal vein. This finding can be easily appreciated on gray scale imaging in transverse plane. Complete obliteration of lumen on mild compression effectively rules out acute thrombosis.

Augmentation (Fig. 18.4): This refers to increase in the blood flow in the vein when distal limb is compressed by hand. This feature can be seen on both on CDFI and pulsed Doppler and is suggestive of patency of venous segment between site of compression and examination. Weak augmentation may be seen in partial thrombosis, or development of venous collateral in the settings of acute thrombosis. Augmentation should be avoided in patients with acute venous thrombosis because of associated risk of embolism.

Valsalva maneuver (Fig. 18.5): The patient is asked to take a deep breath and bear down. This causes increase in the intra-abdominal pressure and retards the venous return towards the heart. In simple words, patient may be asked to hold breath at the peak of inspiration or to simulate

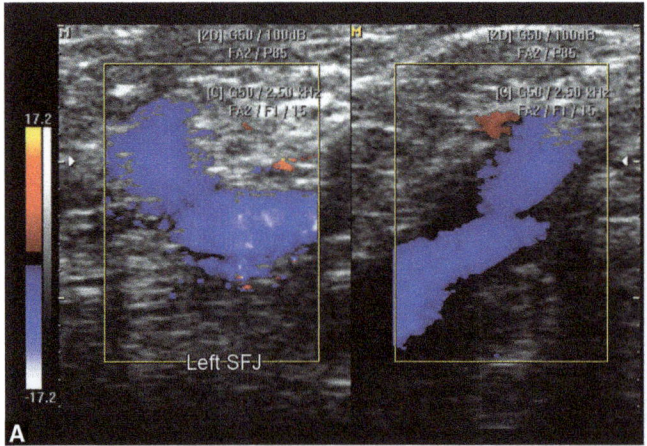 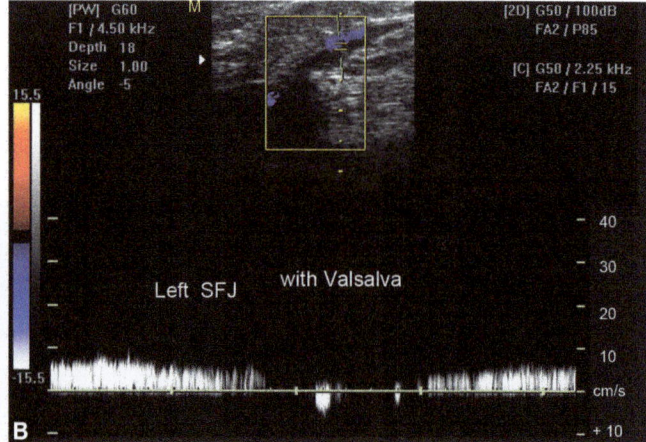

Figs. 18.1A and B: (A) Color Doppler shows similar color flow in common femoral and great saphenous vein; (B) Duplex Doppler shows competent saphenofemoral junction while performing Valsalva.

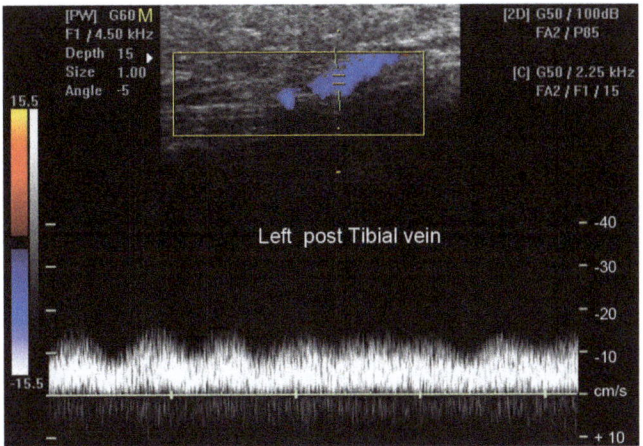

Fig. 18.2: Normal venous waveform; Pulse Doppler image of common femoral vein shows low velocity monophasic flow with respiratory variation (phasicity).

the process of defecation. Pooling of blood occurs in the abdominopelvic and proximal lower extremity veins, causing their dilatation. This feature can be appreciated on gray scale imaging. On CDFI, decrease in color is seen followed by complete cessation. On pulsed Doppler complete cessation of the flow can be documented. A positive test in the femoral veins is indicative of patency of proximal venous system. This maneuver is also used to establish the competence of the saphenofemoral junction. Reversal of color flow and direction of flow is noted in case of incompetent saphenofemoral junction.

LOWER EXTREMITY DEEP VENOUS THROMBOSIS (FIG. 18.6)

Detection of deep vein thrombosis (DVT) accounts for majority of venous system examinations. Detection of

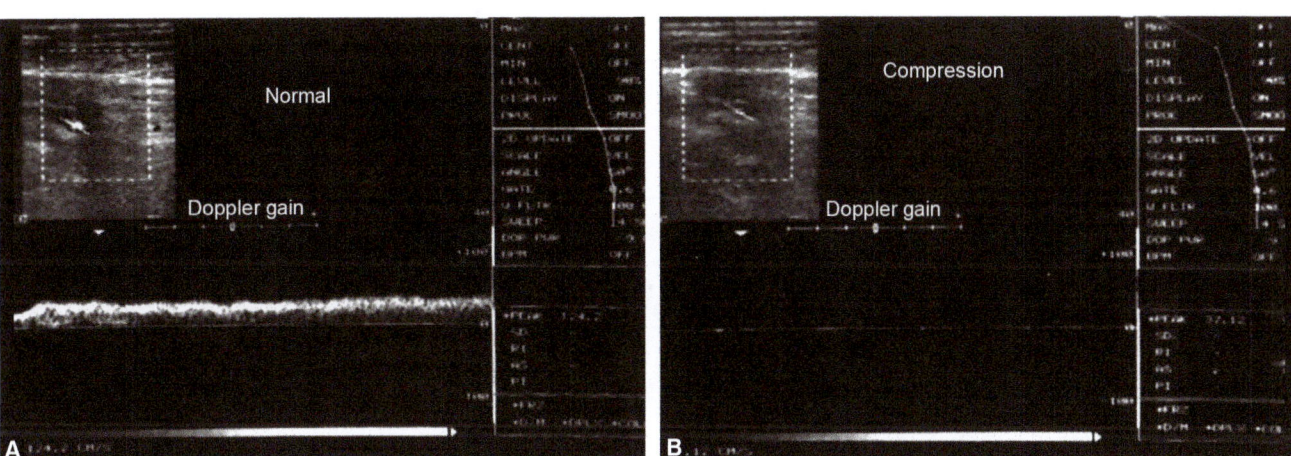

Figs. 18.3A and B: (A) Transverse section through upper thigh shows common femoral vein (arrowhead); (B) On applying gentle transducer pressure, venous lumen is obliterated.

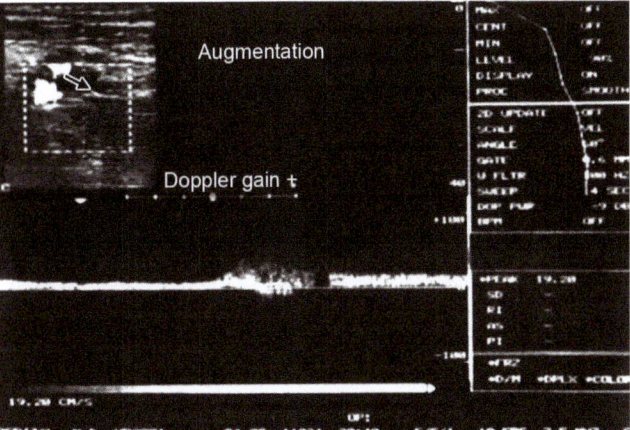

Fig. 18.4: Longitudinal pulse Doppler image femoral vein showing augmentation of blood flow (arrow) on compression of distal lower limb.

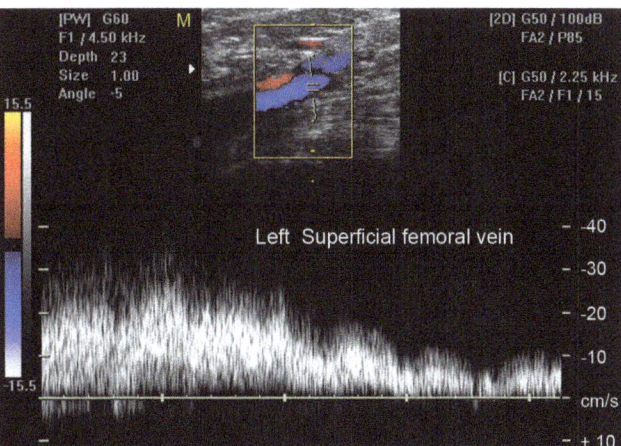

Fig. 18.5: Longitudinal pulse Doppler image of superficial femoral vein showing progressive decrease in venous flow on performing Valsalva maneuver.

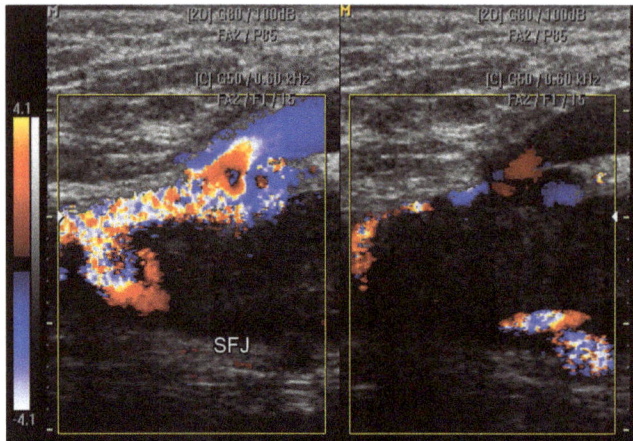

Fig. 18.6: Color Doppler show an intraluminal thrombus in common femoral vein.

KEY POINTS

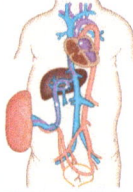

Deep venous thrombosis: sonographic and Doppler findings
- Lack of venous compression, direct visualization of the thrombus. In a thrombus completely filling the lumen, no color is seen on CDFI, no signals are seen on pulsed Doppler interrogation.
- CDFI is better for evaluation of the pelvic veins, adductor canal region and the calf veins.
- Loss of phasicity and absence of normal response on the Valsalva's maneuver suggests obstruction in the proximal venous system.
- Lack of augmentation is seen in obstruction of the distal venous system.
- Partially occluding thrombus is best evaluated with the CDFI.

this entity is important because it can cause pulmonary embolism.

Clinical considerations: Acute deep venous thrombosis is the most common indoor vascular disorder. In the initial stages the thrombus develops in the calf veins. Approximately 40% of these thrombi resolve spontaneously, 40% organize focally. Proximal progression in the popliteal and femoral veins occurs in only 20% of the cases. Acute thrombus is loosely attached and has tendency to embolize. Conditions and factors, which predispose to thrombosis include:
- Prolonged bed rest
- Malignancy, particularly in pancreas, lung or gastrointestinal tract
- Administration of estrogens including oral contraceptives
- Disseminated intravascular coagulation
- Post-partum period, and
- Paralysis.

Symptoms and signs of the deep venous thrombosis consist of pain, swelling, and erythema. These features are however non-specific and may be seen in a large number of local and systemic conditions. Most of the patients are asymptomatic and development of pulmonary embolization may be the first clue to the presence of thrombosis. Lack of specificity of clinical evaluation along with risk of severe life-threatening complication associated with the deep venous thrombosis has prompted search for a non-invasive technique which provides accurate diagnosis in this condition. Impedance plethysmography measures venous capacitance and the rate of venous outflow from the lower extremities. In expert hands it has sensitivity ranging from 87% to 100% and specificity ranging from 92% to 100% for detection of DVT above the knee. Its sensitivity for detection of isolated calf vein thrombosis is 17–33%. Multiple radionuclide techniques have been developed but have not been sufficiently accurate to mandate a role in the diagnostic evaluation. A large number of studies have proven the sonography as the ideal and in most cases the only technique required for the diagnosis. Gray scale US supplanted with Doppler flow assessment has proved to be extremely accurate (sensitivity, 88–100%; specificity, 92–100%) for detection of femoropopliteal DVT and occlusive thrombosis of the external and common iliac veins. One significant limitation of standard Duplex sonography has been the difficulty in identifying and assessing the deep veins of the calf. A second limitation has been the inability to directly image the common and external iliac veins because of their depth from the skin and presence of overlying bowel gas. CDFI vividly displays venous blood flow, thus allowing direct imaging of the entire venous system. Unlike other non-invasive methods, CDFI allows calf veins to be readily examined in most patients. Also evaluation of the abdominal veins is better as compared to other modalities. MRI may detect DVT with equal ease, it also has the additional advantage of assessing deep abdominal and pelvic veins, but its relatively steep cost and limited availability is a major limiting factor.

Sonographic and Doppler Findings

Lack of venous compression is the most sensitive and specific finding with a sensitivity of 93% and specificity of 97%. It is not necessary to compress every continuous millimeter of the venous lumen searching for the clot. In the symptomatic patient, clot usually involves whole or multiple venous segments. Direct visualization of thrombus is a highly specific finding but it is not seen in all cases, as an acute thrombus may be completely anechoic. Increase in the diameter of the thrombosed vein is also seen. Change in venous calibre with respiration and increase in size in

response to the valsalva maneuver is lost. Several pitfalls may occur during venous evaluation include:
- Improper technique
- In patients with large extremities evaluation may be difficult
- Recanalization of the vessel causing residual wall thickening
- Subacute clot may not distend the vein
- Normal valsalva maneuver is seen in partially occluding thrombus; also this maneuver has limited value below the knee.

Gray scale imaging may be unable to visualize some parts of the deep venous system; the problem areas include calf veins, adductor canal where compression is difficult and pelvic veins, which may be obscured by the overlying bowel gas. Pulsed and color Doppler imaging play a significant role in evaluating these areas. Pulsed Doppler should be performed along with gray scale imaging. Absence of flow is seen in cases of thrombosis. Loss of phasicity in a patent segment is suggestive of proximal thrombosis. Lack of augmentation on distal compression, points towards obstruction in the distal venous system. On color Doppler, venous thrombosis is seen as an area of color void (Figs. 18.7A and B). Partial non-occluding thrombus, which may not be detected on gray scale and duplex sonography, is well demonstrated on CDFI. Gray scale imaging along with duplex and color Doppler also help by providing alternative diagnosis in patient with limb swelling, these conditions include Baker's cyst, aneurysm and lymphadenopathy, etc.

When lower extremity venous thrombosis is noted, the upper extent of the clot should be determined. Clot extending above the inguinal ligament necessitates assessment of the pelvic veins and, if necessary, the inferior vena cava to see the upper margin. This information is necessary to determine the site for filter placement and will also provide the documentation of the present extent of the clot. Resolution of thrombus can be seen on sequential studies (Fig. 18.8).

CHRONIC DEEP VENOUS THROMBOSIS

The distinction between acute and chronic thrombus is important because of increased tendency of the acute clot to embolize. Acute clot is more likely to progress proximally. Acute thrombus is usually anechoic or hypoechoic with smooth borders. The vein is enlarged in size. With time the thrombus becomes organized. Chronic occlusion causes wall thickening of the involved segments. These changes lead to poor visualization of the clot and incomplete venous compression. CDFI plays a significant role in differentiation of acute and chronic venous thrombi. The features, which may be observed in chronic DVT, include:
- Irregular, echogenic thickening of vein walls
- Reduced caliber with fragmented color flow
- Atretic venous segments
- Presence of venous collaterals.

UPPER EXTREMITY THROMBOSIS

Thrombosis of the deep veins is the most common abnormality of the upper extremity venous system. Causes of upper extremity DVT include:
- Acute or repetitive trauma

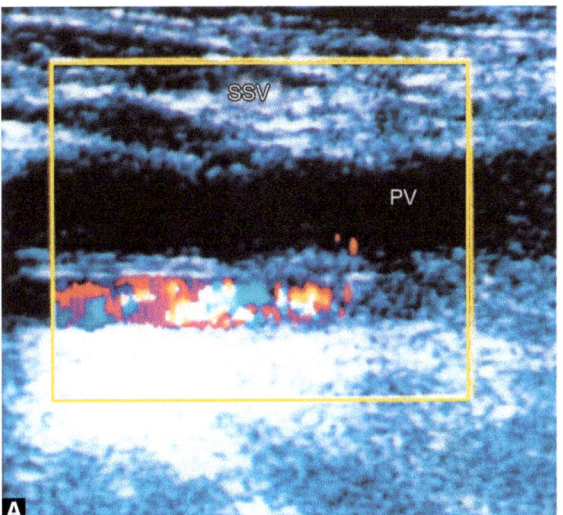
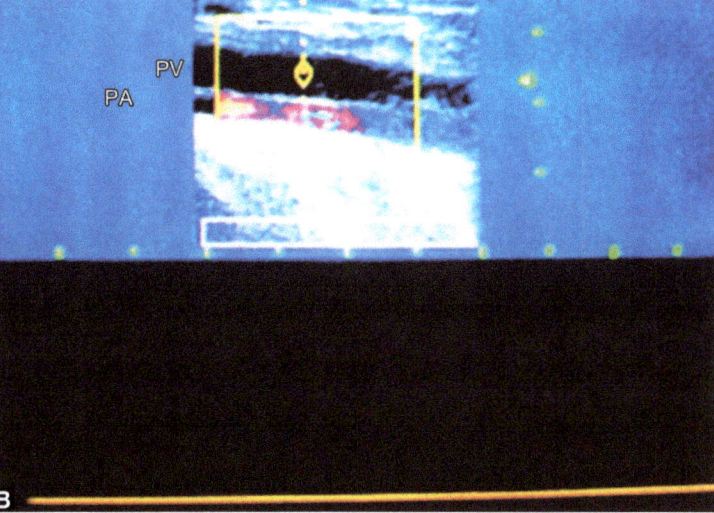

Figs. 18.7A and B: (A) Color Doppler in a patient with limb swelling shows enlarged popliteal vein with absent color; (B) Spectral tracing from the vein revealed absence of flow.

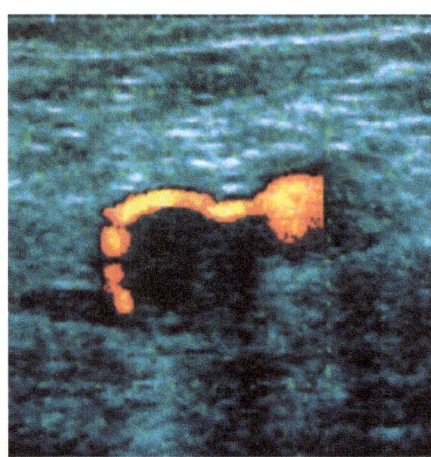

Fig. 18.8: Follow-up power Doppler in a case of deep vein thrombosis shows partial canalization of lumen.

- Vigorous exercise
- Anatomic abnormalities like cervical rib
- Extrinsic compression by malignancy
- Focal infection
- Intravenous drug abuse
- Indwelling central venous catheters.

Only 10-12% of patients with arm DVT develop pulmonary emboli and majority of these are insignificant. Clinical features of DVT in upper limbs are less severe because of development of extensive collateral pathways and lack of hydrostatic pressure. Basic principles for evaluation of the upper extremity are the same as those for the lower limbs. As subclavian and brachiocephalic veins are not easily compressible, evaluation with CDFI assumes more importance. Venous flow is assessed for phasicity, augmentation, and waveform. Features, which may be seen in a case of thrombosis, include:

- Incomplete compression
- Persistent visualization of filling defect on CDFI
- Absence or reduction of transmitted cardiac pulsations
- Abnormal response to the valsalva maneuver
- Detection of large collateral veins

Sensitivity of CDFI for detection of venous thrombosis in upper extremity ranges from 78-100% and specificity from 92-100%. Lower accuracy is a result of technically difficult examination of the upper limbs.

Venous insufficiency: In competence of venous valves may be primary (not preceded by DVT) or it may follow venous valvular damage following DVT (post-phlebitic syndrome). The valvular damage in venous insufficiency leads to valvular incompetence. Incompetence may be intermittent or persistent and may be observed in:

1. Deep venous system
2. Saphenofemoral and/or saphenopopliteal junction and
3. Perforating veins.

KEY POINTS

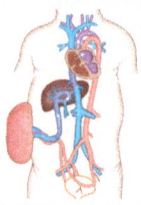

Venous insufficiency
- The patient should be examined in erect position with weight transferred to the opposite limb.
- Proximal veins are evaluated with the Valsalva's maneuver while techniques are better for the distal veins.
- A very short period of flow reversal is normal and should not be construed as an evidence of abnormality.

Venous incompetence is assessed by examining the patient in erect position, facing the examiner, holding onto a support, to provide stability and eliminate unwanted contraction of the leg muscles. The weight of patient is placed mainly on the opposite limb.

Deep venous system: The number of valves in the deep veins increases distally. Hence, proximal valvular damage produces more hemodynamic abnormality. For complete assessment the following veins must be examined:

a. Common femoral vein
b. Proximal superficial femoral vein
c. Distal superficial femoral vein
d. The popliteal vein
e. Proximal and distal posterior tibial vein
f. Proximal and distal anterior tibial vein
g. Proximal and distal peroneal vein
h. Dorsalis pedis vein.

Saphenofemoral junction (Fig. 18.9): It is visualized in the groin, for Duplex evaluation the sample volume should be placed in the proximal great saphenous vein. Sample volume should include entire lumen, by putting the cursors on the inner walls. For examining saphenopopliteal junction, the patient faces away from the examiner and the leg is slightly flexed at the knee. The probe is placed on the skin and its position is adjusted so that three structures can be identified in a sagittal plane. The popliteal artery lying deepest, the popliteal veins lying more superficial to it, and the short saphenous vein most superficial. Because of variation in the anatomy of the saphenopopliteal junction, careful scanning above and below the popliteal fossa is necessary before individual veins can be identified. Other veins that should be identified and scanned for incompetence are the gastrocnemius veins. They drain into popliteal and/or short saphenous veins. They may be confused with short saphenous vein but can be differentiated from it, as they do not reach the subcutaneous tissue plane, as is the case with short saphenous vein.

Perforating veins: It can be identified with real time imaging by scanning transversely along the long and short saphenous

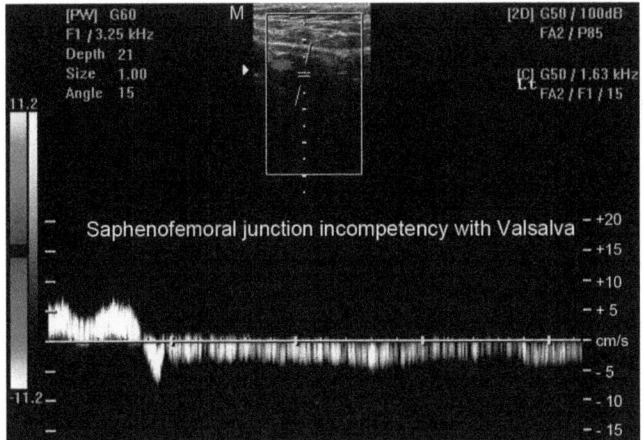

Fig. 18.9: Duplex Doppler shows incompetent saphenofemoral junction while performing Valsalva as revealed by continuous flow in the reverse direction with Valsalva.

veins or the posterior arch of the long saphenous vein. For this examination, the patient stands as described previously or sits on a couch with leg positioned vertically over the edge and the foot resting on a stool on which examiner is sitting facing the patient. Perforating veins can be seen dipping from the superficial veins towards the deep system. The probe is rotated in a manner that the superficial and deep veins are visualized in a longitudinal plane with the perforating vein joining the two. All visualized perforators are not incompetent. The incompetent perforators usually have a large lumen usually more than 3 mm in diameter.

Proximal venous structures like common femoral vein, proximal superficial femoral vein and great saphenous veins are best evaluated using Valsalva maneuver. On performing this maneuver, a normal vein shall show progressive reduction followed by cessation of color on CDFI. In presence of incompetent valves, venous reflux will be seen as change in color, lasting for variable duration, depending upon the degree of valvular incompetence.

Distal augmentation maneuver is more useful for evaluation of distal femoral vein, popliteal vein, posterior tibial vein and saphenopopliteal junction. Brisk distal compression causes increased antegrade flow in the venous system. The compression is then released. A very short period of flow reversal may be seen in normal veins due to effect of gravity, but this reversal ceases, as the returning blood encounters the first competent venous valve.

Incompetent veins have a greater degree of flow reversal, lasting for a longer period of time. On CDFI, this is seen as change in color. On pulse Doppler tracing change in flow direction is seen.

In perforating veins normal direction of flow is from the superficial to the deep venous system. Retrograde flow is prevented by the presence of venous valves. In presence of incompetent perforators, flow augmentation causes reflux of blood from deep to superficial venous system. On CDFI, this is seen as flow towards the transducer placed on the skin (normally coded red). Site of incompetent perforators can be marked on skin to enable surgeon to accurately ligate these veins.

Spectral display may be helpful to quantitate the degree of reflux. It may be graded as follows:

Grade I : reflux lasting for 1–2 sec.
Grade II : reflux lasting for 2–3 sec.
Grade III : reflux lasting for 4–6 sec.
Grade IV : reflux lasting more than 6 sec.

Preoperative saphenous vein mapping: Infrainguinal bypass procedures, that use an autogenous saphenous vein can be aided by a detailed preoperative assessment. Better information about the venous anatomy and any anatomic variations results in improved use of veins and precise planning of the specific surgical procedure for the bypass procedure. Duplex scanning along with CDFI has proved to extremely valuable for saphenous vein mapping.

Technique: Patient's limb is placed in a dependent position by asking him to stand or sit upright with legs unsupported. The examination starts at the knee. A transverse section is used to localize the great saphenous vein and patency is confirmed by compressing it. Probe is then rotated to get a longitudinal image and its position is marked with a small line by using a waterproof marker. The vein is then traced along its entire course. Coupling gel is used sparingly, so that the skin surface can be marked easily.

Tributaries are more easily seen on transverse images, anterior and posterior tributaries are marked 'A' and 'P'. Veins crossing the main system are marked with 'X' at the crossover point. Site of perforators is also marked. If a double system is found their arrangement is recorded.

When the examination is complete, gel is wiped from the skin, the preliminary map made with waterproof marker is traced using permanent marking ink. This imprint lasts for 3–4 days.

Chapter 19

Intravascular Ultrasound: Newer Advances, Current Applications and Future Directions

INTRODUCTION

Catheter-based angiography is still the most valuable modality to make the diagnoses and guide interventional procedures in coronary and peripheral vascular disease. However, it has many limitations, pathologic studies have revealed that angiographic interpretation frequently leads to an under- or overestimation of disease severity.[1-3] Angiography depicts the arteries as a two-dimensional view of the contrast-filled lumen, hence any arbitrary projection can misrepresent the true extent of stenosis, particularly for eccentric lesions.[4] The estimation of degree of stenosis by angiography relies upon comparison with an uninvolved normal segment. Autopsy studies demonstrate that there is no truly normal segment, the disease usually being diffuse in nature. Also, angiography is limited in its ability to assess the disease mechanism and composition of the obstructive lesion.

Over the last few years, intravascular ultrasound (IVUS) has emerged as new technique to assess vascular pathology. It refers to the acquisition of cross-sectional images of the target vessel by an ultrasound probe placed on the tip of an endoluminally positioned catheter.

RATIONALE FOR INTRAVASCULAR ULTRASOUND IMAGING

The application of IVUS to vascular imaging has evolved based upon several characteristics inherent to ultrasound technology. Due to the tomographic orientation of ultrasound, the full circumference of the vessel wall can be visualized and not just a two-dimensional view. This enables comprehensive assessment of angiographically difficult areas such as diffusely diseased arteries, eccentric lesions, ostial stenosis and angiographically fore-shortened segments. Also, measurements are performed using an electronically generated scale, thus offering an advantage over angiographic stenosis estimation which needs to be corrected for radiographic magnification.[4,5]

A unique feature of IVUS is its ability to provide qualitative information about plaque composition and its response to interventional strategies. The consistency of plaque (soft, fibrous, calcific or mixed) and its differentiation from thrombus is well demonstrated by IVUS. Various studies have demonstrated a good correlation between the histopathology of the atheromatous plaque and its echogenicity on IVUS.[6,7]

The IVUS imaging has been used mainly for coronary interventions. The following description focuses on the present day role of IVUS in imaging and intervention in peripheral vascular disease and its applications in the future.

Technical Aspects

The equipment required to perform intravascular ultrasound consists of two major components: a catheter with a miniaturized transducer at its tip and a console containing the electronics necessary to reconstruct the image. Frequency of the ultrasound used is typically centered at 12.5–40 MHz. For peripheral vascular imaging, 20 MHz is the most used frequency. Larger vessels such as the aorta require frequency in the range of 12.5–20 MHz. There are two types of catheter systems: those with an end-hole which are delivered over the guide wire, and those which do not have an end-hole and are introduced directly through the sheath. Larger catheters are introduced through larger guiding catheters and sheaths.

Although the reduction in transducer size results in a decrease in resolution, this is partially compensated for the use of higher frequencies. Typically, the wavelength at 30 MHz is 50 μm, yielding a practical axial resolution of 150 μm.[8] Determinants of lateral resolution are more complicated and depend on imaging depth.

Two basic approaches to transducer design have been evaluated: phased-array and mechanical type. In the phased-array systems, multiple transducer elements (32-64) in an annular array are activated sequentially to generate the image. Mechanical probes use a drive cable to rotate a piezoelectric transducer at 1800 rpm, yielding 30 images per second. The advantages and limitations of the two designs are compared in Table 19.1.

Image Interpretation

A well-defined imaging protocol is vital for proper interpretation of IVUS images in the peripheral vascular tree. A slow pullback of the transducer from the distal to the proximal vessels segments is the optimal way to acquire reproducible information about vessel architecture and catheter orientation. Most centers use a motorized pullback system to withdraw the catheter at a predetermined constant rate. Standard perivascular landmarks and side branches as seen on angiography and ultrasound are used to ensure that repeated measurements (e.g. pre- and post-intervention) are assessed at the same position within the artery.

Normal Arterial Anatomy

The generation of ultrasound images is based on the difference in the acoustic impedance of the layers of the vessel wall. Due to this difference, these layers reflect US differently.

Blood

On IVUS images, blood has a characteristic speckled pattern that is constantly changing in echogenicity with the cardiac cycle being slightly more echogenic during systole.[9] In real time imaging, sometimes the lumen/intima interface may be difficult to distinguish when the blood flow is slow and stagnant, such as proximal to a severe stenosis. In such situations, the increased backscatter from blood may give the false impression of thrombus or plaque. One more reason for increased backscatter from blood may be the incorrect adjustment of the control for near field gain (time gain compensation or TGC). When the TGC is set too high, blood speckle becomes accentuated, masking the lumen/intima border.[10]

KEY POINTS

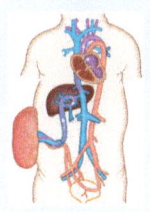

IVUS: General principles
- Very high frequency transducers ranging from 12.5–40 MHz are required.
- Phased array and mechanical type of transducers can be used.
- Large elastic arteries have two layered appearance; muscular arteries appear three layered.

TABLE 19.1: Comparison between phased-array and mechanical IVUS transducers.

Phased-array transducers	Mechanical transducers
1. Can be coupled with smaller catheters	1. Require relatively larger catheters
2. Flexible and hence can be guided into smaller and tortuous vessels with ease	2. Stiffer, hence traversing the aortic bifurcation or reaching the visceral vessels is difficult without the use of guiding catheters
3. Non-uniform rotation in tortuous vessels is not a problem	3. Non-uniform rotation may be a problem due to the presence of a drive cable and moving parts
4. Can be easily incorporated into interventional devices	4. May be difficult to couple with interventional catheters
5. Complex in design	5. Designing is comparatively simple
6. Relatively expensive	6. Less costly

Arterial Wall

The wall of the artery is composed of the intima, internal elastic lamina, media, external elastic lamina, and adventitia (Fig. 19.1). The intima consists of a monolayer of endothelial cells which in itself is beyond the resolution of current ultrasound catheters. However, if there is intimal hyperplasia, it may be detected as a thin echogenic layer (Fig. 19.2).[11] The internal elastic lamina is seen as the innermost thin echogenic layer.[7] Because of its high echogenicity, the actual thickness of the layer may be overestimated (a phenomenon referred to as blooming), which may sometimes make it difficult to distinguish from mild intimal proliferation.[11] The outermost layer, i.e. the adventitia is collagen-rich and is thus bright in appearance.

The echogenicity of the media, depends upon the relative content of smooth muscle on one hand and collagen and elastin on the other. The latter are strongly echoreflective, and in objective terms, the reflectance of collagen is about 1000 times more than that of muscle.[10] The relative composition of the media is different for the

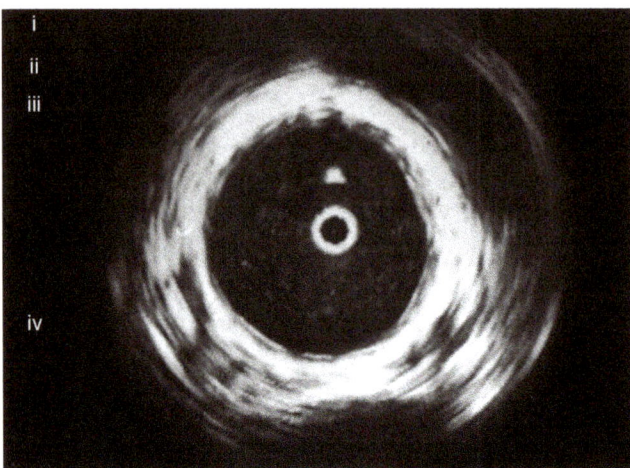

Fig. 19.1: IVUS image in a normal subject: 3-layered appearance (i) Thin inner echogenic layer (internal elastic lamina), (ii) Middle hypoechoic layer (media), (iii) Outermost echogenic layer (adventitia). Blood around catheter seen as speckled pattern.

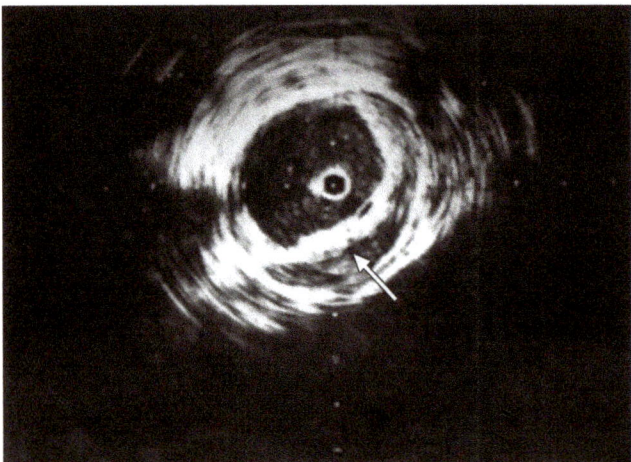

Fig. 19.2: IVUS image showing eccentric increase in thickness of inner layer (arrow)—intimal hyperplasia.

elastic and muscular arteries. The aorta, pulmonary artery, and the proximal segments of the brachiocephalic, carotid, subclavian and common iliac arteries belong to the elastic type. All other arteries such as the coronary, renal and femoral are the muscular type. The media of the muscular arteries is composed largely of smooth muscle cells, and thus it is poorly echoreflective, forming a large acoustic mismatch between the surrounding layers, resulting in a three-layered appearance on the US image.[12] Large elastic arteries have a media that contains a higher relative amount of collagen and elastin which make this layer strongly echoreflective. Hence, the distinction between the three layers is less marked, resulting in a two-layered appearance.[13]

APPEARANCE ON IVUS IN VARIOUS DISEASE STATES

Atherosclerosis: Studies have compared the ultrasound appearance of plaques to histology in freshly explanted human arteries.[13,14] Currently IVUS is the most reliable imaging modality that identifies the composition of arterial plaques.

Gussenhoven et al.[15] proposed that there are essentially four basic relationships between plaque composition and its echogenicity on IVUS: hypoechoic, representing a high lipid content of plaque; soft echoes, representing fibromuscular tissue; hyperechoic, representing collagen-rich (fibrous) plaque; and hyperechoic with lack of through transmission, representing calcium (Fig. 19.3). Hodgson et al.[16] studied IVUS morphology in human coronary arteries and correlated the image obtained with angiography. They classified IVUS images into 5 morphological subtypes: (a) soft, (b) fibrous, (c) calcific, (d) mixed (Fig. 19.4), (e) concentric subintimal thickening. They found that compared with stable angina, patients with unstable angina had more soft lesions (greater lipid content) (74% vs 41%), fewer calcified and mixed plaques (25% vs 59%) and intralesional calcium deposits (16% vs 45%). IVUS demonstrated a greater sensitivity than angiography for identifying unstable lesions (74% vs 40%). These observations have important implications for peripheral vascular disease as well. It is the plaque composition, rather than the stenotic severity, that predicts the vulnerability of a lesion to rupture and produce acute symptoms. This information is most reliably provided by IVUS and no other imaging modality.

Plaque measurements: Atheroma area is determined by planimetry of the intimal leading edge and external elastic lamina (EEM), thus including the media in measurements. The media is included due to two reasons: the spread of ultrasound signal of the intimal plaque into the media, obscuring the trailing edge of the intima (known as 'blooming'), and the media not being consistently seen as a truly sonolucent layer. Measurements performed in this manner have shown a close correlation with histological assessment.[14,15]

Plaque burden or "percent area stenosis" refers to the percentage of the EEM area occupied by the atheroma. This quantitative ultrasound measurements is usually substantially greater than that made on angiography due to two major reasons: the diffuse nature of the disease affecting even the angiographically "normal reference sites", and the expansion of the EEM which occurs as a response to atherosclerosis (known as positive remodeling)[17,18] and maintains a constant luminal area during the early stages (Glagov effect).

KEY POINTS

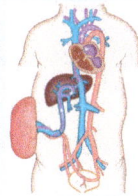

IVUS in atherosclerosis
- IVUS is most reliable method for identification of composition of the arterial plaque.
- Hypoechoic plaque has high lipid content.
- Soft plaque is rich in fibromuscular tissue.
- Hyperechoic plaque mainly contains collagen.
- Hyperechoic plaque with shadowing is mainly composed of calcium.
- Unstable plaques are more reliably identified with IVUS as compared to angiography.

The majority of plaques are seen to be eccentric in location on IVUS studies. This observation has important implications for guiding interventional procedures, particularly for directional atherectomy and other selective plaque removal techniques.

In some vessel segments, instead of vessel expansion, vessel shrinkage may occur, which has been referred to as deremodeling or negative remodeling. This may actually contribute to luminal stenosis. Recently, this phenomenon has been implicated in restenosis after interventional procedures.[19]

Other Disease States

Thrombus: Thrombus is echogenic, and may be difficult to distinguish from a noncalcified fibrous plaque or even stagnant blood. It however, has a typically scintillating or sparkling pattern on real time US examination. The presence of microchannels, and an echodensity of less than 50% of the adventitia is important clues to its correct identification.[20,21]

False lumen: A false lumen may occur spontaneously or commonly following endovascular interventions. Mistaking a false lumen for true lumen can have serious consequences if the former is selected for stent or stent-graft placement (as in aortic dissections). IVUS may help in such situations by: recognition of the characteristic three-layered appearance of true lumen; identification of side branches taking off from the true lumen; and by the slow flowing, more echogenic blood within the false lumen. In addition, flush injections of contrast may at times reveal the echogenic patterns of the contrast to "hang-up" and take longer to evacuate from the false lumen compared to the true lumen.

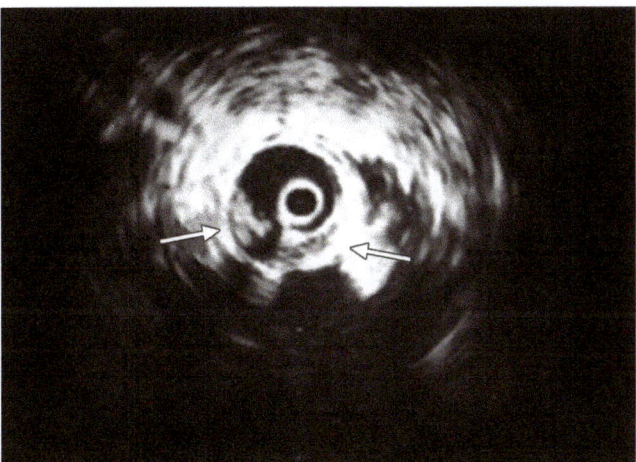

Fig. 19.3: Same patient at another level: fibrous plaque (arrows) with outer echogenic line with distal acoustic shadowing (calcium).

Aneurysm: A true aneurysm is differentiated histologically from a false aneurysm by the presence of media in the former. IVUS can detect the presence of hypoechoic media to distinguish the two entities, although at times the media may be very thinned out.

Nonspecific aortoarteritis: Sharma et al.[22] reported the IVUS imaging findings in aorta in Takayasu's arteritis. They observed that intima is unaffected and remains thin. There is increase in the echogenicity and thickness of the media. The adventitia is also similarly affected with diffuse periarterial fibrosis (Figs. 19.5 and 19.6). Due to these changes, the characteristic three-layered appearance may not be seen at places. There may be calcification. The compliance of the aortic wall may be seen to be lost on real time imaging. Importantly, these changes were observed even in the angiographically "normal" segments of the vessel, emphasizing the diffuse nature of involvement by the disease.

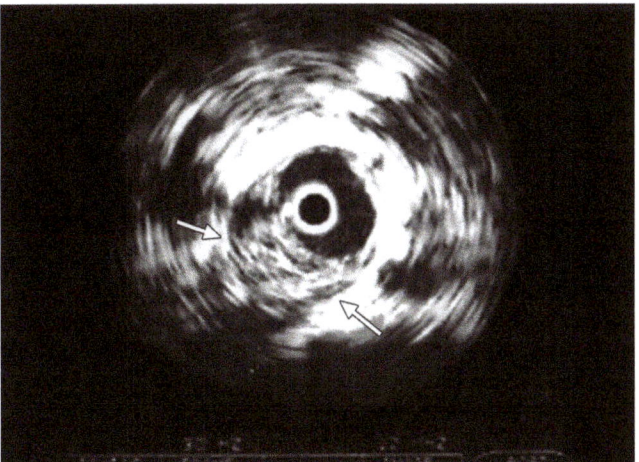

Fig. 19.4: IVUS image of aorta in a 58-year-old male: arrows point to mixed echogenicity plaque.

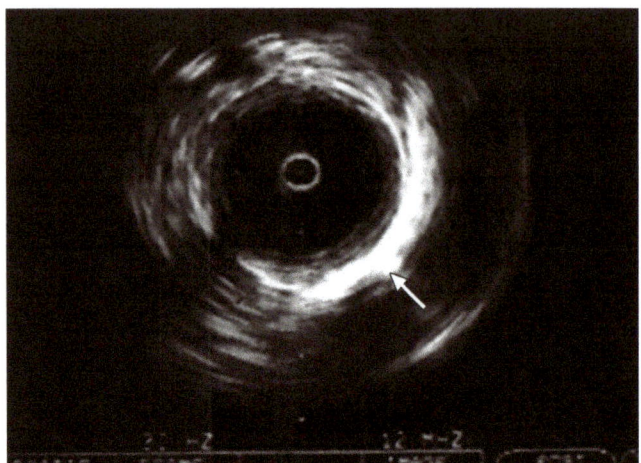

Fig. 19.5: Young hypertensive female: thick echogenic media and adventitia (arrow) with thin innermost layer, suggesting aortoarteritis.

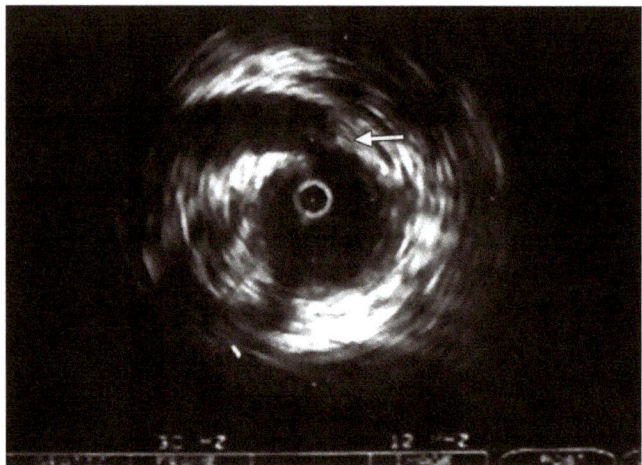

Fig. 19.6: Same patient as in Figure 19.5: Renal artery take-off (arrow) seen in upper part of image with stenosis at its ostium. Aortic wall shows thick echogenic media.

CLINICAL APPLICATIONS

Quantitative ultrasound: Angiography permits only monoplanar assessment of the lumen diameter, while IVUS allows planimetric measurement of the artery lumen as well as the vessel wall area. This leads to underestimation of the disease, as has been consistently demonstrated by various studies.

Balloon angioplasty: A major mechanism of percutaneous transluminal angioplasty (PTA) is the creation of cracks and dissections of atherosclerotic plaques with localized medial dissection. This has been clearly demonstrated by IVUS studies.[23] Concentric lesions that dissected during PTA achieved a greater lumen gain compared to those that did not dissect or were eccentric in location.[24] The detection of a large intimal flap created during PTA mandates a repeat prolonged inflation or stent placement. Hence, the use of IVUS can help determine the end-point of angioplasty.

Accurate determination of balloon size is enhanced by using IVUS to measure vessel diameters. In addition, IVUS can help in selecting an appropriate recanalization technique by virtue of its ability to differentiate a stenosis produced by thrombus, plaque or mural abnormality.

The amount and distribution of calcium may have a significant impact on the outcome of angioplasty procedures.[25] This can be reliably detected by IVUS. Compliant lesions without a definite fibrocalcific structure are more likely to have elastic recoil following PTA, whereas large calcific deposits may predispose to more severe tearing of the vessel wall.

The IVUS is helpful after PTA when pressure gradients still exist despite a satisfactory angiogram as it provides a direct anatomical assessment of the residual stenosis. Angiography consistently underestimates the degree of residual narrowing even when performed in multiple projections.[26]

Stenting: Endovascular stenting is performed for complex lesions, total occlusions, or in cases with suboptimal response or obstructive dissection following PTA. Due to the brightly echogenic appearance of the metal struts, stents are easily recognized on IVUS. IVUS is extremely valuable in assessing the degree of apposition of the stent to the vessel wall, an information not obtained on angiography.[27] In cases with incomplete apposition, balloon dilatation within the stent should be performed. This is important since any space left between the stent and the endothelium will be occupied by thrombus, delaying the ingrowth of the endothelium to cover the inner surface of the stent.

Atherectomy: For atherectomy, it is important to know the location and depth of the plaque as well as the presence of significant calcification. Ultrasound imaging can identify superficial calcium, which is associated with poor tissue retrieval. The sizing of the atherectomy device is crucial, since a device which is undersized will leave a significant residual plaque burden, whereas one that is oversized may share or cut into the media and adventitia, potentially leading to vessel rupture or formation of a pseudoaneurysm. Deep intimal tearing also predisposes to accentuated intimal hyperplasia and significant restenosis following the procedure.[25,28] In this respect, the planimetric information obtained from IVUS is helpful to select the ideal size of the atherectomy device.

The most striking finding from IVUS studies in the context of directional atherectomy is the substantial residual plaque burden following the procedure, consistently demonstrated with IVUS in cases where the angiographic result seems to be optimal.[29] This has called attention to the issue of more aggressive plaque removal on the basis of ultrasound imaging, allowing the safe use of larger burrs with a greater subsequent lumen gain.

Stent graft placement: For endovascular treatment of aneurysms, it is imperative to know the diameter of proximal and distal neck in order to select the correct size of the stent graft. If the device is too small, endoleaks may occur post-procedure from the proximal or the distal end. This sizing is accurately done with the cross-sectional measurement performed with IVUS. Also, during the procedure the complete apposition of the stent struts or hooks to the vessel wall can be confirmed with IVUS imaging. This cannot be accurately assessed with angiography.

For stent graft placed for aortic dissection, the sealing of the site of entry tear is most reliably confirmed only with ultrasound imaging.

Vena cava filter: Whenever technical problems (filter tilting or filter migration) or complications (caval thrombosis or recurrent pulmonary embolism) of filter placement are suspected, IVUS may be used to complement or obviate cavography. It is also possible to perform the entire procedure under ultrasound guidance, since the identification of renal veins is easy with IVUS.

Mechanisms of restenosis-insights with IVUS imaging: In the early years of interventional cardiology, it was believed that the predominant mechanisms of restenosis was intimal hyperplasia. Following angioplasty, this would occur with a deep extension of the dissection, exposing the media to blood and initiating an aggressive platelet response which results in intimal proliferation.[25] With atherectomy, IVUS may sometimes demonstrate a scalloped outline of the lumen, predisposing to increased local turbulence which causes greater platelet aggregation and restenosis.[30] However, Pasterkamp et al.[31] studied peripheral vessels with IVUS and observed that shrinkage of the vessel or negative remodeling was another major mechanism contributing to late lumen loss. In another study on coronary interventions,[32] decrease in the EEM area contributed to 70% of the lumen loss, whereas intimal proliferation was responsible for only 23% of the loss.

The restenotic response occurring following stent place-ment is different in that it is primarily due to neointimal hyperplasia. This is probably because stents can resist the remodeling process.[33] This, combined with the fact that stents result in greater initial luminal expansion, contributes to a lower late restenosis rate with stenting compared to balloon angioplasty or atherectomy.

MISCELLANEOUS APPLICATIONS

- In case of aortic dissection, IVUS has been to be superior to angiography and transoesophageal echocardiography in identifying the points of entry and re-entry.[34]
- Percutaneous fenestration of aortic dissection has been accomplished successfully using IVUS as the guiding imaging modality. Identification of the highly echogenic needle as it passes from one lumen into the other is easily monitored with ultrasound.
- IVUS can be employed for assessing progression of plaque, where it is superior to angiography.[35]
- Tissue characterization is possible with ultrasound imaging based on the differential acoustic impedance properties of the various layers of the vessel wall. This may have a role in patients with Marfan's syndrome (abnormalities in the elastin content) where IVUS may be used for diagnosis and follow-up.[36]
- IVUS has the capability to study the cardiac chambers, wall motion abnormalities and valve movements.[37]
- Endoluminal sonography has been used for evaluation of gastrointestinal and genitourinary tracts as well as tracheobronchial tree to image a variety of abnormalities.[38-40]
  - Uses in the gastrointestinal tract include distinguishing between various submucosal lesions, assessing the severity of esophageal varices and evaluating fibrosis in scleroderma.
  - In the genitourinary tract, endoluminal US has been applied to diagnose upper urinary tract calculi, tumors and mural abnormalities as well as an adjunct to endourological procedures. It has been experimentally employed in the imaging of tubal abnormalities.
  - In the tracheobronchial tree, it has been applied as a guide to biopsy of lymph nodes and tumors not visualized on routine bronchoscopy.

LIMITATIONS OF INTRAVASCULAR ULTRASOUND

1. With the current resolution and processing available with IVUS devices, it may be difficult to differentiate a thrombus superimposed upon plaque from a soft, lipid laden plaque.
2. In tortuous vessel anatomy, there may under or overestimation of disease due to inability to maintain a constant catheter-vessel coaxial alignment.
3. Calcific/fibrous lesions may cause echo drop-outs, hindering the visualizing of underlying plaque.
4. The high cost of equipment may be inhibitory to a majority of interventionists, who are still not comfortable with its use.

FUTURE DIRECTIONS

New and creative areas of IVUS applications are being explored. Doppler capabilities are being incorporated within IVUS catheters to allow for simultaneous hemodynamic assessment of stenosis. Real-time three-dimensional reconstruction of IVUS data, by providing information about spatial relationships of anatomical structures may enhance the capabilities of IVUS.

Continued improvements in transducer design and technology will allow for better resolution and penetration of US waves. Improvements in catheter tractability and steerability should allow for easier catheterization of tortuous vessels and side branches that are presently difficult to select.

One of the key issues, for the future of intravascular US to be incorporated as an integral part of the interventional radiologist's armamentarium is the demonstration of a clear clinical benefit.[41] Two kinds of studies are currently being initiated, those that analyze the effect that IVUS imaging has on decision making of the operator during the therapeutic procedure, and those that evaluate the impact of this modality on the long-term outcome of endovascular interventions. There are also studies engaged in developing and testing prototypes of combined imaging/stent delivery and imaging/atherectomy devices. These would significantly reduce the procedure time and give an "online" assessment of plaque orientation and changes occurring with the device. Ultrasound may have the potential to be used for pulverizing plaque or thrombus, creating a channel whereby a subsequent angioplasty can be performed. It may even be used as a sole therapeutic modality using higher energies, thus bringing down the cost and time of lysis procedures.

Endoluminal sonography, particularly three-dimensional reconstruction algorithms may open new vistas in gastroenterology imaging such as in treatment of inflammatory bowel disease, staging of rectosigmoid neoplasia and pancreatobiliary disease processes. It may be an adjunct to imaging and intervention in endometrial, cervical and prostatic tumors.

REFERENCES

1. Vlodaver Z, Frech R, Van Tassel RA, et al. Correlations of the antemortem arteriogram and the postmortem specimen. Circulation. 1973;47:162-69.
2. Isner JM, Kishel J, Kent KM, et al. Accuracy of angiographic determination of left main coronary arterial narrowing: Angiographic-histologic correlative analysis in 28 patients. Circulation. 1981;63:1056-64.
3. White CW, Wright CB, Doty DB, et al. Does visual interpretation of the coronary arteriogram predict the physiologic importance of a coronary stenosis? N Engl J Med. 1984;310:819-24.
4. Nishimora RA, Welch TJ, Stanson AW, et al. Intravascular US of the distal aorta and iliac vessels: Initial feasibility studies. Radiology. 1990;176:523-25.
5. Davidson CJ, Sheikh KH, Harrison JK, et al. Intravascular ultrasonography versus digital subtraction angiography: A human in vivo comparison of vessel size and morphology. J Am Coll Cardiol. 1990;16:633-36.
6. Yock PG, Linker DT, White NW, et al. Clinical applications of intravascular ultrasound imaging in atherectomy. Int J Cardiac Imag. 1989;4:117-25.
7. Tobis JM, Mallery J, Mahon D, et al. Intravascular ultrasound imaging of human coronary arteries in vivo. Analysis of tissue characterizations with comparison to in vitro histological specimens. Circulation. 1991;43:913-26.
8. Nissen SE, Yock P. Intravascular ultrasound: Novel pathophysiological insights and current clinical applications. Circulation. 2001;103:604-16.
9. Yamada EG, Fitzgerald PJ, Sudhir K, et al. Intravascular ultrasound imaging of blood. The effect of hematocrit and flow on backscatter. J Am Soc Echo. 1992;5:385.
10. Metz JA, Yock PG, Fitzgerald PJ. Intravascular ultrasound: Basic interpretation. Card Clin. 1997;15(1):1-15.
11. Tobis JM, Mahon D, Goldberg SL, et al. Lessons from intravascular ultrasonography: Observations during interventional angioplasty procedures. J Clin Ultrasound. 1993;21:589-607.
12. Fitzgerald PJ, St. Goar FG, Connolly AJ, et al. Intravascular ultrasound imaging of coronary arteries. Is three layers norm? Circulation. 1992;86:154-58.
13. Nishimura RA, Edwards WD, Warnes CA, et al. Intravascular ultrasound imaging: In vitro validation and pathologic correlation. J Am Coll Cardiol. 1990;16:145-54.
14. Gussenhoven EJ, Essed CE, Lancee CT, et al. Arterial wall characteristics determined by intravascular ultrasound imaging: as in vitro study. J Am Coll Cardiol. 1989;14:947-52.
15. Gussenhoven WJ, Essed CE, Frietman P, et al. Intravascular echographic assessment of vessel wall characteristics: A correlation with histology. Int J Cardiac Imag 1989;4:105-16.
16. Hodgson J MCB, Reddy KG, Suneja R, et al. Intracoronary ultrasound imaging. Correlation of plaque morphology with angiography, clinical syndrome and procedural results in patients undergoing coronary angioplasty. J Am Coll Cardiol. 1993;21:35-44.
17. Glagov S, Weinsenberg E, Zarins CK, et al. Compensatory enlargement of human atherosclerotic arteries. N Engl J Med. 1987;316:1371.
18. Kakuta T, Curries JW, Haudenschild CC, et al. Differences in compensatory vessel enlargement, not intimal formation, account for restenosis after angioplasty in the hypercholesterolemic rabbit model. Circulation. 1994;89:2809.
19. Kimura T, Kaburagi S, Tamura T, et al. Remodeling of human coronary angioplasty or atherectomy. Circulation. 1997;96:475-83.

20. Chemarin-Alibelli MJ, Pieraggi MT, et al. Identification of coronary thrombus after myocardial infarction by intracoronary ultrasound compared with histology of tissues sampled by atherectomy. Am J Cardiol. 1996;77:344.
21. Lee DY, Eigler N, Fishbein MC, et al. Identification of intracoronary thrombus and demonstration of thrombectomy by intravascular ultrasound imaging. Am J Cardiol. 1994;73:522.
22. Sharma S, Sharma S, Taneja K, et al. Morphological mural changes in the aorta in non-specific aortoarteritis (Takayasu's arteritis): Assessment by intravascular ultrasound imaging. Clin Radiol. 1998;53:37-43.
23. Isner JM, Rosenfield K, Losordo DW, et al. Percutaneous intravascular US as adjunct to catheter-based interventions: Preliminary experience in patients with peripheral vascular disease. Radiology. 1990;175:61-70.
24. Fitzgerald PJ, Yock PG. Guide Trial Investigators: Discrepancies between angiographic and intravascular ultrasound appearance of coronary lesions undergoing intervention. A report of Phase 1 of the Guide trial. J Am Coll Cardiol. 1993;134A:738-44.
25. Steele PM, Chesebro JH, Stanson AW, et al. Balloon angioplasty: natural history of the pathophysiological response to injury in a pig model. Circ Res. 1985;57:105-12.
26. Ehlrich S, Honye J, Mahon D, et al. Unrecognized stenosis by angiography documented by intravascular ultrasound. Cathet Cardiovasc Diagn. 1991;3:198-201.
27. Yock PG, Fitzgerald PJ, Linker DT, et al. Intravascular ultrasound guidance for catheter-based coronary interventions. J Am Coll Cardiol. 1991;17:39B-49B.
28. Backa D, Polnitz AV, Nerlich A, et al. Histologic comparison of atherectomy biopsies from coronary and peripheral arteries, abstracted. Circulation. 1995;82(Suppl III): III-324.
29. Matar FA, Mintz GS, Pinnow E, et al. Multivariate predictors of intravascular ultrasound end points after directional coronary atherectomy. J Am Coll Cardiol. 1995;25:318-24.
30. Tobis JM, Mallery JA, Gessert J, et al. Intravascular ultrasound cross-sectional arterial imaging before and after balloon angioplasty in vitro. Circulation. 1990;80:873-82.
31. Pasterkamp G, Wensing PJ, Post MJ, et al. Paradoxical arterial wall shrinkage may contribute to luminal narrowing to human atherosclerotic femoral arteries. Circulation. 1995;91:1444-49.
32. Mintz GS, Kent KM, Pichard AD, et al. Contribution of inadequate arterial remodeling to the development of focal coronary artery stenosis: an intravascular ultrasound study. Circulation. 1997;95:1791-98.
33. Painter JA, Mintz GS, Wong SC, et al. Serial intravascular ultrasound studies fail to show evidence of chronic Palmaz-Schatz stent recoil. Am J Cardiol. 1995;75:398-400.
34. Ayala D, Chandrasekaran K, Ross J Jr, et al. MHz intravascular ultrasonography in the diagnosis of aortic dissection: Comparison to trans-esophageal echocardiography and aortography (abstract). Circulation. 1993;88:0522.
35. Hausmann D, et al. Accuracy of intravascular ultrasound to assess progression of experimental aortic atherosclerosis (abstract). Circulation. 1993;88:2699.
36. Recchia D, et al. Quantification of abnormal aortic elastin content and organization in Marfan syndrome with ultrasonic tissue characterization (abstract). Circulation. 1993;88:3119.
37. Pandian NG, et al. Intracardiac echocardiography: current developments. Int J Card Imag. 1991;6:207-19.
38. Liu JB, Goldberg BB. Endoluminal vascular and nonvascular sonography: past, present and future. Am J Roentgenol. 1995;165(4):765-74.
39. Liu JB, Goldberg BB. 2-D and 3-D endoluminal ultrasound: vascular and nonvascular applications. Ultrasound Med Biol. 1999;25(2):159-73.
40. Goldberg BB, Liu JB, Merton DA, et al. Endoluminal US: experiments with nonvascular uses in animals. Radiology. 1990;175(1):39-43.
41. Fitzgerald PJ, Yock PG. Mechanism and outcomes of angioplasty and atherectomy assessed by intravascular ultrasound imaging. J Clin Ultrasound. 1993;21:579-88.

20
Chapter

Role of Color Flow and Doppler in Obstetrics, Gynecology, and Infertility

INTRODUCTION

Doppler ultrasound offers a very efficient noninvasive technology to study the circulatory system. This method allows an insight into uterine, ovarian, tubal, and other important pelvic vessels. The excellent reproducibility of the technique and the ability to visualize smallest of the vessels in the ovary, uterus, endometrium, and conditions such as ectopic pregnancy makes it an excellent diagnostic tool with high degree of accuracy. The sensitivity and specificity of the diagnosis is increased and great help is obtained in the evaluation of gynecological malignancy.

The technology of color flow imaging deals with two points:
a. Imaging problems
b. Clinical uses.

IMAGING PROBLEMS

When the first color flow imaging was used, the images were too fascinating and different from the gray scale and Duplex images that many thought that it was not ultrasound. Yet like Duplex and B mode imaging, color flow has its own problems despite the bright and dynamic images. These are as follows:
1. *Tissue attenuation:* Muscle, fat, plaque, and connective tissue rapidly attenuate signals. Though, these signals are very small, the echo signals from blood vessels are smaller.
2. *Accurate blood flow sampling:* It will depend upon pulsed Doppler sample volume geometry. The same flow will have a different frequency mix as the sample volume shape changes.
3. *Color flow imaging system:* It detects moving blood in color. This is easy to do when blood is the only echo source within the scanning field, which obviously is not leading to a complex mixing of signals at blood vessel interface. Strong tissue signals mix with peak blood signals. The walls are not always still either. The technology must be able to adequately separate moving blood from sometimes moving soft tissues. It must also separate different patterns in blood movements.

Color flow scanning takes us away from conventional imaging approaches to vessels and organs in the sense that B-mode imaging traditionally seeks out the specular reflections of a structure. The ultrasound beam is perpendicular to the flow pattern in the vessel; on the other hand Doppler needs an angle away from 90°, preferably less than 60° for greatest accuracy (Fig. 20.1A).

CLINICAL USES

Color flow imaging specifically visualizes the vascular system. The word "vascular" not only includes the heart, carotids or aorta but a huge system spread all over the body with systemic, neural, and hormonal controls. The vascular system of the body responds to stress, trauma, drugs, and hosts a very complex biochemistry for clot and thrombus formation. A successful vascular image system must be able to portray changes due to normal regulation, drugs, and diseases. It must also do more than just put color on the display. Hence, if a color flow imaging has to function as an effective clinical tool it must be able to detect disease and evaluate the extent of the disease.

Hence, in the arterial and venous system, color flow imaging should be able to tell us the condition of the wall,

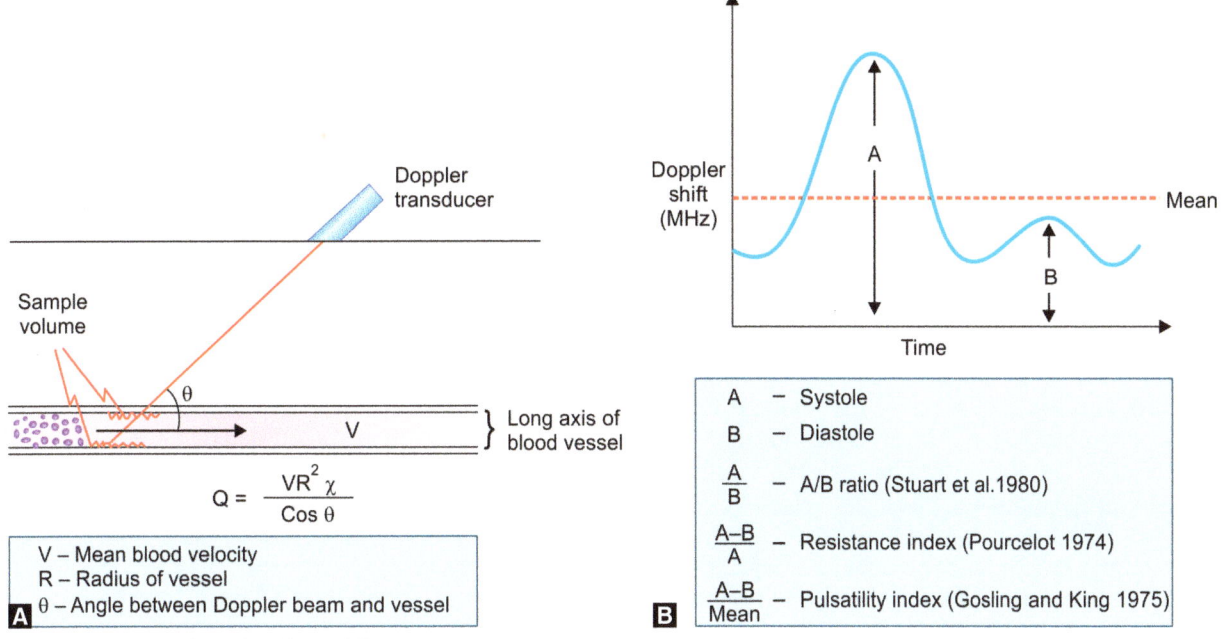

Figs. 20.1A and B: (A) Doppler measurement of blood flow; (B) Flow velocity waveform.

the lumen (stenosis), the intima, should be able to detect a plaque, predict the blood flows and over, and above it should be able to identify neovascularization.

The Doppler Signal

When an ultrasound beam is transmitted towards the blood flow in a vessel, it is scattered in all directions and back scattered to the transducer. The moving RBC causes Doppler shift of the scattered ultrasound. This velocity of blood flow can be determined using certain equations, if the values of the angle and of the Doppler signal are known. The processing of the Doppler signal unrolls sequential steps of amplification, demodulation, spectral processing, and display (Fig. 20.1A).

The spectral analysis of Doppler signal involves processing, quantification of the frequency and power content of the signal. The vertical axis of the sonogram shows the magnitude of the frequency shift and horizontal axis represents the temporal change. Brightness of the spectrum is an indication of power of the spectrum.

In order to quantify the volatile resistance, various indices have been proposed (Fig. 20.1B).

1. $\text{PI (Pulsatility Index)} = \dfrac{\text{Peak Systolic Velocity} - \text{End Diastolic Velocity}}{\text{Mean Velocity}}$

(Gosling and King 1975)

2. $\text{RI (Resistance Index)} = \dfrac{\text{Peak Systolic Velocity} - \text{End Diastolic Velocity}}{\text{End Diastolic Velocity}}$

(Bourcelot 1974)

3. $\text{Systolic/Diastolic Ratio} = \dfrac{\text{Peak Systolic Velocity}}{\text{End Diastolic Velocity}}$

(Stuart et al. 1980)

The higher the value of these indices more the impedance to blood flow and perfusion of the particular area. In order to understand the pathological features of different gynecological conditions one has to know about the indices of various vessels.

How the Color Image is Formed?

Color images are of two types: (i) Asynchronous and (ii) Synchronous imaging. In asynchronous imaging, the gray scale and Doppler information are gathered at different times. In contrast, synchronous imaging information is gathered simultaneously.

Asynchronous Color Flow Imaging

Two images are produced during scanning and are later superimposed. The gray scale comes from a real time image. The Doppler image comes from steering another ultrasound beam at an angle to the array (0–45°). The image is composed in a digital scan converter. Two different frequencies can be used for the two image components; a system could have gray scale at 5 MHz and color at 3 MHz.

Synchronous Color Flow Imaging

Simultaneous processing for amplitude, phase and frequency is achieved by the same echo signal. This technology is so different that it is known as angiodynagraphy. The linear array sends a dynamically focused beam, which is perpendicular to the vessels. This is good for imaging but not for Doppler. To provide the Doppler angle needed to visualize blood flow, a wedge stand off site between the array surface and the skin surface. The image is divided into a set of sample bits, which are same in the field of view. Within this site the system looks at the echo signal amplitude in one path, at the phase and frequency in the other.

The machine now builds the image on a pixel basis, testing exit for evidence of motion and its direction. If motion exits at a pixel, it is colored, otherwise it takes on a gray scale proportionate to the echo signal strength. Having set out the image formation the next step is color coding of the pixels, in which motion was detected.

Color Coding the Information

'Gray's Anatomy' color code is used by all of the color flow imaging systems. Flow in one direction is red, and in the opposite direction, it is blue. Now, because all of us are tuned to the fact that all red vessels are arteries and blue vessels are veins, it is all too easy to read the image the wrong way. Even the most skilled readers fall prey to this reading error from time to time. It is to be noted and clarified that color indicates and represents existence of motion and direction of flow, not the vessel type. Color shows where flow exists in the image and its direction with respect to the transducer.

COLOR DOPPLER IN GYNECOLOGY

Main Uterine Vessels

The color Doppler signal from the main uterine vessels may be seen in all patients lateral to the cervix. The small branches of uterine artery can be followed by searching the corpus ascending along the lateral wall (Fig. 20.2). Waveform analysis shows high velocity and high resistance flow. The RI depends on the age, phase of menstrual cycle and any special condition such as pregnancy or tumor.

RI of uterine artery is as follows:
a. In early proliferative phase 0.88 + 0.04 (Fig. 20.3A)
b. Secretory phase 0.84 + 0.04 (Fig. 20.3B)
c. Radial vessels 0.78 + 0.10 (Fig. 20.3C)
d. Spiral vessels 0.54 + 0.03.

Ovarian Vessels

It is difficult to visualize the ovarian vessels but an experienced operator, using modern color Doppler unit can detect them in most patients in the lateral upper pole of the ovary (Figs. 20.4A to C).

Color flow is usually not prominent, velocity is low and resistance varies according to the menstrual cycle. A low velocity, high impedance pattern is seen during the follicular phase. At ovulation, there is maximum increase in the velocity and RI decrease, reaching a dip of 0.44 + 0.09 four to five days later and slowly increases by 0.04–0.05 before menstruation.

Active ovary : RI 0.44 + 0.09
PSV (27 + 10 cm/sec)
Inactive ovary : RI 0.76 + 0.22
PSV (8.9 + 3.8 cm/sec)

Iliac Flow

The common and external iliac arteries show plug flow, a window under the waveform and a reversed component during diastole. The internal iliac vessel in contrast has a parabolic flow with an even distribution of velocities within the waveform.

Ovarian Masses

Neovascularization

The importance of neovascularization remains in the hypothesis that increased cell population must be preceded by the production of new vessels. Such abnormal vascular morphology can be used as a valuable marker for the presence of a malignant tumor. New vessels are continually produced at the periphery of the tumor and act as marker for continued growth and proliferation. The amount and vascularity of the stroma vary greatly in different tumors. In general, rapidly growing tumors particularly sarcomas have

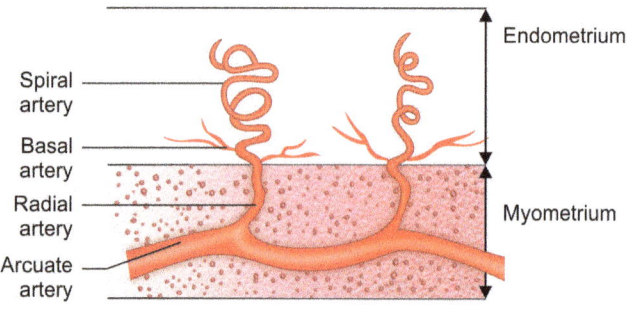

Fig. 20.2: Vasculature of uterine wall.

Role of Color Flow and Doppler in Obstetrics, Gynecology, and Infertility | **185**

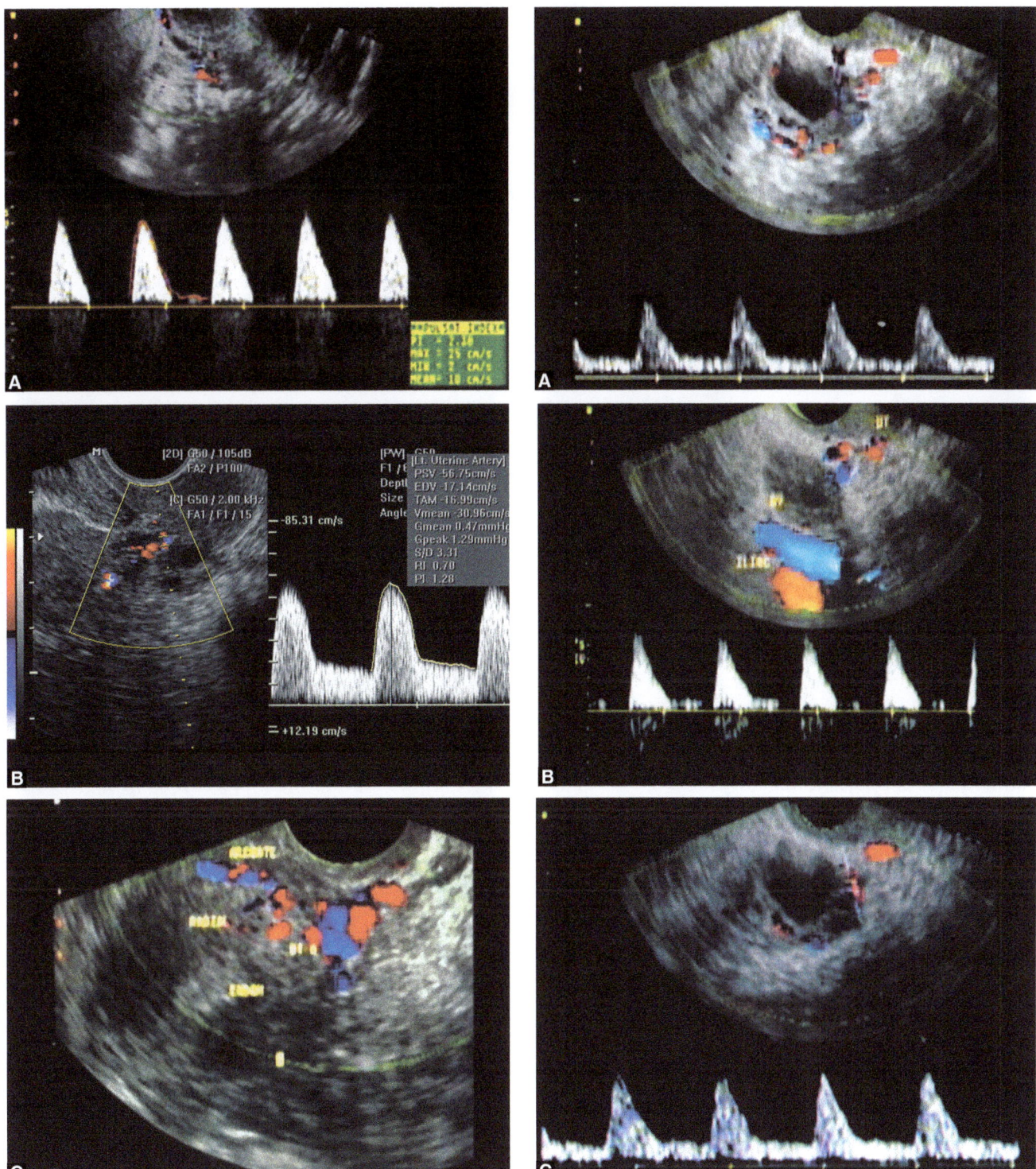

Figs. 20.3A to C: (A) Uterine artery waveform during the early proliferative phase; (B) At day 10 of menstrual cycle; (C) Color Doppler showing uterine, arcuate and radial artery.

Figs. 20.4A to C: (A) Ovarian arterial flow pattern. Intrastromal color flow is also noted; (B) Ovarian branch of uterine artery; (C) Spectral waveform of the ovarian artery.

a highly vascular stroma with little connective tissue. More slowly growing tumors are less well vascularized.

Intratumoral blood flows displayed on Color Doppler image indicate that there is flow rapid enough to be detected. The presence of AV communications should be an important factor that produces sufficient velocity above the minimal threshold on Color Doppler Imaging. The technique may be helpful in demonstrating pelvic tumors with rapid blood flow and in providing hemodynamic information. Color Doppler can also depict the hemodynamic characteristic of the tumor, allowing echo sources of the hypoechoic zones to be separated into compartment, vessels and the blood pooling or hemorrhage surrounding them.

The goal of transvaginal color Doppler sonography should be to identify ovarian tumors which are not significantly enlarged. TV-CD is a non-invasive method and its diagnostic sensitivity, specificity and accuracy seem to be clinically good enough for it to be a potential technique for use in a screening program.

Several authors have attempted to improve their diagnosis of ovarian cancer by considering the flow characteristics using the RI or PI. Kurjak and Zalud used an RI of 0.4 as a cutoff and found that all 624 benign masses had an RI of >0.4 and that 54 of 56 cancers had an RI of less than 0.4. However, there is a considerable overlap between benign and malignant impedance and it is now generally becoming recognized that we must consider the morphology in addition to the impedance estimate.

The other lesions which demonstrate low impedance high diastolic flow are tuboovarian abscesses, actively hemorrhagic corpus luteum (Fig. 20.5A), and some dermoids (Fig. 20.5B). If the waveform has a diastolic notch, the possibility of it being benign is more. Malignant tumors tend to demonstrate color flow in the central portion, increased flow is seen in the papillary excrescences or in irregular areas of the wall in a malignant mass.

In endometriosis low impedance flow is seen when there is hemorrhage in the menstrual phase of cycle.

Fibroids

Color flow Doppler and spectral Doppler findings are variable in uterine fibroids reflecting their natural history with growth followed by episodes of degeneration. The vascularity in fibroids is typically peripheral with very high velocities and low resistance (Figs. 20.6A to C). In contrast the center of fibroids is often avascular and necrotic. The vascularity is usually inversely related to the amount of calcification within the fibroid. Areas of degeneration are usually devoid of vascularity.

A pedunculated fibroid can simulate an ovarian cancer. On endovaginal color flow copious vascularity may be seen with perfusion characteristics identical to those in ovarian cancer. The pitfall can be avoided by demonstrating the connecting pedicle.

There is an increase in blood flow and a decrease in impedance in both uterine arteries in patients with fibroids. The degree of vascularity of a fibroid can determine how the patient should be managed, i.e. when myomectomy should be offered and by which route, whether GnRH agonists should be given or when hysterectomy should be performed. As a general rule of thumb vascularity of fibroids is greater.

In contrast to fibroid, adenomyoma usually shows higher central vascularity with lower RI values.

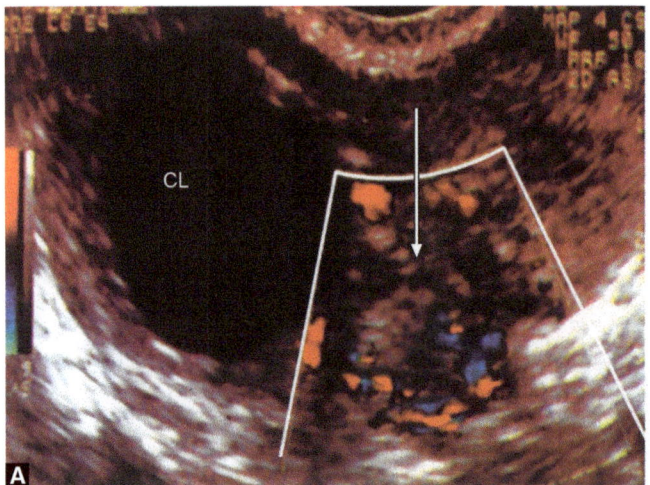
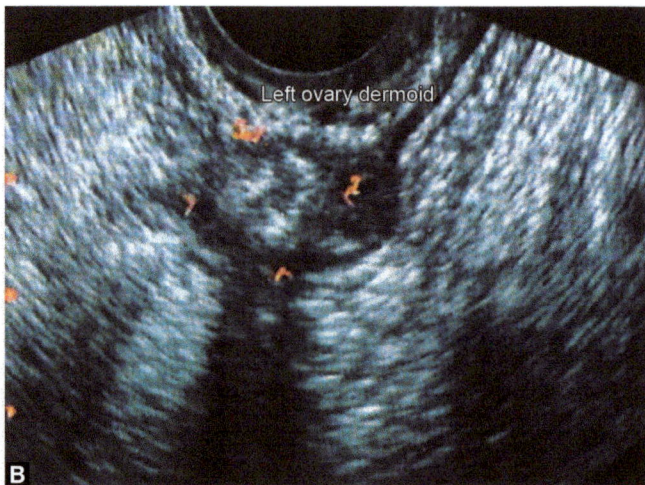

Figs. 20.5A and B: (A) Color flow pattern of the corpus luteum; (B) Gray scale image showing an ovarian dermoid.

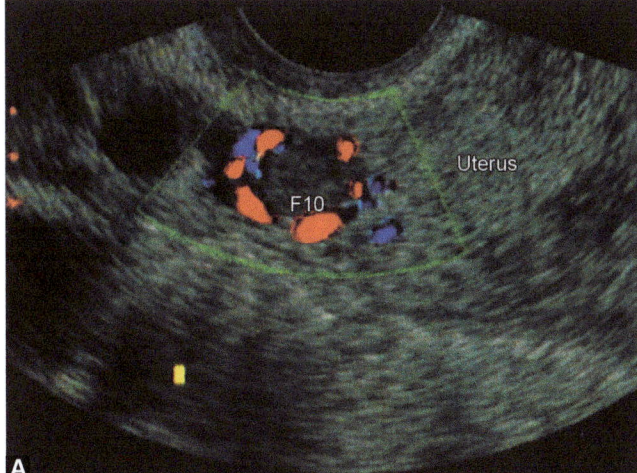
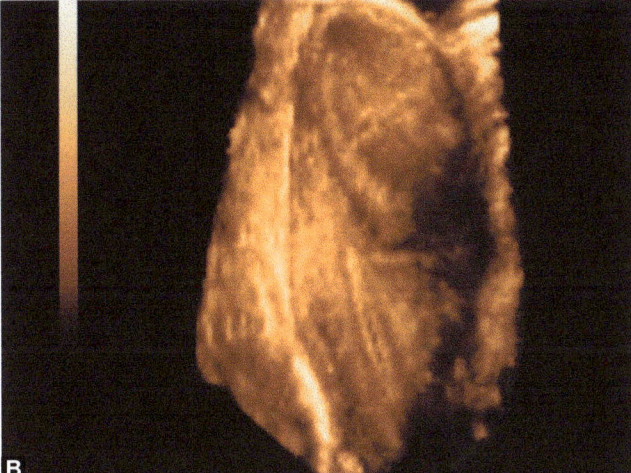
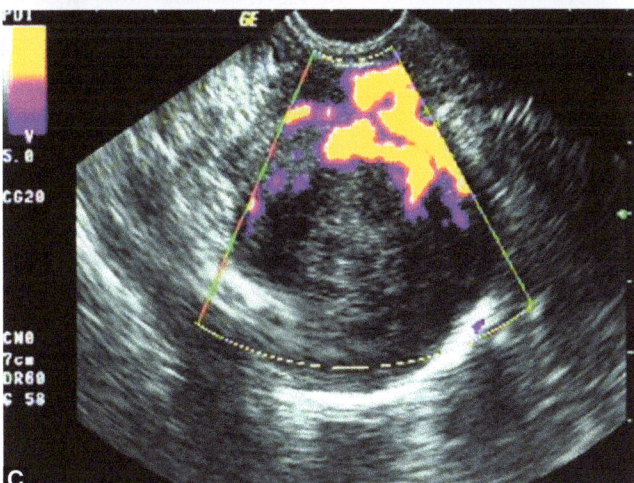

Figs. 20.6A to C: Color Doppler demonstrates peripheral vascularity in a fibroid; (B) 3D image of a uterine fibroid; (C) Power Doppler demonstrates peripheral vascularity in a fibroid.

KEY POINTS

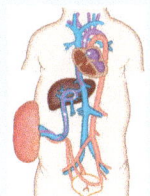

- Normal uterine arteries-low velocity and high resistance flow. Resistance varies with period of menstruation.
- In-active ovarian flow is low velocity. with high resistance, active ovarian flow is high velocity with low resistance.
- Malignant lesions more commonly show central vascularity with low impedance, high diastolic flow.
- Fibroids show peripheral vascularity with low impedance, high diastolic flow.
- Fibroids show peripheral vascularity with high resistance flow.
- In ovarian torsion, no visible arterial flow. Endometriosis show scattered flow patterns. High resistance flow is seen within the hilar vessels.
- High velocity, low impedance flow is seen in molar pregnancy due to extensive arteriovenous communications.

Premenopausally and on HRT

Adnexal Ovarian Torsion

One of the major applications of color Doppler is in the diagnosis of ovarian torsion. Although ovary has a dual blood supply, torsion typically affects flow from both ovarian artery and from abdominal branch of uterine artery. The typical appearance is enlarged ovary, which may demonstrate irregular solid areas related to hemorrhage which may precipitate torsion initially. There is no visible arterial flow within the ovary and high resistance flow in hilar vessels. This early diagnosis can save the organ and allow laparoscopic untwisting which is a relatively simple procedure.

Endometrioses (Fig. 20.7)

Color Doppler may demonstrate flow within these apparent solid structures thereby confirming the diagnosis. The vessels at the periphery of the endometriotic cyst show relativity high vascular impedance. If inflammatory changes occur there may be altered flow showing reduction in impedance to flow (D/D malignancy).

Gestational Trophoblastic Disease (Figs. 20.8A and B)

These include molar pregnancy (both partial and complete), invasive mole and choriocarcinoma. Patients with moles usually present in early pregnancy as a threatened abortion and serum HCG levels are found to be greater than 100,000 U/L. Examination of the uterus by endovaginal ultrasound discloses echogenic contents, and the application of color flow shows these contents to be highly vascular with placenta like flow. If a normal gestation is seen within uterus, the serum hCG should be repeated because errors in dilutions are not uncommon and may lead to erroneously high serum level.

Color is extremely helpful in possible recurrence. Myometrial invasion or invasion of adnexa may be seen by the application of color flow. Moles have extensive arteriovenous communications, which account for high velocity, low impedance flow. Choriocarcinoma displays a typical color coded 'hot' area representing pre-existing and newly formed blood vessels. All these vessels show high velocity low impedance blood flow signals.

Gestational Trophoblastic Tumors

There is reduction in the resistance indices of uterine artery Doppler spectra—This pattern correlates well with aggressive trophoblastic tumors and with prognosis. Those tumors exhibiting high resistance index value require massive chemotherapy and fewer treatment cycles.

Ectopic Pregnancy

The advent of color Doppler to TV probe has improved the diagnostic accuracy to almost 98%. Color flow imaging shows classical "fire ring" with trophoblastic flow pattern (Figs. 20.9A to C). Also color flow help in monitoring medical treatment with methotrexate and in planning medical treatment.

Pelvic Congestion Syndrome

The association between chronic pelvic pain, dyspareunia and pelvic varices has been termed pelvic congestion syndrome. There is dilatation of pelvic veins with congestion of the ovaries with resultant ovarian swelling and cyst formation, occasionally there may be vulvar and leg varices. In advanced cases, there may be dilatation of the uterine plexus of veins within the uterine parenchyma. Dilated pelvic veins can be seen in the absence of symptoms and not all patients with characteristic congestion exhibit the typical ultrasound appearance. Large serpiginous pelvic veins of a diameter >4 mm with flow velocities <5 cm/sec in association with cystic ovaries are characteristic. Similarly reversed flow during valsalva which is usually transient, is maintained in this condition with reverse flow of 2 cm/sec or greater.

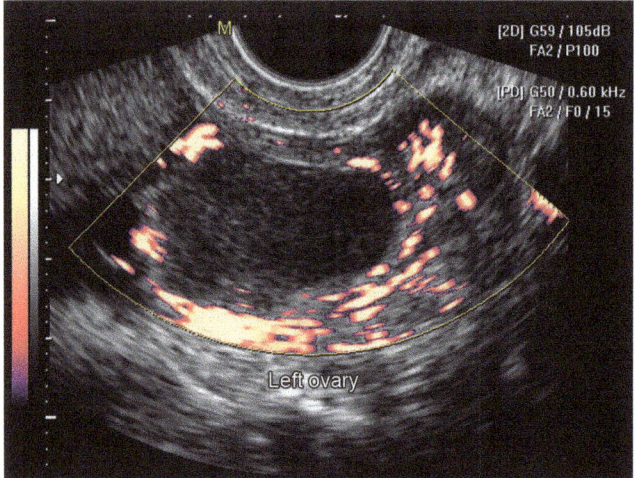

Fig. 20.7: Power Doppler demonstrates peripheral vascularity in an endometrioma of ovary.

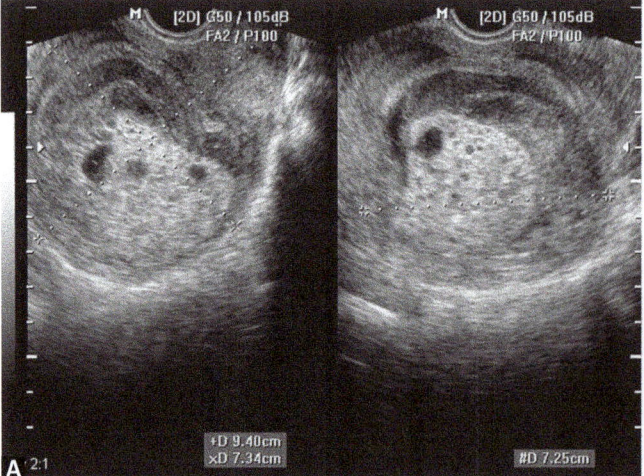

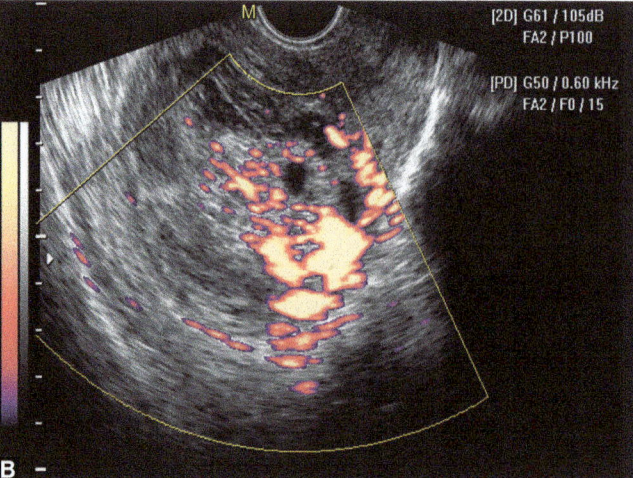

Figs. 20.8A and B: (A) Gray scale image shows hydatiform mole; (B) Power Doppler image shows high vascularity around hydatiform mole.

Role of Color Flow and Doppler in Obstetrics, Gynecology, and Infertility | **189**

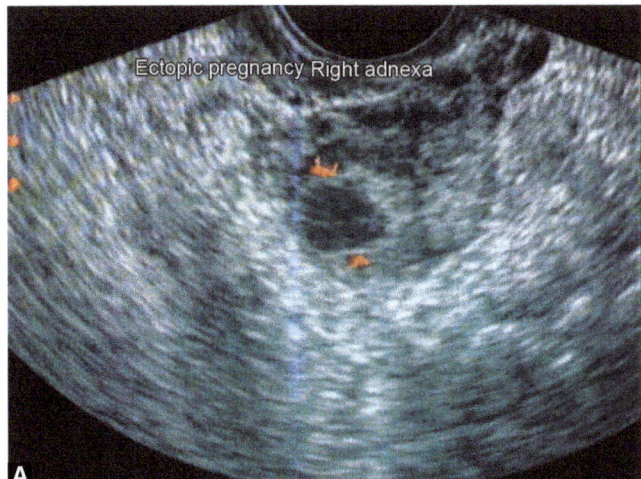

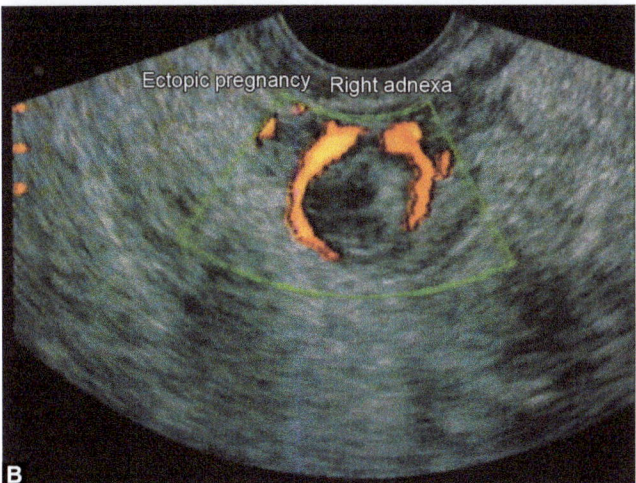

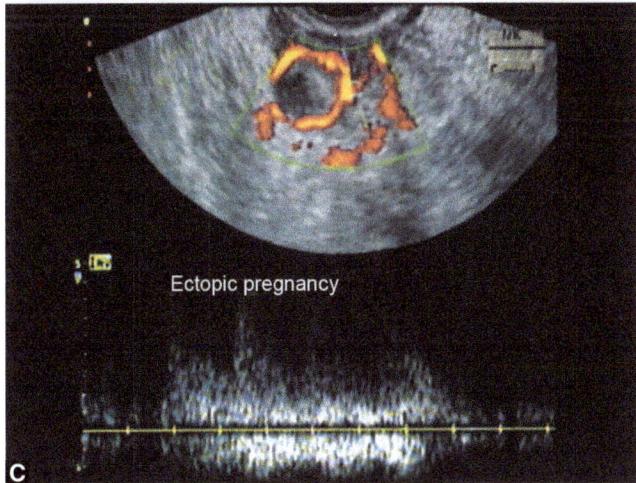

Figs. 20.9A to C: (A) Ectopic pregnancy—Gray scale image showing a complex right adnexal mass; (B) Ectopic pregnancy—On color Doppler "ring of fire" appearance is seen; (C) Ectopic pregnancy—Duplex Doppler demonstrates trophoblastic flow pattern.

Color Doppler sonography is excellent for the diagnosis of uterine and ovarian plexus varicosities. It differentiates arteries from veins.

Malignant Uterine Tumors

Uterine sarcomas appear as in homogeneous mass with increased tumor vascularity showing low impedance flow. In addition, peak systolic velocity also shows a decline from normal. Abnormal blood vessels are seen in all cases with sarcoma, whereas only 30% of fibroids show abnormal vessels. Richly vascularized necrotic and large uterine myoma has to be properly evaluated for its blood flow in order to differentiate from sarcomas.

Endometritis and Endometrial Carcinoma (Figs. 20.10A and B)

Endometritis results from infection, trauma such as D and C, prolonged labor, premature rupture of membranes or retained products of conception. Endometritis may be associated with considerable hyperemia, this may be of the low impedance pattern described in endometrial carcinoma (Taylor, et al.). In patients with postmenopausal bleeding due to endometrial carcinoma, the mean PI was 0.91 with a range of 0.31-1.49 (Bovine et al.). Women with other causes for postmenopausal bleeding had a mean PI of 3.83 with a range of 1.95-6.40. Unfortunately due to the confusion with similar flow found in both hyperplasia of endometrium and in endometritis the value of this ratio is not clear. In practice any postmenopausal woman presenting with endometrial thickness of >6 mm needs to undergo biopsy (Fig. 20.11).

It has recently become apparent that tamoxifen may also be associated with some significant endometrial abnormalities. From the NCI report, it appears that the risk of endometrial cancer in patients receiving tamoxifen is approximately three times that of normal population.

Intrauterine Polyp (Figs. 20.12A and B)

The diagnosis of intrauterine polyps can be difficult without invasive procedures. Even with endovaginal ultrasound, polyps can be easily missed unless fluid is instilled into the uterine cavity to outline them. Endovaginal color flow can be helpful where the vascular pedicle can be demonstrated (Fig. 20.12C). This feature differentiates it from endometrial blood clot which is devoid of vascularity.

Uterine Arteriovenous Malformation (UAVM)

These are usually secondary to dilatation and curettage of the endometrial cavity. It is characterized by a central

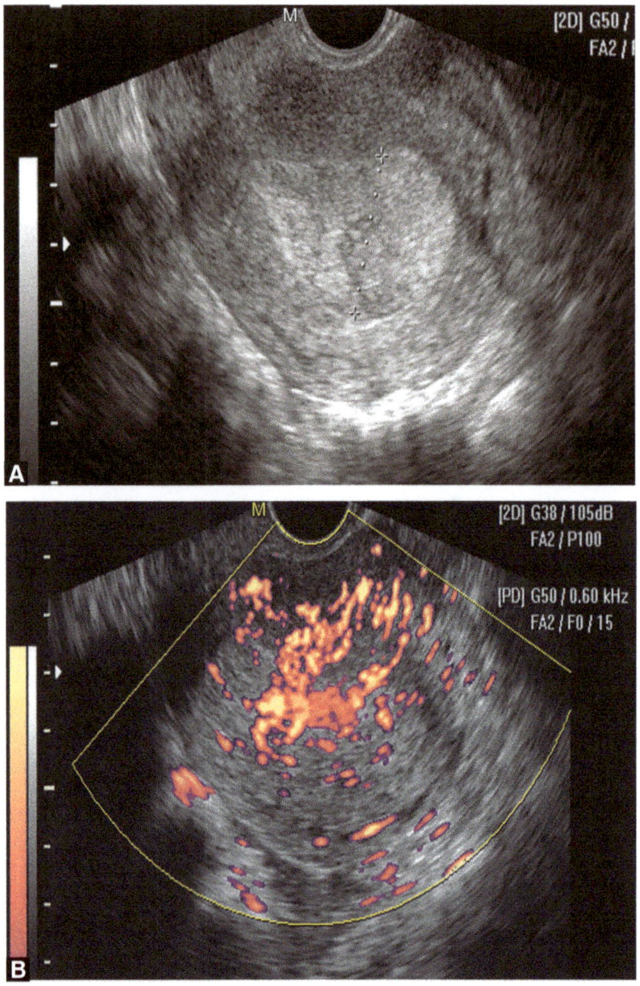

Figs. 20.10A and B: (A) Gray scale image shows endometrial carcinoma presenting as increased endometrial thickening; (B) Power Doppler image shows high and haphazard vascularity in endometrial carcinoma.

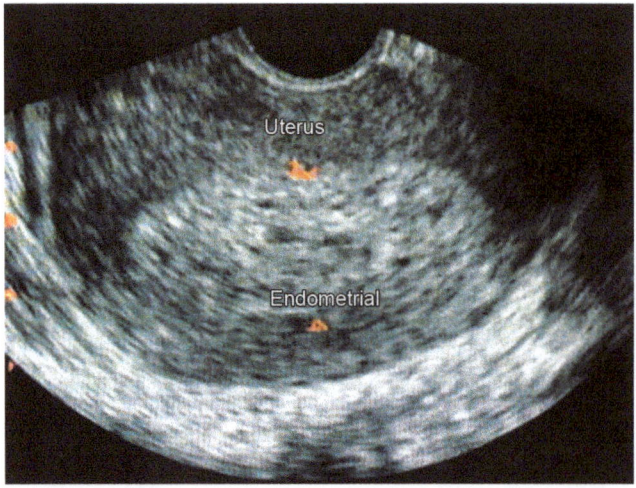

Fig. 20.11: Increased endometrial thickness in a case of endometrial hyperplasia.

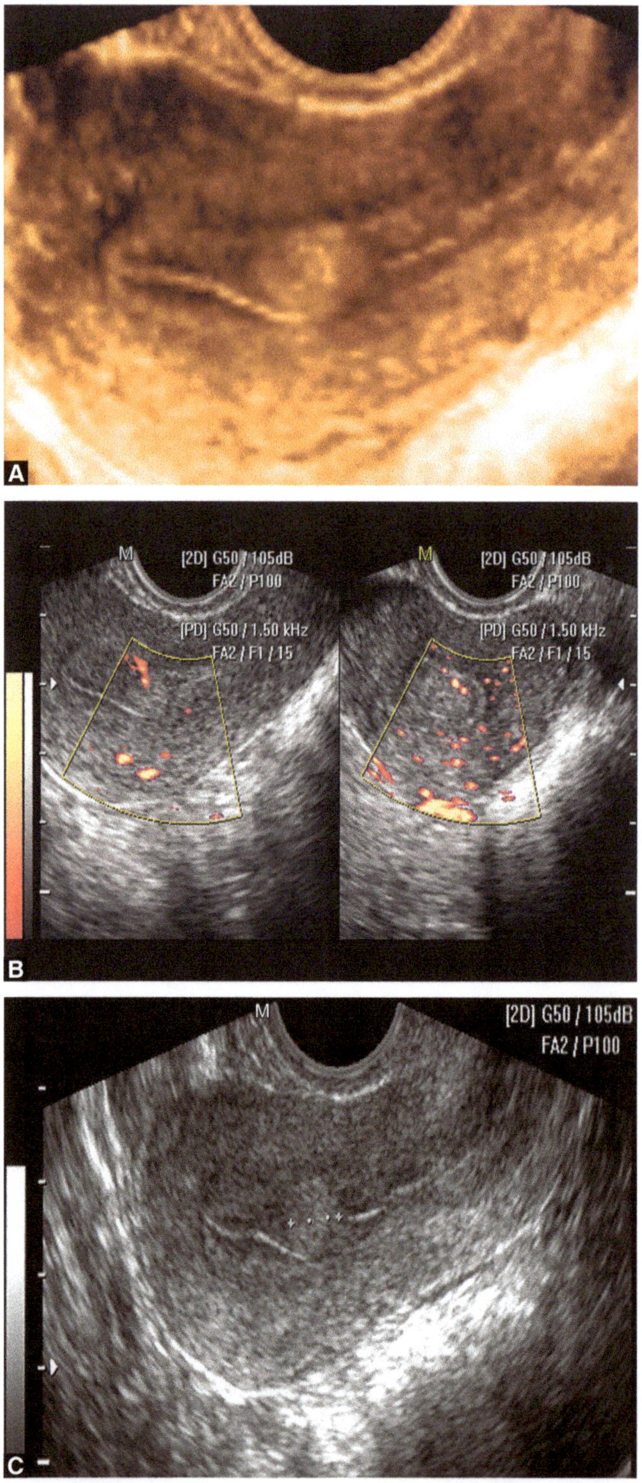

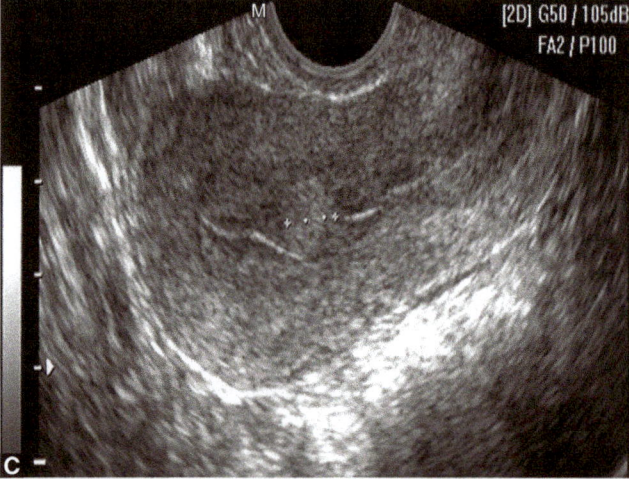

Figs. 20.12A to C: (A) 3D image shows endometrial polyp; (B) Power Doppler image shows vascularity in endometrial polyp; (C) Endometrial polyp seen as a localized echogenic lesion in the endometrium.

niche and peripheral area showing multiple dilated and tortuous vascular channels of arterial and venous origin. This is usually accompanied with dilatation of the uterine and pelvic venous plexus and low resistance, pregnancy like flow in the uterine arteries.

Carcinoma of the Cervix (Figs. 20.13A to C)

Doppler appears to have little applications in the diagnosis of carcinoma of the cervix. However, cervical carcinoma can be seen on endovaginal ultrasound and neovascularity can be demonstrated.

Sonosalpingography

Tubal patency study by fluid injection through the cervical cannula and observation of fluid dynamics through the fallopian tube and fluid collection in the pelvis is a common, non-invasive and useful test. Color Doppler helps easy identification of flow of fluid through the tubes and also facilitates location of free spill of fluid into the peritoneal cavity (Waterfall Sign).

During the same procedure if 200–250 cc of fluid is injected via the Foley's, then the adnexa and POD can be evaluated for adhesions.

ROLE OF COLOR DOPPLER IN INFERTILITY

Introduction

The advent of transvaginal color Doppler sonography has added a new dimension to the diagnosis and treatment of infertile females. Color Doppler innovation is a unique non-invasive technology to investigate the circulation of organs like uterus and ovaries. Dynamic changes occur almost every day of the menstrual cycle in a reproductively active female. These events are picked up very well by transvaginal color Doppler and definite conclusions can be drawn regarding the diagnosis, prognosis, and treatment of infertile patients. As the vaginal probe lies close to the organs of interest various vessels supplying these structures can be studied in detail like the uterine artery, ovarian artery and their branches.

Study of Menstrual Cycle by Color Doppler

It is very important to study the whole of the menstrual cycle by transvaginal color Doppler during the evaluation of infertility. It provides vital information about follicular dynamics like blood flow to the growing follicle, the vascular supply of the endometrium and corpus luteum vascularization which are very important for a successful outcome in terms of pregnancy.

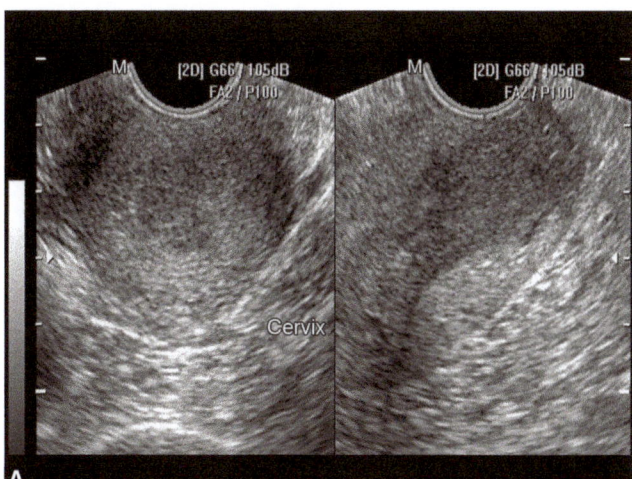
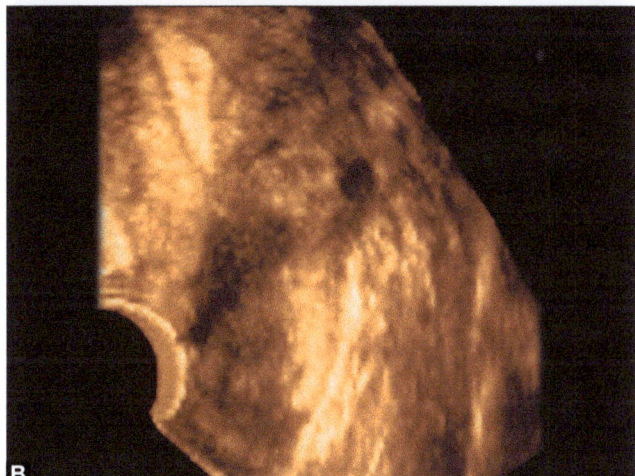
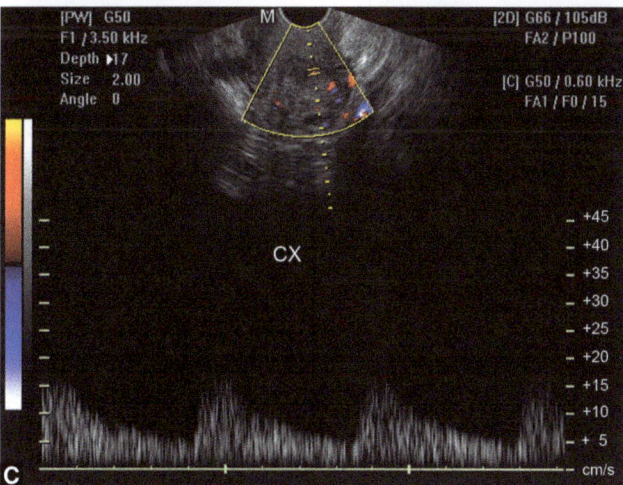

Figs. 20.13A to C: (A) Gray scale image shows hypoechoic mass in cervix; (B) 3D image shows mass in cervix; (C) Color Doppler image shows vascularity in cervical mass with low resistance flow.

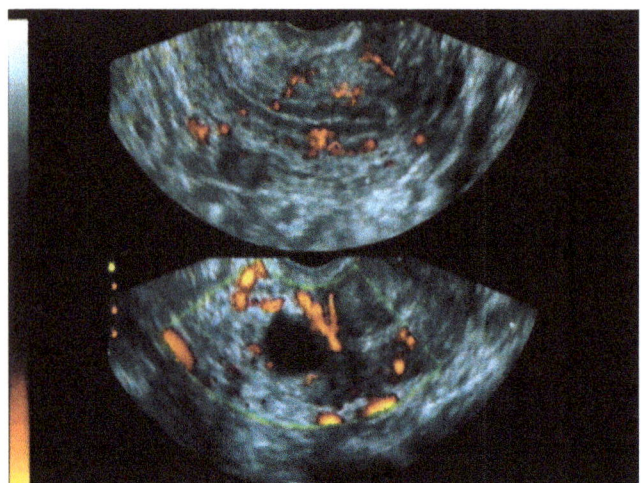

Fig. 20.14: Color Doppler showing ring of angiogenesis around the dominant follicle of the ovary. Vascularity is also seen in the endometrium.

Changes in the Ovary

The ovaries are situated on either side of the uterus and measure about 2.2–5.5 cm in length, 1.5–2.0 cm in width, and 1.5–3.0 cm in depth and are recognized by the presence of follicle of different sizes. The blood supply is by ovarian artery via the infundibulopelvic ligament and ovarian branch of the uterine artery. There is anastamosis between the two sources of blood supply. The primary and secondary branches of the ovarian artery grow along with the development of the follicle. Dominant follicle within the ovary can be recognized by transvaginal color Doppler by day 8th or 10th of the cycle by a ring of angiogenesis around it, when compared to the subordinate follicles which do not demonstrate this (Fig. 20.14). These vessels become more abundant and prominent as the follicle grows to about 20–24 mm in size.

The phases are described as early follicular (Day 5–7), late follicular (Day 11–13), early luteal (Day 15–17) and late luteal (Day 26–28). In general the index values are high in the early part of menstrual cycle and fall as ovulation approaches. According to Kurjak et al. the RI in the early proliferative phase is 0.54 +/− 0.04 and declines the day before ovulation (LH Peak) when it is about 0.44 +/− 0.04.

This is the best time for administration of surrogate hCG. The increase in peak systolic velocity with a relatively constant is a particularly interesting finding that might herald impending ovulation. It is hoped that information on ovarian perfusion may be used to predict ovulation and to investigate ovulatory dysfunction. The lowest RI values were obtained during the mid luteal phase (RI 0.42 + 0.06) with a return to higher vascular resistance (0.50 + 0.04) during the late luteal phase.

The dominant ovary corpus luteum show a low impedance waveform with a RI of 0.39–0.49, characteristic of blood flow in early pregnancy (Fig. 20.15). The contralateral ovary shows a high impedance flow with a RI of 0.69–1.00 characteristic of non dominant ovary (Kurjak et al.). If the ovary having corpus luteum shows high RI (> 0.50) it is associated with nonviable outcome.

Luteal Phase Changes in Ovarian Vascularity

The functional capacity of the corpus luteum is assessed by the low impedance flow and the abundance of vessels around it. Mature corpus luteum is a highly vascularized structure with a low RI of 0.44 +/− 0.04. In patients with corpus luteum deficiency the vascularity is not optimal and the RI is raised to around 0.59, with decreased diastolic flow. If pregnancy occurs then low RI of 0.50 continues.

Secretory Changes in the Endometrium

Michael Applebaum in his study with transvaginal color Doppler divided the endometrium and periendometrial areas into 4 zones. In the study conducted by him no pregnancy was reported in IVF patients unless vascularity was demonstrated in Zone III or IV prior to transfer.

Doppler Assessment of Uterine and Ovarian Flow in Infertility and IVF

Goswamy et al. found absent diastolic flow during the ovulatory phase in infertility patients and with severe problems and even reversal of diastolic flow.

Role of Ultrasound and Color Doppler in Endometrial Evaluation

Ultrasound (TVS) offers a simple, reliable, reproducible, quick, and noninvasive method for assessing the female pelvis.

Uterine Perfusion (Fig. 20.16)

The uterine artery gives rise to the arcuate arteries which are oriented circumferentially in the outer third of the myometrium. These vessels give rise to the radial arteries, which after crossing the myometrium-endometrium border, further branch and give rise to the basal arteries and the spiral arteries.

The RI in the uterine artery hovers around 0.88 ± 0.04 until day 13 of the 28 day menstrual cycle (Figs. 20.17 and 20.18). Increased uterine artery impedance is seen 3 days after the LH peak (day 16). This is explained by increased contractility and compression of vessels traversing the uterine wall which decrease their diameter and consequently cause higher resistance to flow. Lowest blood flow impedance

Role of Color Flow and Doppler in Obstetrics, Gynecology, and Infertility | 193

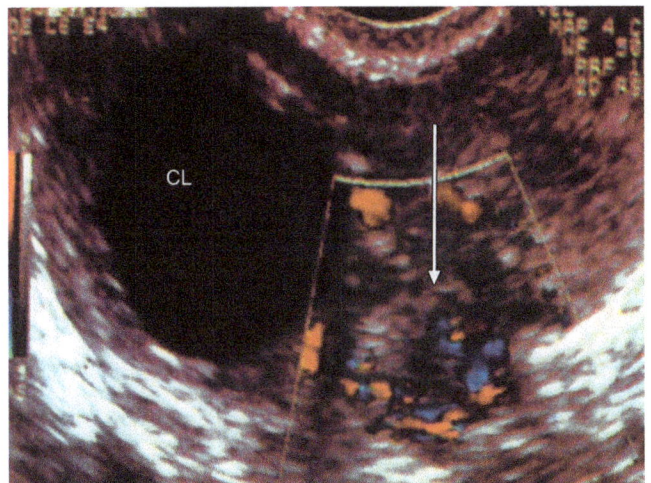

Fig. 20.15: Color Doppler image of corpus luteum.

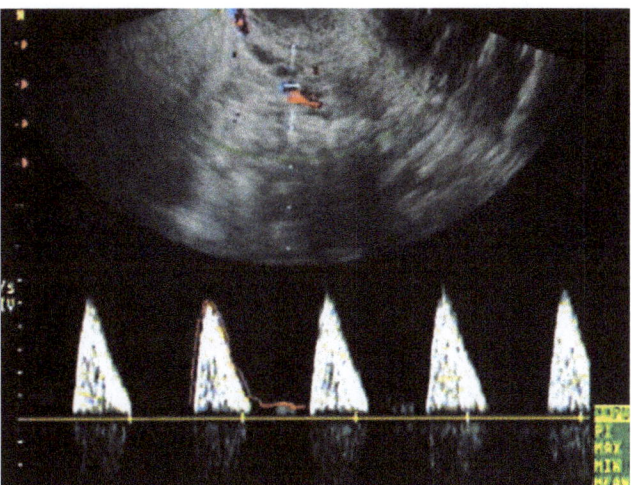

Fig. 20.17: Uterine artery flow at second day of menstrual cycle.

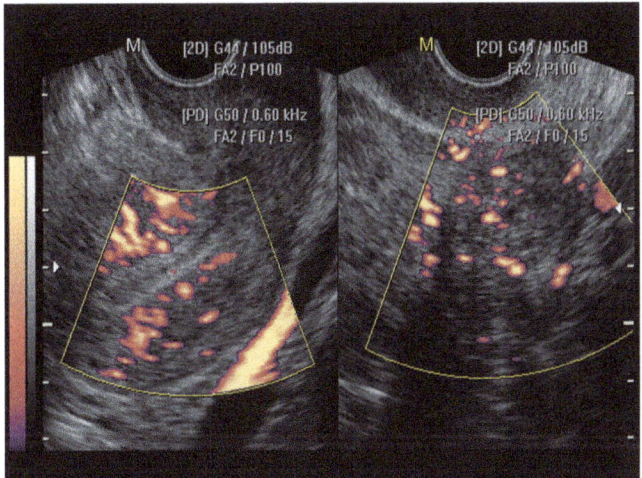

Fig. 20.16: Power Doppler image shows vascularity reaching up to the endometrium.

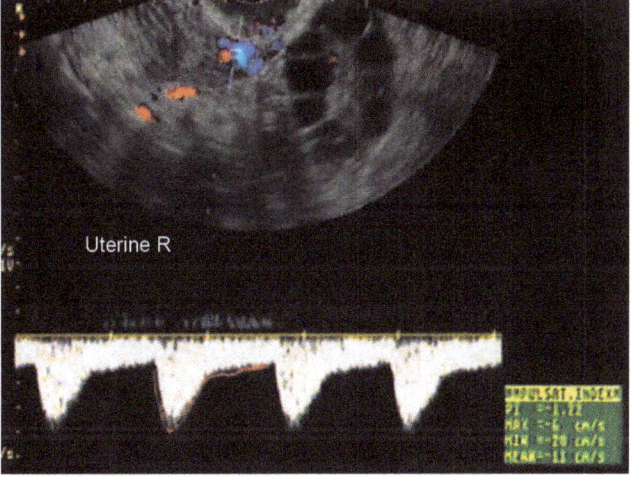

Fig. 20.18: Uterine artery flow at day ten showing low impedance flow.

occurs during peak luteal (RI = 0.84 + 0.04) during which implantation is likely to occur. RI of radial vessels is 0.78 + 0.10.

Like RI, PI values have also found significance in several studies on infertile females conducted by Kurjak et al. Their studies revealed that in subfertile and infertile females, the PI values are higher than 2.5. PI values greater than 3.0 are associated with poor outcome.

Blood flow velocity waveform changes in the spiral arteries during normal ovulatory cycles are characterized by lower velocity and lower impedance to blood flow than are those observed in the uterine arteries with larger diameter. It seems that features of endometrial blood flow may be used to predict the implantation success rate and to reveal unexplained infertility problems more precisely than evaluation of the main uterine artery alone.

Changes in the Endometrium

Michael Applebaum in his study with transvaginal color Doppler divided the endometrium and periendometrial areas into 4 zones. In the study conducted by him no pregnancy was reported in IVF patients unless vascularity was demonstrated in Zone III or with in Zone III or IV prior to transfer.

Zone 1 : 2 mm thick area surrounding the hyperechoic outer layer of the endometrium.
Zone 2 : The hyperechoic outer layer of the endometrium.
Zone 3 : The hypoechoic inner layer of the endometrium.
Zone 4 : The endometrial cavity.

Ultrasound Technique for Uterine Biophysical Profile

To perform the UBP special care should be taken. The following guidelines are recommended: (Applebaum 1996).

1. To determine the presence of a 5-line appearance, information from both the transabdominal and transvaginal studies may be useful. For example, although a 5-line appearance may be noted transabdominally, it may not always be possible to see it endovaginally due to uterine position (and vice versa). In this case, a 5-line appearance is considered to be present and endometrial vascular penetration may be estimated when performing the endovaginal study.
2. Perform the Doppler study slowly—The flow of blood in the endometrium is of low velocity, it may take time for the ultrasound machine to register the presence of blood flow and create the image. If one sweeps through the endometrium too quickly, flow may not be seen. Additionally endometrial blood flow has a mercurial personality—it may appear as if it comes and goes. It may also appear in some areas and not others. Do not observe hastily.
3. Endeavor to make the endometrium as specular a reflector as possible. Use the techniques of manual manipulation of the anatomy and probe pressure to achieve this.
4. Scan endovaginally both coronally and sagittally. There may be a difference in how well the blood flow is imaged.
5. When measuring the endometrium in the A-P dimension, try to obtain the value when no contraction affecting it is present. Contractions may affect this value. Also when possible, obtain the measurement in a standard plan such as when both the endometrial and cervical canals are continuous.

The Uterine Biophysical Profile

In our experience, certain sonographic qualities of the uterus are noted during the normal mid-cycle. These include:
1. Endometrial thickness in greatest AP dimension of 7 mm or greater (full-thickness measurement).
2. A layered ("5 line") appearance to the endometrium.
3. Blood flow within zone 3 using color Doppler technique.
4. Myometrial contractions causing a wave-like motion of the endometrium.
5. Uterine artery blood flow, as measured by PI, less than 3.0
6. Homogeneous myometrial echogenicity.
7. Myometrial blood flow seen on gray-scale examination (internal to the arcuate vessels).

The uterine scoring system for reproduction ("USSR") comprises evaluation of the following parameters:
1. Endometrial thickness (full-thickness measured from the myometrial-endometrial junction to the endometrial-myometrial junction).
2. Endometrial layering (i.e. a 5-line appearance).
3. Myometrial contractions seen as endometrial motion.
4. Myometrial echogenicity.
5. Uterine artery Doppler flow evaluation.
6. Endometrial blood flow.
7. Gray-scale myometrial blood flow.

Each parameter is scored as follows:
1. Endometrial thickness
   a. <7 mm = 0
   b. 7-9 mm = 2
   c. 10-14 mm = 3
   d. >14 mm = 1
2. Endometrial layering
   a. No layering = 0
   b. Hazy 5-line appearance = 1
   c. Distinct 5-line appearance = 3
3. Myometrial contractions (seen as wave-like endometrial motion high-speed playback from videotape)
   a. < 3 contractions in 2 minutes (real time) = 0
   b. > = 3 contractions in 2 minutes (real time) = 3
4. Myometrial echogenicity
   a. Coarse/inhomogeneous echogenicity = 1
   b. Relatively homogeneous echogenicity = 2
5. Uterine artery Doppler flow
   a. PI-2.99-3.0 = 0
   b. PI-2.49 = 0
   c. PI <2 = 2
6. Endometrial blood flow within Zone 3
   a. Absent = 0
   b. Present, but sparse = 2
   c. present multifocally = 5
7. Myometrial blood flow internal to the arcuate vessels seen on gray-scale examination
   a. Absent = 0
   b. Present = 2

The values assume a technically adequate ultrasound examination with no abnormalities of uterine shape or development, no other gross uterine abnormalities (e.g. significant masses) and a normal ovarian cycle (e.g. without evidence of ovarian-uterine discordance). A male factor component to the infertility is not present.

In our limited experience (Applebaum)[1] with this system thus far, a USSR "perfect score" of 20 has been associated with conception 100% of the time. [The number of patients in which we predicted successful conception cycles based upon the UBP and USSR perfect score was 5. The group included 2 spontaneous cycles (non-IVF, non-IUI), 2 IUI and 1 IVF]. Scores of 17-19 (10 patients) have been associated with conception 80% of the time. Scores of 14-16 (10 patients) have a 60% chance, while scores of 13 or less (25 patients) have resulted in no pregnancies.

Absent endometrial flow, despite highest values for the other parameters, has always been associated with no conception.

ROLE OF TRANSVAGINAL COLOR DOPPLER IN OTHER CONDITIONS ASSOCIATED WITH INFERTILITY

Luteinized Unruptured Follicle

This condition is recognized by serial ultrasonography to monitor the growth of follicle, with failure to see expected changes at the time of ovulation.

The typical blood flow pattern seen in the corpus luteum is absent.

In LUF syndrome, no difference in terms of intraovarian RI was obtained after the LH peak. Similar RI values were obtained during the follicular and luteal phases (0.55 ± 0.04 Vs 0.54 ± 0.06). There was no difference between the sides in terms of intraovarian vascular resistance.

Luteal Phase Defect

This is due to decreased vascularization of corpus luteum. The three to seven folds increase in blood supply is necessary to deliver the steroid precursors to ovary and removal of progesterone as shown in experimental animals.

In the LPD group no difference was obtained in terms of intraovarian RI during the follicular phase. The mean RI throughout the luteal phase (0.56 ± 0.04) was significantly higher compared to that in the normal women. Fushemole did not show any difference between the easly, middle and late luteal phase. In the LPD group, differences occurred in terms of intraovarian RI between the sides.

Fibroid

To define the borders of fibroid color Doppler is of real help as the vascular supply at the periphery of the leiomyoma can be delineated very well. Good vascularity denotes a favorable response to GnRH if used before laparoscopic surgery.

Endometriosis

On gray scale scan endometrioma is seen as a hypoechoic, well defined, intraovarian mass with homogeneous low level internal echoes and variable posterior acoustic enhancement. Color Doppler may demonstrate the flow around and not within the endometriotic cyst.

Tubal Causes

During active phase of PID low impedance blood flow signals are usually detected and after effective antibiotic therapy flow tends to return to normal. In the absence of this change surgery is indicated.

Polycystic Ovarian Disease (PCOD) (Fig. 20.19A)

Contrary to the normal ovarian blood flow which is seen around the growing follicle PCOD subjects show abundantly vascularized stroma. It has been shown in several studies that presence of vascularity in the ovaries detected on CDFI or PDI before 8 days of menstrual cycle is highly suggestive of vascularized ovarian stroma which is an indirect evidence of PCOD. Waveforms obtained from the ovarian tissue showed a mean resistance index of 0.54 without cyclical change between repeated examinations.

Patients of PCOD with RI less than 0.54, if gonadotropins are administered will land into ovarian hyperstimulation syndrome.

Uterine Factor

The possibility of decreased uterine blood flow may be associated with infertility as already discussed in preceding paragraphs. Presence of reverse diastolic flow in uterine arteries is a negative marker. Gowswamy et al. depicted in their study that uterine artery indices which were high in failed IVF cases improved after the patients were put on oral estrogen therapy and pregnancy rate improved when compared to those who did not get this treatment.

Color Doppler in *In Vitro* Fertilization

Color Doppler could prove valuable in the prediction of the response of patients to ovarian stimulation in assisted conception, assessment of oocyte quality based on perifollicular flow and parameters influencing implantation following embryo transfer.

a. *Prediction of patient response to ovulation stimulation:* It is seen that women with greater ovarian stromal peak systolic blood flow velocity have increased intraovarian perfusion (Fig. 20.20). Thus, in response to the same dose of gonadotrophin administration, a larger amount is delivered to the target cells. In women with PCOD ovaries a higher stromal blood flow velocity is seen not only at the baseline scan but also during the entire menstrual cycle Color Doppler therefore offers valuable information regarding the dose of gonadotrophin required for successful ovarian stimulation in assisted conception.

   In a stimulated cycle resistance of the intraovarian vessels measured by transvaginal color Doppler correlates well with number of follicles, that is those with more than 15 mm size. This correlation exists

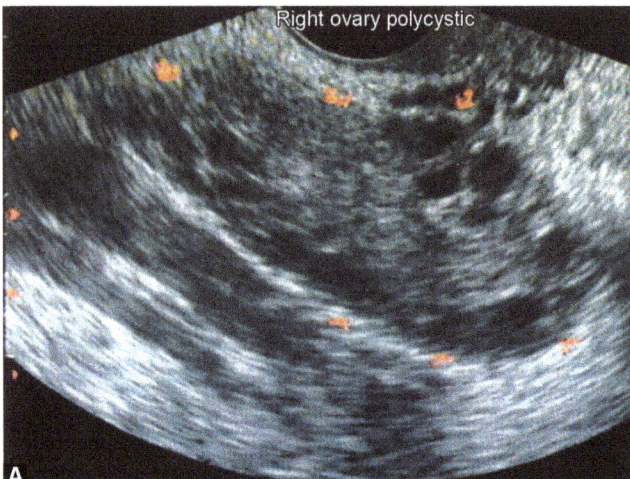

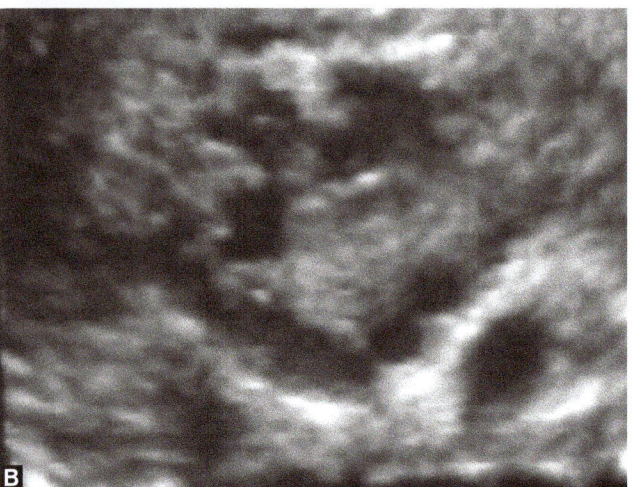

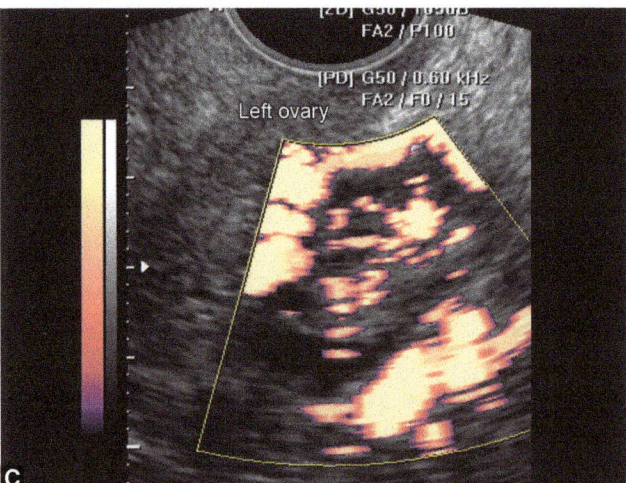

Figs. 20.19A to C: (A) PCOD: gray scale image showing an enlarged right ovary (volume: 28.78 mL) with small peripheral follicles and increased stromal echogenicity; (B) Gray scale 3D image shows a polycystic ovary; (C) Power doppler image shows high vascularity in echogenic stroma of polycystic ovary.

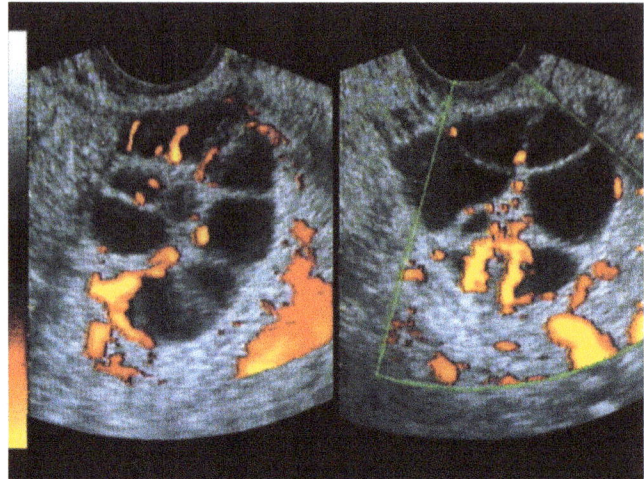

Fig. 20.20: Intraovarian perfusion seen in a case of ovarian stimulation.

even during the early follicular phase, when follicular recruitment and development have just started. This suggest that vascularization of the follicles may play a role in their maturation from early follicular phase onwards. This study in the early follicular phase can prevent ovarian hyperstimulation syndrome (OHSS).

b. *Color Doppler and its contribution towards in vitro fertilization:* During stimulation protocols color Doppler ultrasound has its greatest contribution in monitoring follicular development and guiding oocyte harvesting procedures. The use of color Doppler ultrasound can occasionally be of help as it avoids accidental puncture of iliac vessels and also vessels on the surface of ovary.

c. *Follicular characteristics assessment in predicting oocyte quality:* A rapid rise in blood flow velocity in the perifollicular and ovarian stromal vessels is seen at the time of LH surge. These changes are as a result of neoangiogenesis occurring during late follicular development. A marked increase in peak systolic velocity around the follicle, in the presence of a relatively constant pulsatility index could be a sign of follicle maturity and herald impending ovulation. Administration of hCG resulted in a rapid increase in peak velocities. Nargund et al. showed that oocytes obtained from highly vascularized follicle were of higher quality and were more likely to fertilize and result in pregnancy. From the available data, it appears that assessment of perifollicular vascular perfusion could lead to a better selection of oocytes and ultimately a higher pregnancy rate.

d. *Implantation:* Steer et al. noted that the lowest uterine artery PI was found 9 days after the LH peak, which is consistent with maximum uterine perfusion at the time of peak luteal function and expected implantation.

They also showed that uterine artery impedance was different in the mid luteal phase in women with subfertility compared with those with normal fertility. They grouped the patients according to whether the PI was low (1-1.99), medium (2-2.99) or high (>3.0). There were no pregnancies in high PI group and the PI was significantly lower in women who become pregnant as compared with those who did not.

In a recent work by Campbell it is possible to calculate the probability of pregnancy by using PI values of uterine artery on the day of embryo transfer. Highest probability of pregnancy was predicted for patients who had medium values for PI. Those with high PI had failure rate up to 35%.

The ability to predict implantation before the administration of hCG allows the clinician the option to delay giving hCG until the uterine artery PI improves. An alternative approach would be to try to improve uterine perfusion by the administration of glyceryltrinitrate (GTN). It has been suggested that administration of GTN may increase pregnancy rates in women with poor uterine perfusion.

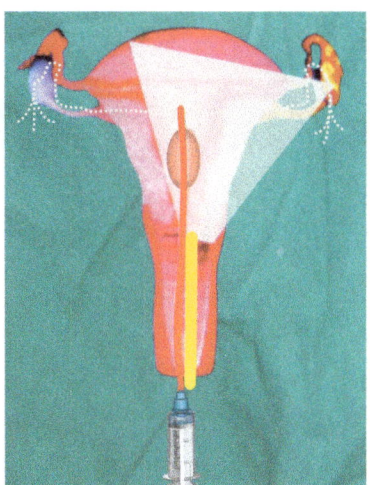

Fig. 20.21: Sonosalpingography technique.

Conclusion

The role of this new modality in the evaluation of an infertile female is becoming more important as various centers are coming out with a multitude of studies indicating its superior accuracy and excellent reproducibility.

TUBAL EVALUATION

Introduction

Endosonography as a tool for checking the patency of fallopian tubes was an expected development with great strides taken within the field of gynecology. Sonosalpingography also known as 'Sion Test' used transvaginalsonography to confirm the tubal patency by visualizing the spill of fluid from the fimbrial end of fallopian tubes (Figs. 20.21 and 20.22). Fallopian tubes are isoechoic and cannot be normally seen on ultrasound unless pathological or fluid surrounds the tubes. We propose to perform this test not as a substitute for hysterosalpingography or laparoscopy but as a noninvasive, cheap outdoor screening procedure in patients of infertility.

Sonosalpingography

We used this test as a basic screening test for evaluating tubal patency in all.

Number 8 Fr. Foleys catheter, is put inside the uterine cavity the bulb is inflated with 2 mL of distilled water. Prior to procedure the patient is asked to evacuate the

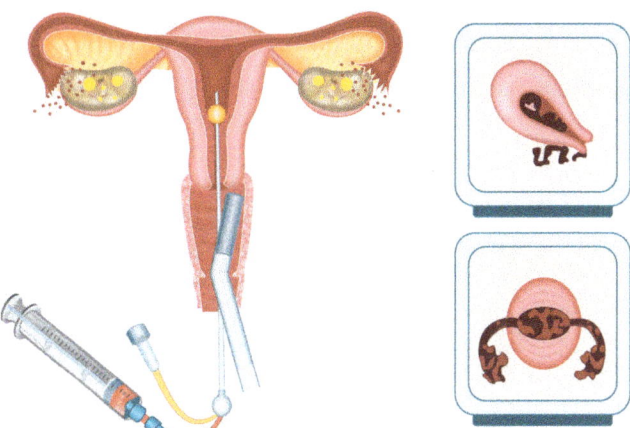

Fig. 20.22: Sonosalpingography with echovist.

bladder and baseline vaginal scan is performed. 20-60 mL of solution containing ciplox, hylase, and dexamethasone is taken in 50 mL catheter tip syringe and pushed via Foleys catheter and spill is studied from the fimbrial end (Figs. 20.23A and B).

We have done the 'Sion Procedure' in the patients of suspected pelvic factors. In this we have flooded the pelvis using the same fluid about 200-300 mL, pushed via foley's catheter and visualized the fallopian tubes (Fig. 20.24).

Aims and Objectives

The present study was conducted with the aim to study the tubal patency using sonosalpingography as a first screening method. The patients were further followed up by hysterosalpingography and laparoscopy. 'Sion Procedure' was done in only suspected cases having adhesions and tubal pathology.

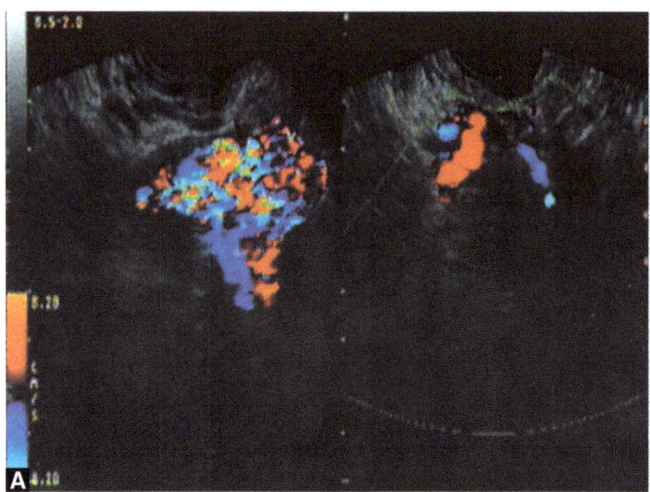
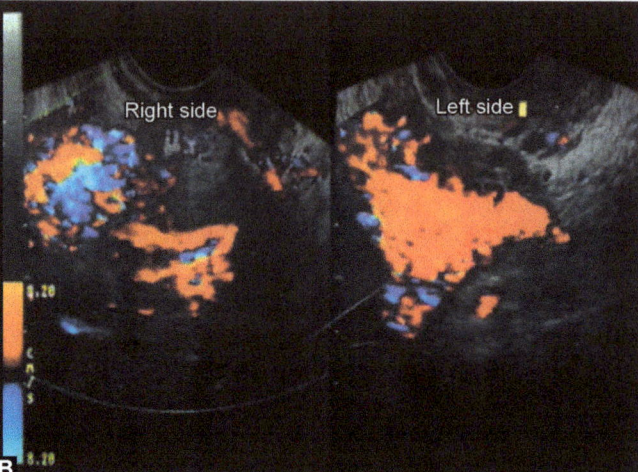

Figs. 20.23A and B: Spill from the fimbrial end on both sides confirming the tubal patency.

Observations (Tables 20.1–20.5)

Results and discussions: As it is very evident from the above tables that sonosalpingography is a good noninvasive screening test for judging the tubal patency. The findings of sonosalpingography were further confirmed by hysterosalpingography. In patients where a tubal pathology was suspected, Sion procedure was done and we found that out of 25 patients of suspected pelvic factor problem 5 had adhesions, 2 had fimbrial pathology. The same group of patients were further followed up by diagnostic laparoscopy and we could additionally pick one more case of adhesions. Since last 6 years we are evaluating all cases of infertility by color Doppler (Medison 7700 and Voluson 530 D).

Optimal Conditions for Embryo Transfer

The lower the PI value in uterine artery the more the chances of pregnancy. Steer et al. have shown that if PI is > 3 before ET no pregnancy results.

Conclusion

The role of this new modality in the evaluation of an infertile female is becoming more important as various centers are coming out with a multitude of studies indicating its superior accuracy and excellent reproducibility.

COLOR DOPPLER IN RELATION TO OBSTETRICS

The minimum frequency of transducer should be 7.5 MHz in early pregnancy (up to 8 weeks) and 5 MHz in 9–13 weeks pregnancy. The vaginal probe should have dynamic focusing and produce minimal artifacts. The transducer

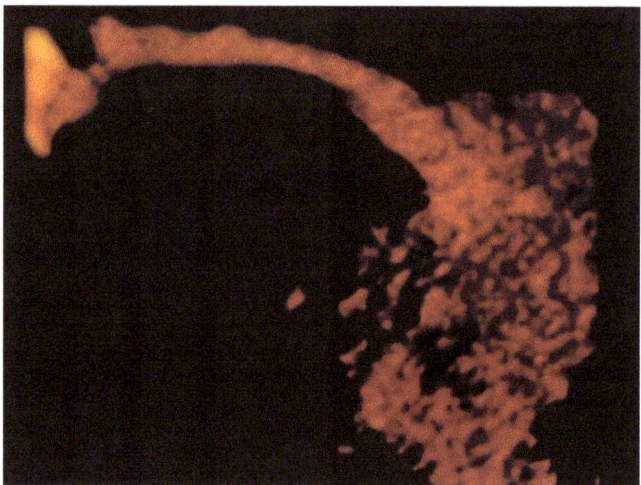

Fig. 20.24: 3D color tubes.

TABLE 20.1: Case distribution.

Total cases	Infertility		Positive	Sion test	Negative	Sion test
	Primary	Secondary				
200	160	40	135	10	25	30

TABLE 20.2: Negative Sion test (n = 55).

Total cases	Hysterosalpingography	
	Tubal block	Patent tube
55	51	4

TABLE 20.3: Laparoscopy.

Total cases	Diagnostic laparoscopy	
	Tubal patency	Tubal block
20 selected randomly	17	3

TABLE 20.4: Sion procedure suspected pelvic factor.

Cases	Adhesions	Fimbrial path	Normal
25 random	5	2	18

TABLE 20.5: Suspected pelvic factors (n = 25) laparoscopy.

Cases	Adhesions	Fimbrial path	Normal
24	6	2	16

KEY POINTS

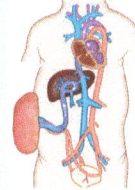

I. Color Doppler in infertility
- Doppler indices of ovarian and uterine perfusion change with the phases of menstrual cycle.

Ovarian artery
- Follicular phase — Low velocity, high impedance pattern, RI (early proliferative phase) = 0.54±0.04
  Day 8–10, dominant follicle shows a ring of angiogenesis around it
- At ovulation — High velocity, low impedance flow
  RI (a day before ovulation) = 0.44±0.04
  PSV = 27±10 cm/sec
- Luteal phase dominant ovary with corpus luteum shows RI = 0.39–0.49
  RI > 0.5 has a nonviable outcome.

Uterine artery
- High velocity, high resistance flow
- RI depends on age and phase of menstrual cycle
- RI (proliferative phase 1–13 days) = 0.88±0.04
- RI (day 16, i.e. 3 days after LH surge) increases
- RI (peak luteal phase) = 0.84±0.04 (leads to successful implantation)

Uterine Biophysical profile (UBP)
- Done during mid cycle phase
- USSR scores the following parameters to determine the success of natural or artificial conception:
  - Endometrial thickness
  - Endometrial layering
  - Myometrial contraction
  - Uterine artery Doppler flow
  - Endometrial blood flow within zone 3
  - Myometrial blood flow to arcuate vessels on gray scale
  - Score of 20–100% conception
  - Score of 13 or less-No conception occurs

II. TVCD in Other Conditions Associated with Infertility
- Intraovarian RI remaining same before and after LH peak signifying luteinized unruptured follicle
- RI (luteal phase) of 0.56±0.04 (more than in normal women) suggests a luteal phase defect
- Good peripheral vascularity in fibroid denotes a favorable response to GnRH
- In PCOD, there is vascular stroma which shows mean RI of 0.54 with no cyclical changes
- Role of Doppler in *in vitro* fertilization: the dose of gonadotropin directly corresponds to the ovarian stromal PSV, the marked increase in PSV around follicle and a constant pulsatility index signifies follicle maturity and impending ovulation, 9 days after LH peak showed lowest uterine PI (i.e. maximum uterine perfusion) and good chances of implantation.

SSG/ Sion Test
- Non invasive modality to assess the tubal patency
- 20–60 mL of solution (ciplox, hylase, and dexamethasone) is instilled via a Foley's catheter placed in the uterine cavity
- Visualization of spill from the fimbrial end establishes tubal patency
- Flooding the pelvis with 200–300 mL of fluid helps in detecting adhesions.

should have color sensitivity to demonstrate small vessels with low velocity blood flow, which characterize the trophoblast. An update Duplex Doppler or a triplex Doppler capability is essential for displaying Doppler waveforms and for calculating the resistance index (RI) and pulsatility index (PI) and also the A/B ratio (peak systolic/end diastolic ratio).

The same is achieved after 14 weeks by TAS. Although no significant difference has been obtained in the value of these indices in clinical practice, but most workers prefer Pourcelot index (PI) over RI. Decreased values of RI reflect less peripheral vascular resistance.

Changes in Pregnancy

1. Gravid uterus shows a generalized increase in vascularity in the myometrium.
2. The decidua (endometrium) shows no evidence of flow before implantation.
3. An area of vascularity is demonstrated in the hyper echoic decidua on day 26–28 post-LMP (implantation site signal).
4. Chorionic sac stage (29–34 days) is characterized by multiple areas of vascularity in the decidua trophoblast layers and adjacent myometrium.
5. CDS picks up diastolic flow of small vessels with low impedance characteristic of trophoblastic invasion even before embryo is sighted (Fig. 20.25).
6. Once embryo is seen (34–39 days) a distinct color signal is seen in its cardiovascular system and is referred to as the embryonic heart beat.
7. As the embryo grows, cardiovascular system will be seen on CDS-the aorta, vena cava, intracranial, and hepatic circulation. The umbilical cord, placenta vitelline (yolk sac) circulation becomes visible at 8-9 weeks gestation (Figs. 20.26A and B).
8. Triplex TV-Doppler (color flow plus duplex) can determine various indices in the pelvic vessels during the first trimester.

Problems in Acquiring and Interpreting the Waveforms

Artifactual Loss of End Diastolic Frequencies

This may be due to:

a. A high angle between the ultrasound beam and the vessel that results in very low frequencies disappearing below the height of the vessel wall filter. If end-diastolic frequencies appear absent one should reduce the vessel wall filter to its lowest setting (usually 50 Hz) or remove it if possible. Then one should alter the angle of the probe relative to maternal abdomen and if end diastolic frequencies are still absent one should then attempt to obtain the signal from a different site within the uterus as this is likely to result in a different angle of insonation. One should also ensure that fetus is not breathing by demonstrating a smooth waveform of the umbilical vein in the opposite channel. We do not report absence of end

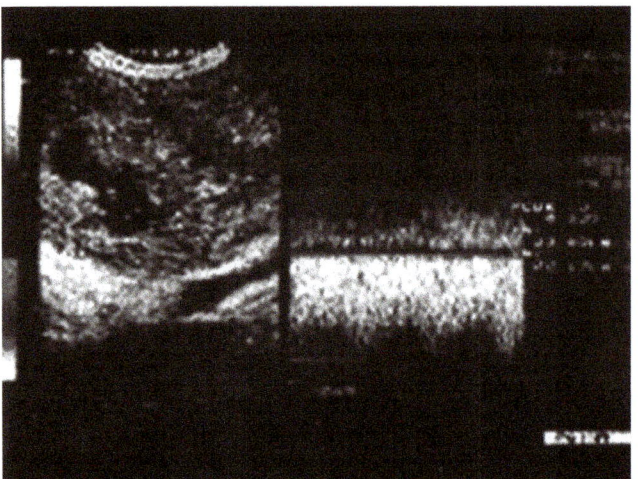

Fig. 20.25: Trophoblastic flow detected in early pregnancy reveals low impedance pattern.

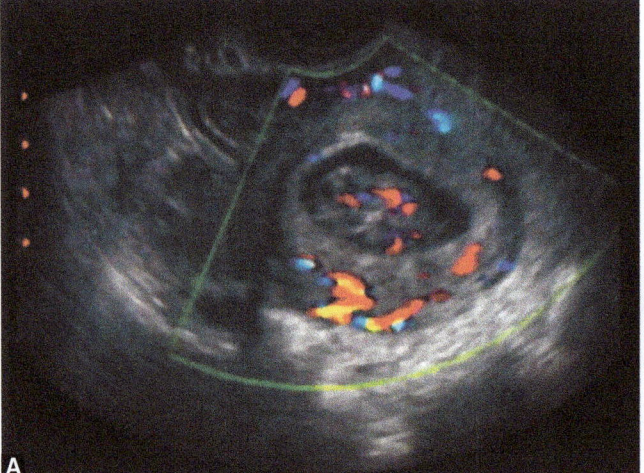
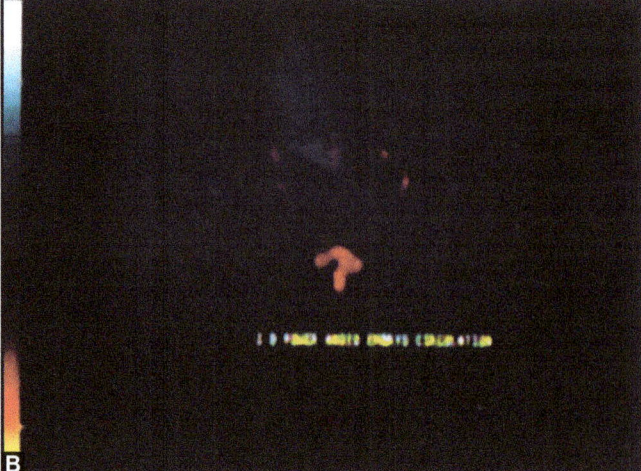

Figs. 20.26A and B: (A) Color Doppler at nine weeks of gestation; (B) 3D power angio of the uterus showing early embryonic circulation.

diastolic frequencies until this has been demonstrated on two successive days. The alternative is to submit the woman to a Duplex, pulsed Doppler examination.
b. *Fetal breathing movements*: These cause wild fluctuations in the signal from umbilical artery and are readily recognizable by being unable to demonstrate a steady state in the umbilical vein that is recorded in the other channel. After a little practice, they can also be recognized from the arterial signal. The only course to take if the fetus is breathing, is to wait until this stop.

Failure to Obtain a Signal

This may be due to:
a. *Incorrect machine settings:* This is usually recognized by having a signal that is not displayed on the screen. First one must check that the frequency range is not too high or low-4 MHz is a good starting point. If the screen is still blank then turn up the gain slowly. If the screen is saturated with white noise then turn the gain down slowly until the waveform appears. If there is still no visual signal then ensure that balance setting is not turned to one extreme such that one channel of the spectrum analyzer is obliterated.
b. Fetal death.
c. Maternal obesity.
d. Oligohydramnios.

In the latter three situations, use a real time transducer to check that the fetus is still alive and then to locate a loop of cord. Mark the spot on the maternal abdomen with a finger and then replace the real time transducer with the Doppler probe. One cannot undertake real time imaging and acquire Doppler signals simultaneously, as the signals interfere with each other. In pulsed Doppler machines the real time imaging is usually frozen when the Doppler signal is being acquired.

Duplex Evaluation in Normal and High Risk Pregnancy

Fetal growth depends on a study supply of nutrients and oxygen from the mother; a normal uteroplacental and fetoplacental circulation is necessary for this to occur. In recent years, however Doppler ultrasound has given us a non-invasive method of evaluating blood flow in the fetoplacental and uteroplacental circulation in normal and complicated pregnancies.

Uteroplacental Circulation

During pregnancy there is hyperplasia and hypertrophy of the uterine wall and the arterioles elongate and coil (Fig. 20.27). At the base of placenta there is thinning of endometrium with invasion of trophoblast. The

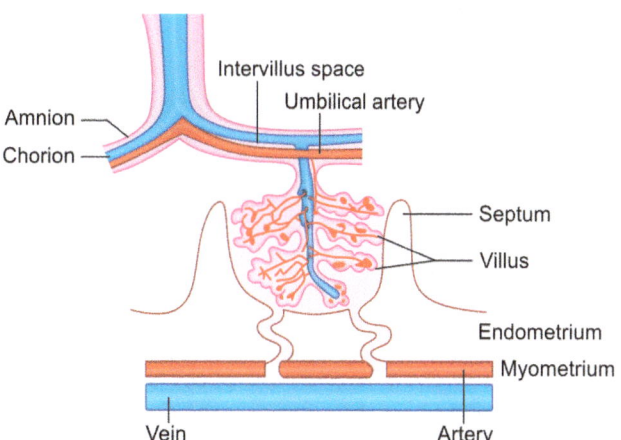

Fig. 20.27: Line diagram showing normal uteroplacental vasculature.

trophoblastic invasion leads to stripping off the muscular elastic coat of spiral arteries by the 20th postmenstrual week. This decreases the resistance to blood flow progressing from the radials artery into the intervillous spaces. The pressure falls about 70–80 mm in the former to 10 mm Hg in the latter.

Fetoplacental Circulation (Fig. 20.28)

The branches of the umbilical artery and umbilical vein radiate out from the site of insertion of the cord along the fetal surface of placenta beneath the amnion. Branches of the artery along with an accompanying vein penetrate the chorionic plate and enter the main stem chorionic villi. There they divide to supply individual chorionic villi. It is at this level that the exchange of nutrients and waste products takes place between the fetal and maternal circulations. The unit composed of the main stem chorionic villus and its branches is called the "Fetal Cotyledon". It is this capillary bed that produces the most resistance to pulsatile blood flow. As pregnancy advances, the size of the chorionic villi increases, whereas their number decreases. This is accompanied by a reduction in the thickness of the tissue layer between the fetal capillaries and the maternal intervillous spaces. These changes allow for more efficient exchange between the two circulations. The fetal circulation is characterized by a high blood flow and a low vascular resistance. Umbilical blood flow increases with gestational age and pressure gradient driving the blood from the descending aorta through the placenta and back to inferior vena cava.

Umbilical flow velocity waveforms before 14 weeks of gestation are typically characterized by the absence of end diastolic velocities. Diastolic flow is incomplete until 14 weeks of gestation. After this, pan diastolic frequencies are consistently present. Intraplacental waveforms with fetal

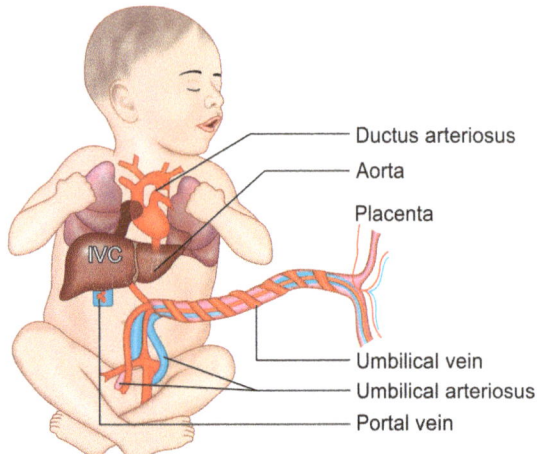

Fig. 20.28: Line diagram showing normal fetal circulation.

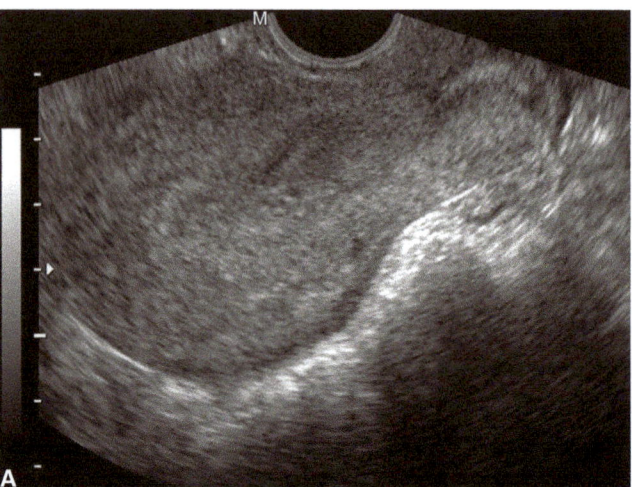

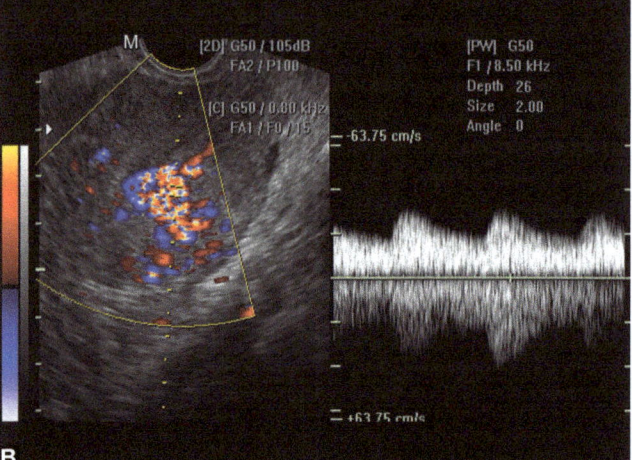

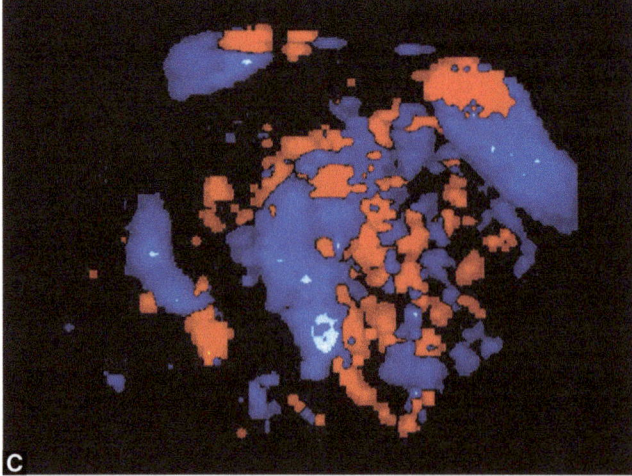

Figs. 20.29A to C: (A) Gray scale image showing a bulky uterus with echogenicity at 3rd postabortal week indicating possible incomplete abortion; (B) Color doppler showing high vascularity in the region of increased echogenicity with low resistance flow confirming incomplete abortion; (C) 3D angiographic image shows the vascular channels associated with incomplete abortion.

characteristics can be identified and clearly differentiated from the beginning of the 2nd trimester.

The appearance of end diastolic frequencies in the umbilical circulation coincide with an abrupt and significant increase in uterine artery peak systolic velocity together with presence of continuous intervillous flow within the placenta. The establishment of the intervillous circulation may be associated with change in the pressure gradient due to the expansion of the intervillous space and/or with modification in blood gases and metabolite concentrations which in turn may explain the rapid appearance of end diastolic frequencies in the umbilical circulation.

Abnormal 1st Trimester

Color flow can be used very effectively in:
1. *Complete versus incomplete abortion (Figs. 20.29A to C):* Dillon et al. reported that 24 hours after an abortion persistent placental flow was seen in half the patients, which resolved spontaneously over the next few days. Although, there are several possible ways to interpret these findings, the most likely explanation is that many therapeutic abortions are incomplete and spontaneously proceed to completion without further intervention. Thus, the decision about further intervention following therapeutic abortion should be made on the basis of patients symptoms and signs and not on the ground of demonstration of intrauterine placental flow alone. However, there should be no placental flow 1 week after an abortion and demonstration of low impedance flow indicates the need for D and C. The intrauterine appearances are unimpressive for retained products. However, the presence of low impedance flow correctly predicted retained product of conception and indicated the need for repeat D and C. It should be stressed that

clinical correlation is important for correct diagnosis because endometritis can give rise to similar low impedance endometrial flow as described earlier.

2. *Ectopic pregnancy:* The process of ectopic placentation is morphologically similar whether it occurs in the uterus or in the fallopian tube (Fig. 20.30). The chorion villi with the intervening intervillous space are well seen within the fallopian tube. High velocity, low-impedance flow is seen in the tubal mass. On color flow a solid adnexal mass shows pronounced vascularity, which identifies it as an ectopic gestation (Figs. 20.31A and B).

Care must be exercised in the differentiation between placental flow in the tube and luteal flow in the ovary. In 85% of ectopic gestations, the pregnancy is on the same side as the corpus which can be used to guide the initial examination. Women are also accurate at realizing their ectopic by the side of their pelvic pain. In practice, it is necessary to identify the ovary by its specific morphology and to look for a vascular area, usually medial to the side of luteal flow, which can therefore be identified as the ectopic gestation.

Taylor et al. showed in his series of ectopic pregnancy, no placental flow was detected in about 18% of cases. These avascular ectopics probably represent nonviable gestations. It is notable that they display low serum hCG values indicating the limited activity of the trophoblast failing to thrive in the hostile environment of the tube. Such gestations may be especially suitable for medical therapy.

3. *Recognition of pseudosac (Fig. 20.32):* A pseudosac displays the normal high impedance flow from the endometrium, whereas the abnormal gestational sac shows the high velocity, low impedance flow of the placental interface. It should be noted that the absence of an embryo does not affect the presence of placental flow because placental flow results from pressure gradient between the maternal tubal arteries and the low resistance of the intervillous space. This depends on trophoblastic activity and not on the presence of fetus.

4. *Molar pregnancy (discussed earlier).*

Second and Third Trimester

In second and third trimester of pregnancy color flow offers a very exciting avenue to study umbilical and placental hemodynamics. Along with fetal circulation this has proved to be very useful in assessing IUGR fetus and fetal anomalies.

Indications for umbilical artery waveform:
- Assessment and continued monitoring of the fetus that has been demonstrated to be small for gestational age on real time ultrasound

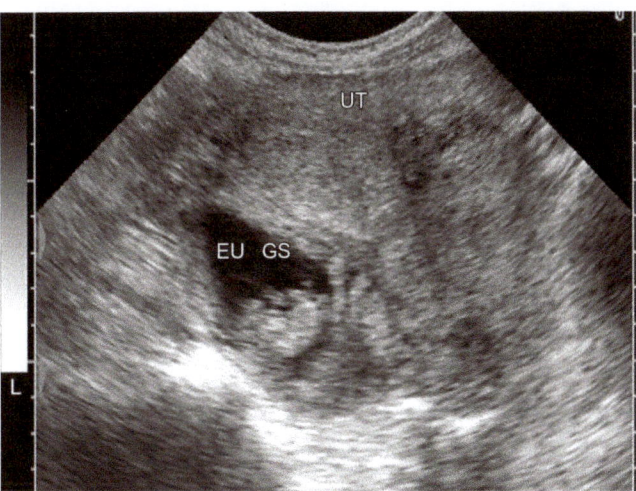

Fig. 20.30: Gray scale image showing small ectopic gestation.

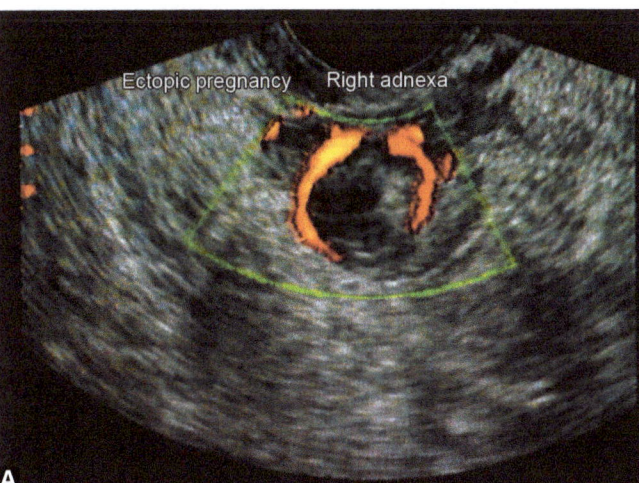
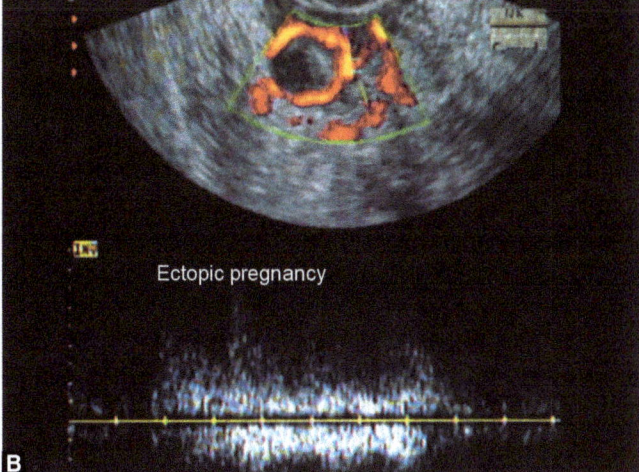

Figs. 20.31A and B: (A) On color Doppler "ring of fire" appearance is seen in ectopic gestation; (B) Duplex Doppler demonstrates trophoblastic flow pattern.

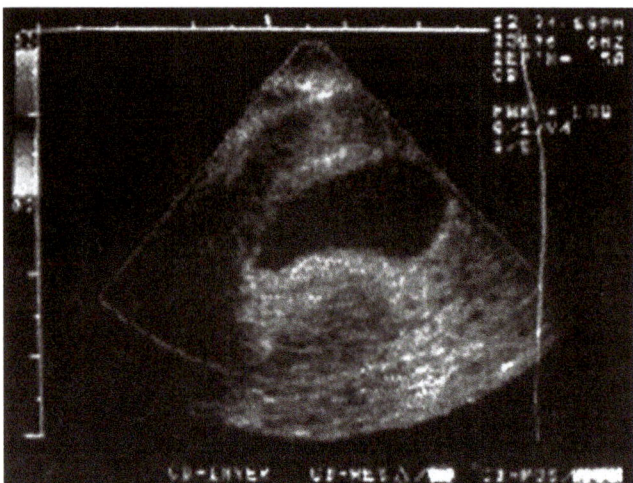

Fig. 20.32: Gray scale image showing an empty gestational sac.

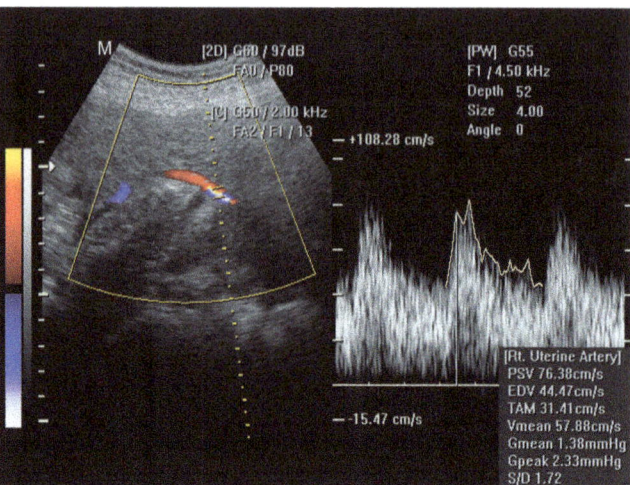

Fig. 20.34: Flow pattern of uterine artery in pregnancy.

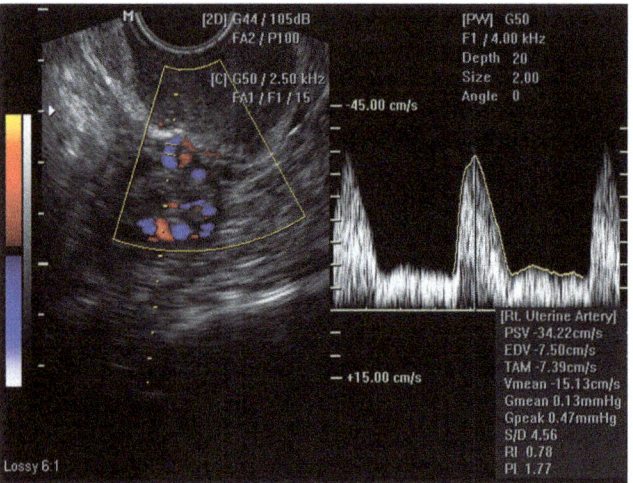

Fig. 20.33: Flow pattern of uterine artery in nonpregnant state.

- Assessment of the fetus of a mother with systemic lupus erythematosus (SLE) and PET
- In conjunction with uteroplacental waveforms in the assessment of oligohydramnios
- Assessment of differing of sizes or growth patterns in twins.

The following are specially examined:

1. *Uterine artery (Figs. 20.33 and 20.34):* Diastolic Notch of uterine artery disappears by 24 weeks (Figs. 20.35A and B) and RI drops from 0.84–0.56 RI of radial branch is 0.33 and that of spiral branch is 0.32. The placentation process continues until 24–26th week of pregnancy, after which there is only a small decrease in values in the main uterine branch reflecting the sum of the radial and spiral vessels. If the notch has not been lost by 24–26 weeks most women will develop a hypertensive complication of pregnancy. After delivery, the uterine artery does not return to its pre-pregnant level for 4–6 weeks.

Impaired uterine artery flow velocity is identified by (a) Persistent abnormal index (b) A persistent notch (c) A significant difference between the indices in two vessels. The upper limit of S/D ratio is approximately 2.6 and the difference between two vessels should not exceed 1.

Adverse outcomes associated with abnormal uterine artery flow velocity include (a) pre-eclampsia (b) Fetal growth retardation and its sequelae.

2. *Umbilical artery:* With the aid of color flow, the umbilical arteries can be detected as early as 6–8 weeks (Figs. 20.36A and B). Doppler flow velocity profile shows only the systolic or ventricular component. By 20 weeks, all fetuses should have end-diastolic flow (Fig. 20.37). As pregnancy advances there is increasing end diastolic flow velocity with lesser changes in systolic peak velocity. A mature umbilical artery flow velocity waveform is usually achieved by 28–30 weeks but some fetuses may show a delayed maturation such as in twins. The indices are highest at the fetal abdomen and are lowest at the cord insertion into the placenta. Those at the mid cord or placental insertion are clinically reliable. Normal resistance index ranges from 0.5–0.7 and S/D ratio is ≤3. Both the umbilical arteries should be evaluated with at least two readings from each artery to avoid errors in analysis.

Absent end diastolic velocity is clearly abnormal and S/D ratio > 4.0 is probably going to stay in the elevated range. Decreased diastolic flow (RI > 0.7) indicates early placental insufficiency (Figs. 20.38A to C). When there is a reversal of flow, it may be a clinical emergency because most of these fetuses die within two weeks (Fig. 20.38D).

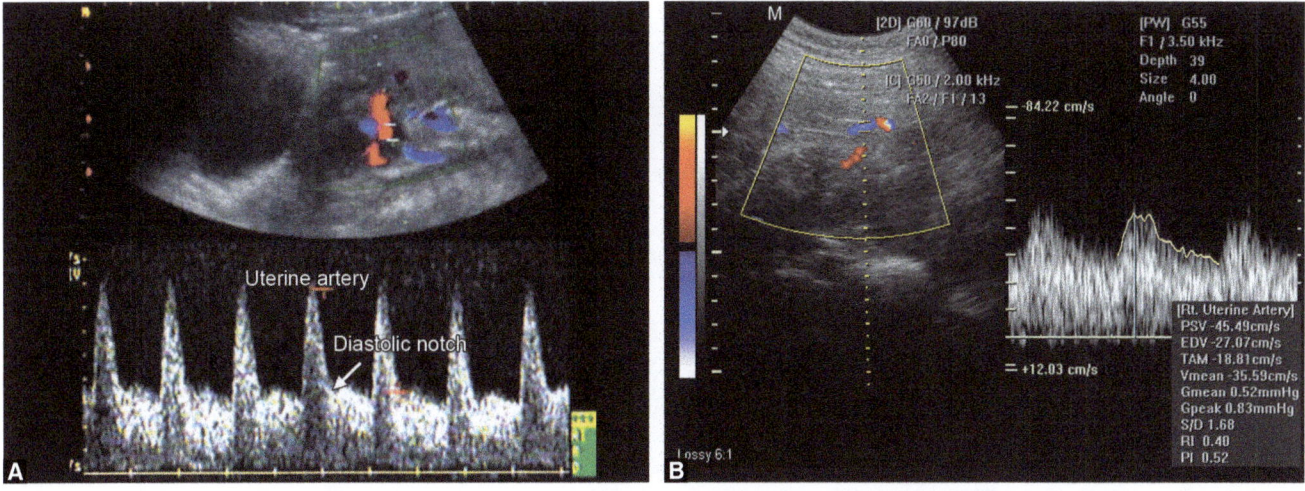

Figs. 20.35A and B: (A) Uterine artery flow pattern before 24 weeks of gestation shows a diastolic notch; (B) The notch normally disappears by 24–26 weeks of gestation.

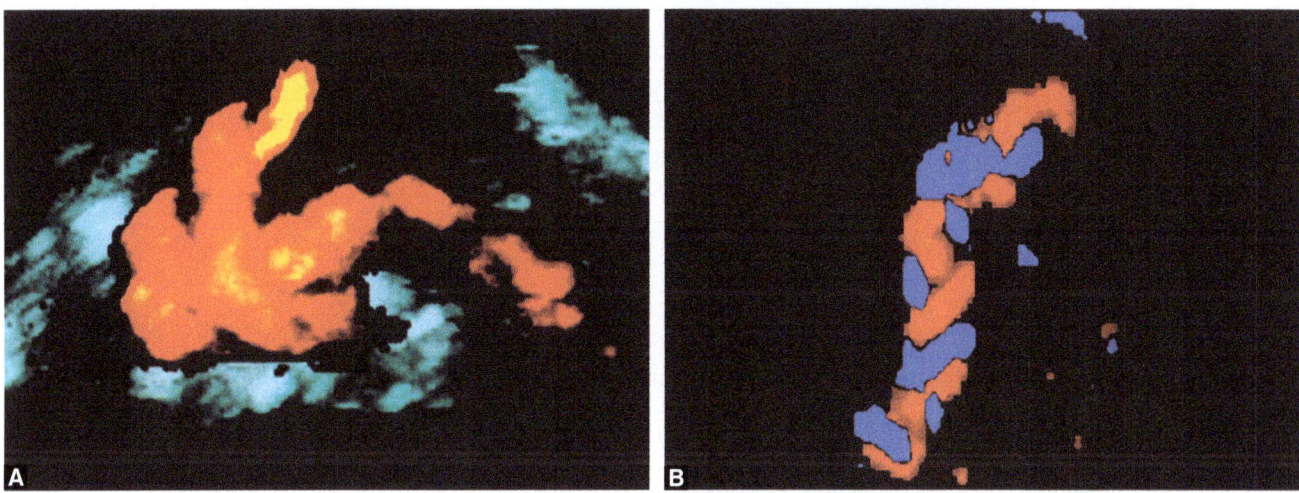

Figs. 20.36A and B: (A) Power Doppler at 7 weeks showing two arteries and one vein in the umbilical cord; (B) 3D angiographic image shows a three vessel cord.

3. *Fetal descending thoracic aorta (Figs. 20.39A and B):* Normal flow wave pattern shows an RI = 0.82 ± 0.1 and a PI = 1.83 ± 0.3 (Fig. 20.40).

    Significance of aortic flow is that there is increase in RI and PI of growth retarded fetuses. High PI is suggestive of fetal acidemia.

    Absent end-diastolic flow is suggestive of perinatal complication such as respiratory distress syndrome, necrotizing enterocolitis, renal failure.

4. *Fetal middle cerebral artery (Figs. 20.41 and 20.42):* Normal resistance index of MCA is > 0.7 and pulsatility index is > 1.3. Fetus with mild hypoxia (reduced umbilical artery flow velocity) will dilate its cerebral vessels as compensatory response (brain sparing effect- RI < 0.7) seen in asymmetrical growth retardation. The middle cerebral artery on both sides should be examined as the values on one side may be affected

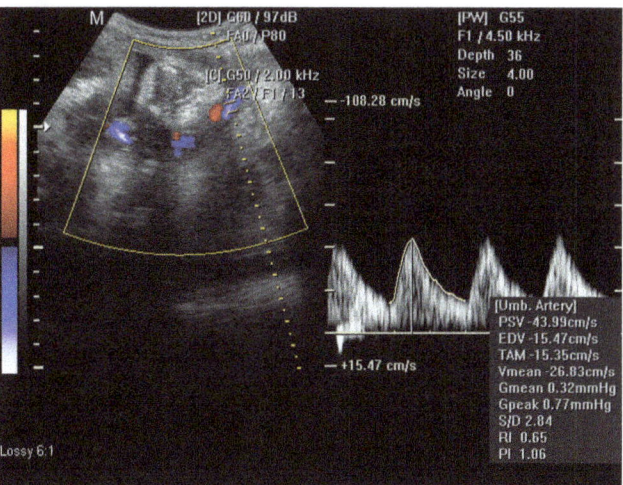

Fig. 20.37: Normal umbilical artery flow pattern reveals a low resistance flow.

206 | Textbook of Color Doppler Imaging

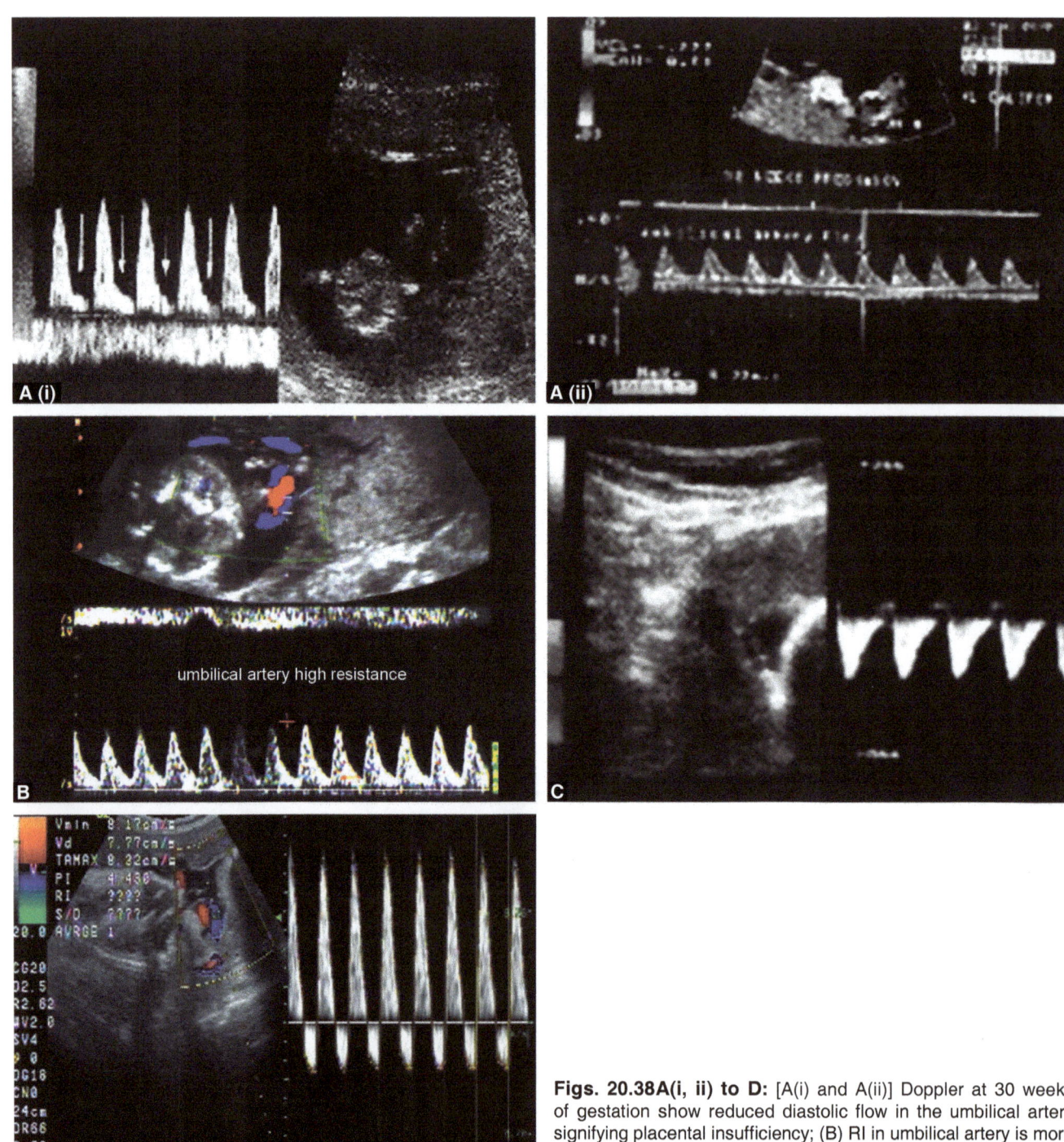

Figs. 20.38A(i, ii) to D: [A(i) and A(ii)] Doppler at 30 weeks of gestation show reduced diastolic flow in the umbilical artery signifying placental insufficiency; (B) RI in umbilical artery is more than 0.7 indicating decreased diastolic flow; (C) Umbilical artery waveform in a case of IUGR; (D) Reversal of diastolic flow in umbilical artery signifying impending fetal death.

Role of Color Flow and Doppler in Obstetrics, Gynecology, and Infertility

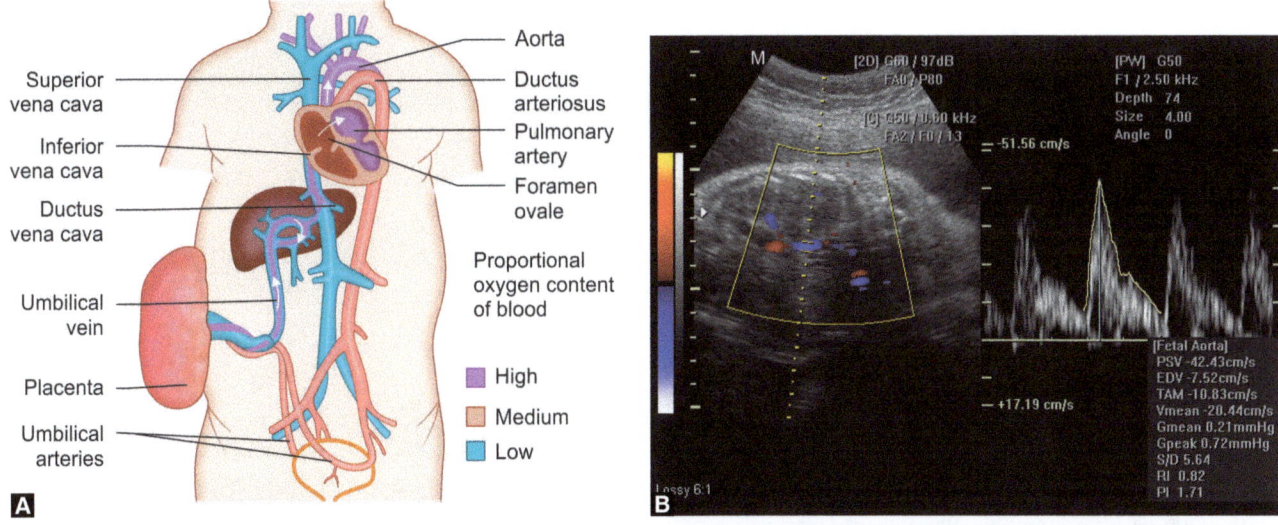

Figs. 20.39A and B: (A) Line diagram showing normal fetal vasculature; (B) Normal flow pattern in fetal aorta.

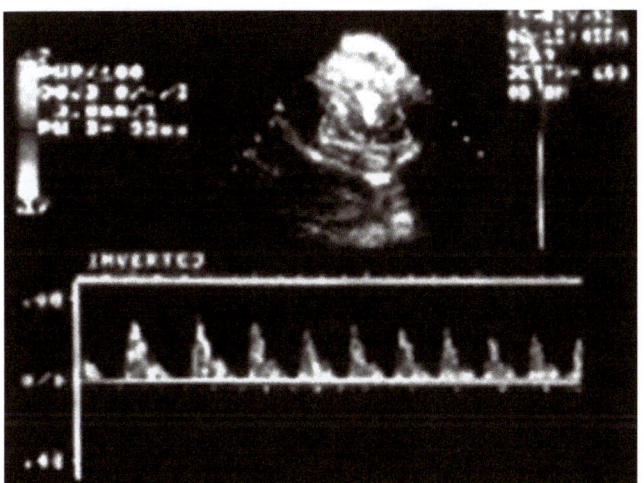

Fig. 20.40: Flow pattern of aorta in IUGR showing loss of end diastolic flow.

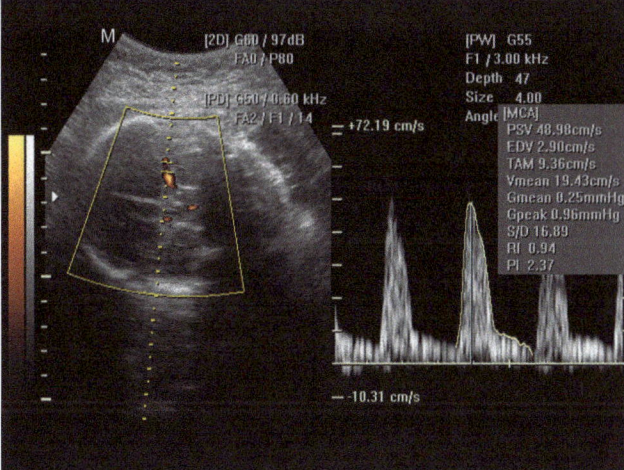

Fig. 20.42: Duplex Doppler showing fetal middle cerebral artery.

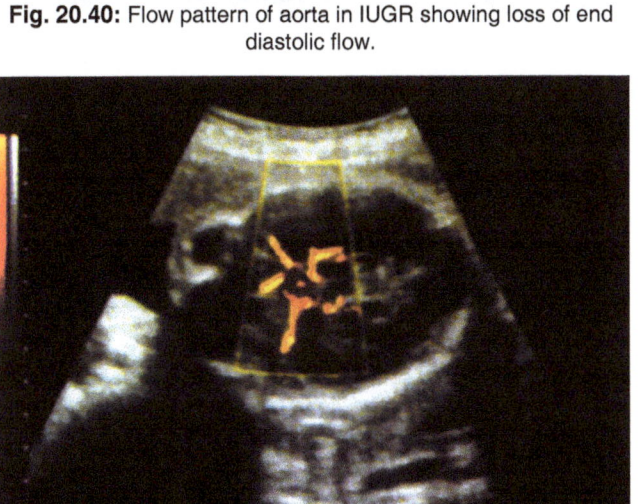

Fig. 20.41: Doppler showing fetal circle of Willis.

first than another. When hypoxia worsens the cerebral vessels lose their autonomic reactivity and return to previous state. This is an alarming sign. The preterminal flow pattern shows absent diastolic flow in the umbilical artery, aorta, vena cava, and umbilical vein pulsations.

In the growth retarded fetus that appears normal, the first question to ask is, what is the state of umbilical and uterine circulation? The next question is, is the fetus hypoxemic? This is determined by middle cerebral Doppler. The fetus with significant reduction of umbilical flow should have dilated cerebrals. If it does not, it is critically ill or not hypoxic. If it is not hypoxic, it may have congenital heart disease and the reduced peripheral flow is caused by reduced forward flow, not increased resistance. Careful evaluation of the heart then becomes imperative.

5. *Fetal venous circulation:* Doppler evaluation of fetal venous circulation especially of the ductusvenosus, hepatic veins and umbilical veins gives an idea of fetal hypoxic and acidotic state (Figs. 20.43A to C). Absent diastolic velocities and reversal of blood flow in ductus venous is an absolute indication of delivery (Fig. 20.43B).
6. *Fetal echocardiography:* A detailed fetal echo study will reflect earliest changes in the fetal circulation (Fig. 20.44).

Limitations of Umbilical Artery Waveform

Umbilical artery waveforms are of little or no value as a screening test for the small for gestational fetus and do not appear to predict unexplained antepartum stillbirths. They are also not predictive of placental abruption.

The role of umbilical artery waveform is not established in fetuses of insulin dependent diabetes and fetal death has been reported within 24 hours of obtaining normal umbilical artery waveforms from the fetus of such women. The place of umbilical artery waveforms in antepartum hemorrhage and preterm labor or rupture of the membranes is unknown.

Interpretations of Waveforms

1. In the absence of acute incident such as a placental abruption, a small for gestational age fetus with normal umbilical artery waveforms will not develop loss of end diastolic frequencies within a 7-day period so that monitoring may be performed weekly.
2. Only 10% of fetuses that are demonstrated to be asymmetrically small for gestational age on real time ultrasound will demonstrate loss of end diastolic frequencies at any time during their pregnancy.
3. Loss of end diastolic frequencies is associated with an 85% chance that the fetus will be acidotic.
4. The finding of a symmetrically small for date fetus with absent and diastolic frequencies in the umbilical artery but with normal uteroplacental waveforms suggest the possibility of a primary fetal cause for the growth retardation such as a chromosomal abnormality or a TORCH virus infection.
5. Fetuses demonstrating absence of end diastolic frequencies but which are managed along standard clinical lines have a 40% chance of dying and at least a 25% morbidity rate from necrotising enterocolitis, hemorrhage or coagulation failure after birth. The time between loss of end diastolic frequencies and fetal death appears to differ for each fetus. Following loss of end-diastolic frequencies there are no other reliable changes in the waveform that help in deciding when to deliver the baby.

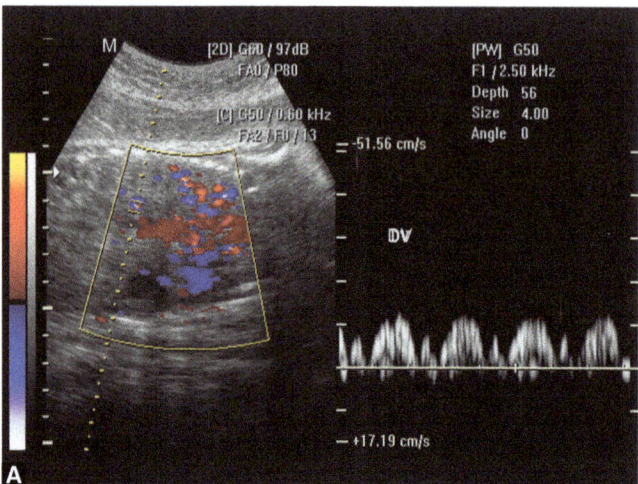

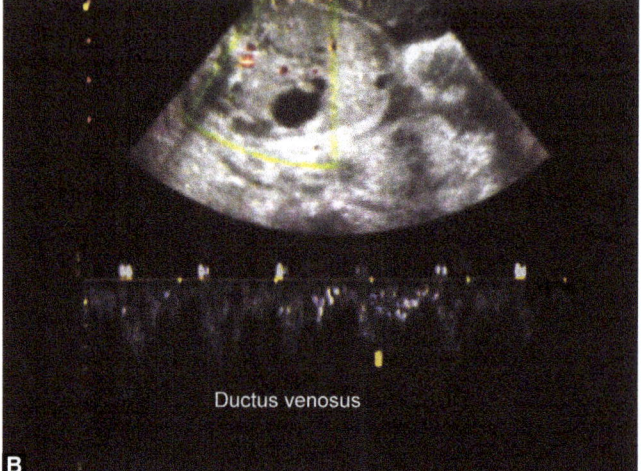

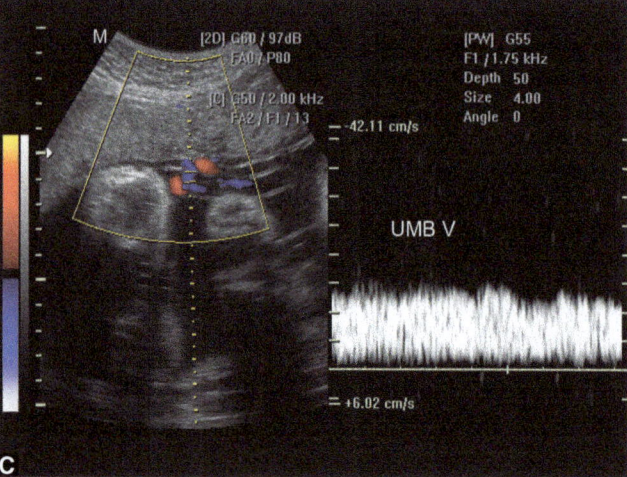

Figs. 20.43A to C: (A) Duplex Doppler showing normal pulsatile flow in ductus venosus; (B) Increased reversed flow in ductus venosus in fetal distress; (C) Duplex Doppler shows normal flow pattern in umbilical vein.

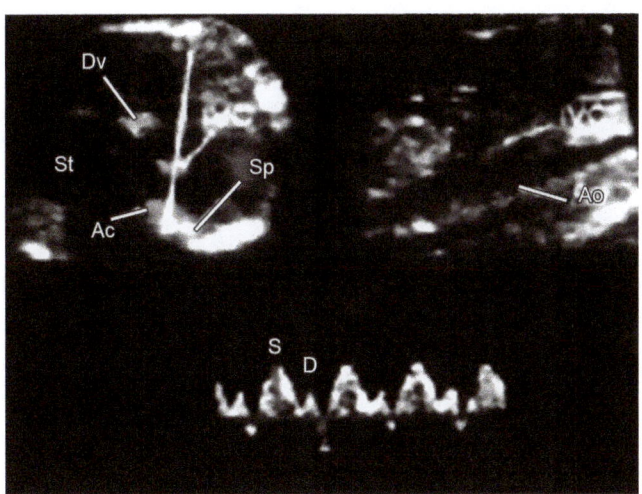

Fig. 20.44: Fetal echocardiography.

KEY POINTS

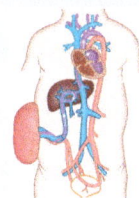

- 7.5 MHz is used in early pregnancy (up to 8 weeks) and 5 MHz in 9–13 weeks of pregnancy. TVS is used after 14 weeks.
- Gravid uterus shows generalized increase in vascularity of myometrium, an areas of vascularity is demonstrated in the hyperechoic decidua on days 26–28 post-LMP (Implantation site signs).
- Placental flow even after 1 week of therapeutic abortion is an indication for dilatation and curettage.
- A solid adnexal mass with pronounced vascularity showing high velocity, low impedance flow suggests and ectopic gestation.
- Pseudosacs display high impedance flow.
- Uterine diastolic notch is seen normally up to 20–22 weeks after which it disappears. Persistence beyond 4 weeks of gestation with high RI suggests pre-eclampsia, IUGR and placental abruption.
- Umbilical artery flow pattern > 26 weeks of gestation show RI < 0.70 and PI < 1.5. Reduced/absent/reversal of diastolic flow indicate IUGR.
- Normal flow pattern show RI = 0.82 ± 0.1 and PI = 1.83 ± 0.3 in descending thoracic aorta. Increased resistance suggests IUGR.
- Middle cerebral artery show brain sparing effect (increased diastolic flow in IUGR)

6. Reversed frequencies in end diastole are only observed in a few fetuses prior to death. This finding should be considered as a preterminal condition. Few fetuses if any will survive without some form of therapeutic intervention.
7. Loss of end diastolic frequencies precedes changes in the cardiotocography by some 7-42 days in fetuses that have been shown to be small for gestational age on real time ultrasound. In the absence of maternal hypertension many centers would toco monitor small for gestational age fetuses solely with Doppler ultrasound. The occurrence of CTG deceleration not related to contractions, together with absent end diastolic frequencies carries an extremely poor prognosis.

Current Recommendations

It is probably reasonable for the clinicians to deliver all small for gestational age fetuses that present with absent (Reversed) end diastolic frequencies after 28 weeks. In units with neonatal intensive care facilities the perinatal mortality for infants that are more than 28 weeks gestation is less than 10% with about a 6% chance of handicap in survivors. If these fetuses are managed along standard clinical lines a mortality rate of about 40% with a 25% chance of severe handicap can be expected.

At less than 28 weeks gestation these fetuses should probably be referred to a regional center for detailed studies of the fetal circulation and possibly cordocentesis with an aim to therapy that may improve fetal oxygenation and growth.

CONCLUSION

Today the advent of color flow imaging, Doppler and power angiography have opened up a new diagnostic horizon for understanding physiology and vascular pathology of gynecology, infertility and uteroplacental and fetal circulation.

The diagnostic ability with use of Doppler in routine practice has increased (Tables 20.6 to 20.8).

TABLE 20.6: Data analysis 5 years MNMH—Agra.

Total deliveries	6500
Ultrasound scans	4320
Diabetes	87
PIH	213
High risk patients	456
Abnormal Doppler	123
IUFD and perinatal deaths	65
NICU admissions	125

TABLE 20.7: Doppler in IUGR and perinatal salvage.

Parameter	Normal	Abnormal	
• All IUGR	R	91.67%	69.4%
	M	87%	60%
• > 1300 g	R	100%	93.7%
	M	95%	90%
• < 1300 g	R	50%	20%
	M	40%	18%

TABLE 20.8: Doppler indices and perinatal mortality.

• Normal uterine and umbilical	Nil
• High umbilical resistance	10%
• Absent diastolic umbilical flow	40%
• Abnormal uterine and umbilical	65%
• Abnormal ductus	90%

"See better with sound
Use color to improve your image
Explore the 3rd and 4th Dimension
Practice better medicine with better images"

BIBLIOGRAPHY

1. Kurjak A, Zalud I. Doppler and Color Flow Imaging. Transvaginal Ultrasound. Mosby Year Book (Ch-15). 1992; pp.285-94.
2. Bourne TH. Transvaginal color Doppler in gynaecology. Ultrasound Obstet Gynecol. 1991;1:359-73.
3. Taylor KJW, Peter NB, Wells PNT. Clinical Applications of Doppler Ultrasound, 2nd edition. Raven. 1995.
4. Kujak A, et al. Transvaginal color Doppler in pelvic tumor vascularity: Lesions teamed and future challanges. Ultrasound Obstet Gynecol. 1995;6:145-9.
5. Peter W Callen. Ultrasonography in Obstetrics and Gynaecology, WB Saunders Company Ltd. 2007.
6. Steer CB, et al. Transvaginal color Doppler imaging of the uterine arteries during ovarian and menstrual cycles. Human Repord. 1990;5: 391-95.
7. Campbell S. Ultrasound in obstetrics and gynaecology: Recent advances. In: Clinics in Obstetrics and Gynaecology. WB Saunders Company Ltd, p. 10: 1983.

Gray Scale Ultrasonography and Color Doppler Study in Fracture Healing

Fracture healing starts from hematoma formation around fracture site to its organization followed by early callus, bone callus, and finally its remodeling. Derangement in this chain can occur at early stage to result into abnormal union or malunion. The basic method to monitor the fracture healing is by conventional radiograph but recently developed non-invasive, non-radiation technique, i.e. ultrasound, provides reliable information regarding healing process like:
1. It may quantitate the state of fracture healing.
2. Early diagnosis of disturbed union.
3. Time of exact surgical intervention.
4. Treatment/diagnostic procedure is performed without adding further trauma to fracture site.

After the recent advancement in ultrasonographic technique, Goldberg et al. (1975)[1] have advocated its extensive use. Real time ultrasonography using high frequency linear array transducer is the best imaging procedure for evaluation of osseous and soft tissue pathology of extremity.

EXPERIMENTAL STUDY

Rabbits have been used for the purpose and fracture has been created in bilateral ulna and followed them for 6-8 weeks. In union group the abnormal mobility persisted for about 3rd to 4th week though in 2nd week there was mild resistance to mobility which progressively increased and after 4th week fracture was no longer mobile. The bony swelling that appeared around 3rd week due to callus formation, increased in size and then slightly decreased in size which was because of remodeling defect. The fracture union and remodeling were completed in rabbits by 8 weeks (Table 21.1).

CLINICAL STUDY

Thirty-eight patients of present study, including delayed union (5), nonunion (8) and fresh fractures (25) were studied. In normal union group patients for about 10 days

TABLE 21.1: Comparison of US and radiographic findings with duration.

Days after surgery	Healing phase evaluated	Radiographic findings	Ultrasonography findings
5–7 days	Stage of organized hematoma	Clear-cut fracture line, no callus	Hypoechoic gap
10–14 days	Stage of early callus	Fracture line visible No e/o callus	Hyperechoic shadow in fracture gap and around it indicating early callus
17–20 days	Stage of bridging callus	Haziness of fracture indicating early callus	↑ in amount and intensity of shadow, hyper-reflecting line indicating bridging callus
24–28 days	Stage of union	Callus seen bridging the fracture ends	↑ in intensity of hyper-reflecting line
5–8 weeks	Stage of remodeling	Initial increase in amount of callus and later reorganization	Not much ↑ in hyperechogenicity minimal remodeling could be assessed

following fracture treatment neither the radiographic nor the USG showed any evidence of callus formation. But between 2nd and 3rd week USG revealed hyperechoic area in the fracture gap, at this stage there was no evidence of new bone formation in the radiograph. At 5-6 weeks time increase in number and intensity of hyperechoic spots were noted which were more in the center than at periphery. Radiography at this stage revealed fuzzy fracture margin indicative of fracture healing. Scan at the time of 8-12 weeks showed increase in intensity and number of hyperechoic spot or zones bridging the fracture gap (Figs. 21.1A and B). Radiograph at this stage showed well-formed bridging callus, which appeared increasing until the fracture line was obscured and remodeling has started. The fracture, which was treated with intramedullary nail, revealed delayed union on radiograph but USG was able to predict the callus formation. Intramedullary nail was discernible in the earlier stage of fracture healing which was obscured in later stage through all the three portals, due to callus obstructing the entry of ultrasound waves. Five cases had evidence of delayed union with feature of nonvisualisation of callus formation either on radiography or on USG even at 8-12 weeks. The site studied were femur (1), tibia (2), humerus (1), and radius (1). At 12 weeks there was steady increase in hyperechoic foci at fracture site and no callus on radiograph (Figs. 21.2A and B).

The cases of nonunion did show some callus at early stage but the progress was arrested. And USG also showed some hyperechoic shadows at early stage but progress in term of amount and intensity was absent. The cases of nonunion to start with USG revealed a gap between fracture ends with hypoechoic zone in between (Figs. 21.3A and B).

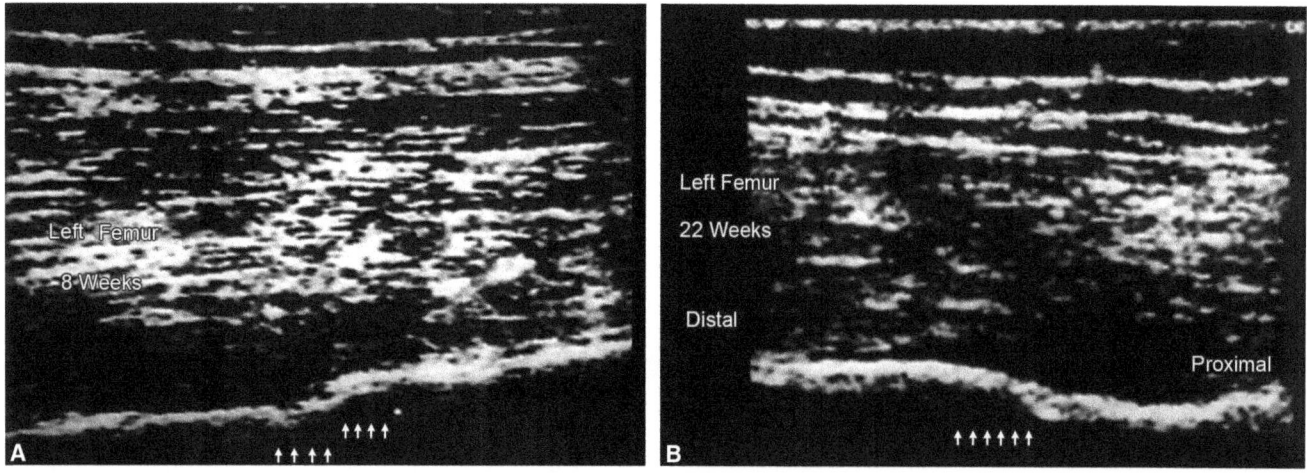

Figs. 21.1A and B: USG scan at 8–12 weeks interval shows increased intensity and number of hyperechoic spots (zone) bridging the fracture gap. Radiograph also revealed bridging callus.

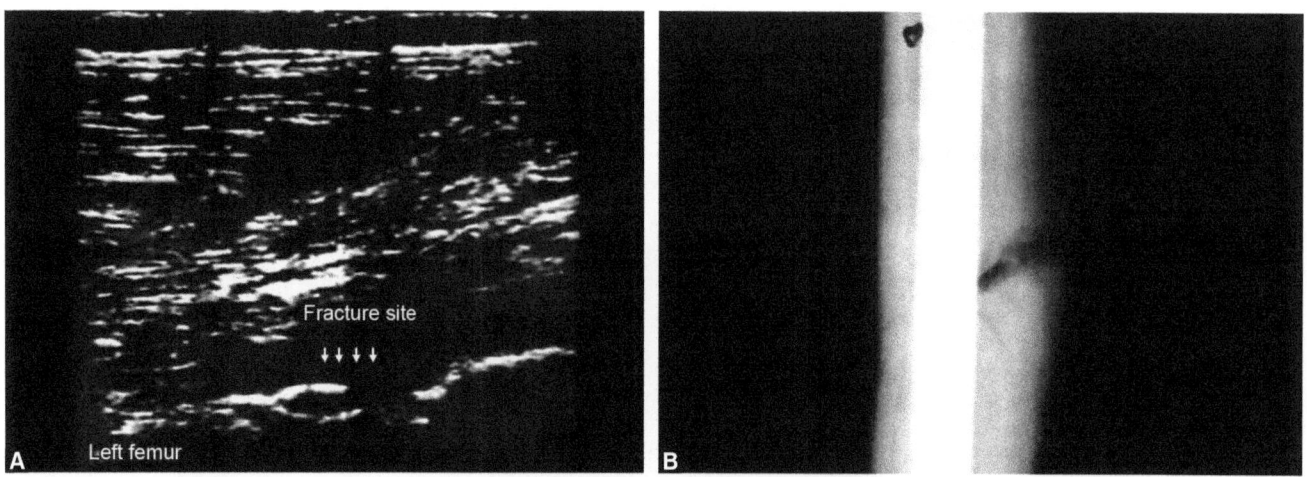

Figs. 21.2A and B: USG shows hyperechoic zone but radiograph did not reveal any evidence of callus formation in a case of delayed union.

Routine radiography does not permit the minor changes in fracture healing during early stage while the ultrasonography through its potential of early assessment of the presence or absence of callus at the fracture site can be used to predict the need for secondary surgical procedure.

Color Doppler was employed to optimize detection of weak and slow flow signals expected from small vessels. Sagittal and axial scan were employed with caution not to have more pressure by transducer to the tissue to avoid obliteration of small superficial vessels. Color Doppler was only able to image anterolateral and anteromedial side of fracture while gray scale sonography could utilize all the three portal, i.e. anterior portal also.

In control subject the bone surface appeared smooth specular reflector with acoustic shadowing. No Doppler signals were observed on periosteal surface or within surrounding tissue.

At first examination (10 days after trauma) gray scale sonography demonstrated a small hypoechoic hematoma surrounding the fracture site. The flow signals were not detected by color Doppler imaging at this stage except a few scattered color dots within periosseous soft tissue 1–2 cm from fracture. Special analysis from periosseous soft tissue varied with RI ranging from 0.51–0.81 visible at the level of periosteum. Within the fracture site small color dots could be appreciated with RI in same range.

Second examination (6 weeks) revealed absence of hematoma, there was increase in flow signals within the periosseous soft tissue with small linear vessel (approx. 1 mm in diameter) 0.40–0.65.

Third examination (10 weeks) had flow signals in small tortuous vessel at the fracture site. The signals had RI ranging from 0.32–0.51.

Fourth examination (15 weeks) showed small hyperechoic streaks at fracture site. Persistence of vascular flow with RI of 0.40–0.63, was also observed.

Fifth examination (18–19 weeks) showed a well-developed callus with good flow on earlier examination and flow signal around it had almost completely disappeared.

Sixth examination (24 weeks) showed no flow either within or around the healed lesion except for small color dots in periosseous soft tissue RI from color dots 0.50–0.77. Fracture cases of delayed union had no flow in fracture site or in periosteum at earlier examination but of small vessels in periosseous tissues successive exam revealed few color dots within fracture site with gradual increase of RI

KEY POINTS

Normal union

- 10 days — Radiograph/USG not helpful.
- 2–3 wks — USG—hyperechoic area in fracture gap.
- 5–6 wks — Increased in number and intensity of hyperechoic spots—more in center than periphery. Radiograph—normal.
- 8–10 wks — Increased in intensity and number of hyperechoic spots or zones bridging the fracture. Radiograph—positive.

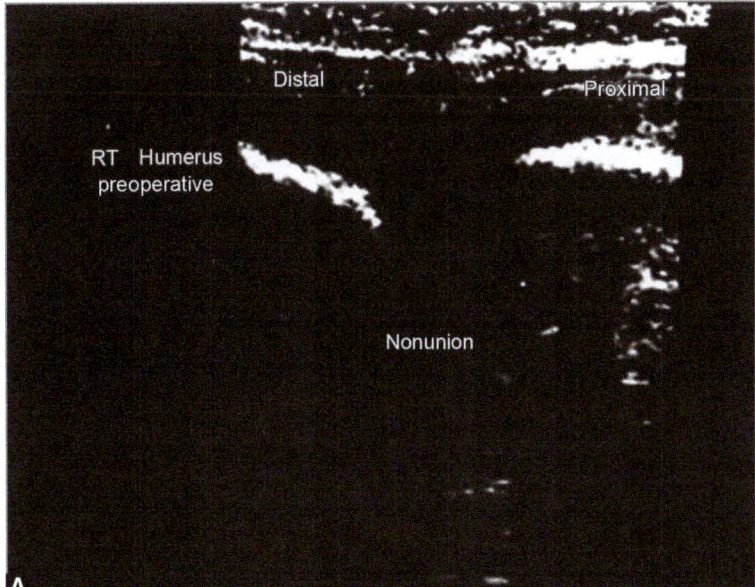 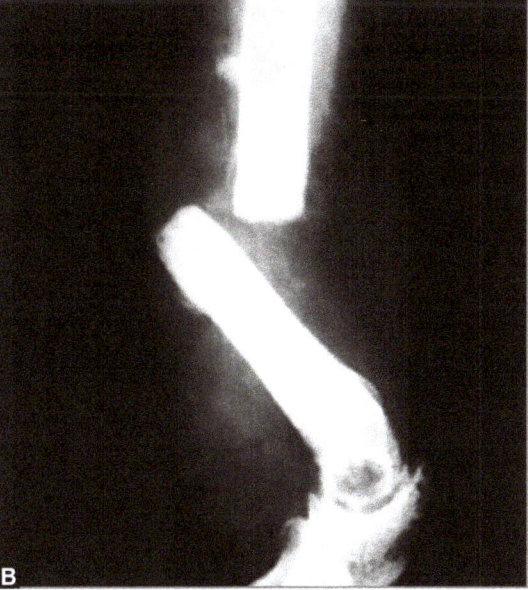

Figs. 21.3A and B: In a case of non-union USG as well as radiograph revealed no evidence of callus formation.

KEY POINTS

Color Doppler

- 10 days — Not much helpful except few scattered color dots within 1–2 cm periosseous soft tissue. RI-0.51 to 0.81.
- 6 weeks — Increase in flow signals within and periosseous soft tissue with small linear vessel (approx. 1 mm in diameter). RI–0.40 to 0.65.
- 10 weeks — Flow signals in small tortuous vessel at fracture site. RI–0.32 to 0.51.
- 15 weeks — Small hyperechoic streaks at fracture site. RI–0.40 to 0.63.
- 18–19 weeks — Good flow inside. Flow signal around disappeared.
- 24 weeks — No flow within or around. Healed lesions. RI–0.50-0.77.
- Delayed union – RI – 0.70-0.80.

0.70-0.80. Gray scale sonography and radiography did not show sign of callus and labeled as delayed union.

However, venous signals could rarely be seen only in those cases that had well developed callus.

Earliest changes during new bone formation are development of small blood vessels. The capillary surrounding the fracture site shows signs of neoangiogenesis, which is accompanied by osteoblast proliferation, in first week after bone fracture. This process may be identified on gray scale sonography about 3 weeks after fracture while conventional radiography cannot visualize the repair process until 30-40 days after trauma.

Two main vascular phenomena occur after a bone fracture. First, at the time of trauma, the normal blood supply to fracture site is disrupted with formation of hematoma. Then blood vessel rapidly reaches this tissue coming both from peripheral soft tissue to periosteal portion of callus and from medullary circulation endosteal callus. Histologically, newly formed capillaries can be recognized as early as 7 days after fracture and many vessels are seen in 9 days. Presence of many vessels with progressive increase of RI, and development of telesystolic notch within spectral waveform indicates normal callus formation. Identification of only 1 or 2 vascular signals at 4th weeks and lack of development of telesystolic notch were considered sign of delayed fracture healing (Callioada et al. 1993).[2]

Initial decrease in RI inpatient with normal callus development is due to impressive neoangiogenesis during the early weeks after fracture, the neoangiogenesis lowers the resistance through the overall increase in vascular caliber. Gradual increase in resistance is likely related to degree of vascularity decreasing. Patients with delayed healing probably have less angiogenesis and thus higher resistance. In addition, the scarce vascularity in the non-union group makes Doppler evaluation technically difficult. Early demonstration of delayed healing can help guide treatment changes (Caruso et al. 2000).[3] Additional studies are needed to show whether the color Doppler imaging can demonstrate the return of vascularization after change in therapy and whether the patient outcome is affected by the use of this technique. At present, conventional radiography remains the primary technique for evaluating callus formation.

REFERENCES

1. Goldberg. Textbook of Diagnosis Uses of Ultrasound. 1975.
2. Callioada F, Bottinelli O, Sala G. Color Doppler differential diagnosis between normally and delayed healing bone fracture. Radiology. 1993;189:209.
3. Caruso G, Lagalla R, Derchi L, et al. Monitoring of fracture calluses with color Doppler sonography. J Clin Ultrasound. 2000;28:20.

3D and 4D Ultrasound: Principles, Advantages, and Applications

Ultrasonography (USG) has been used as an imaging modality for over five decades now. Being a safe, cheap, portable, and easily available it has now become the most widely used imaging modality in clinical practice. There have been constant technical innovations which have introduced newer and advanced aspects of imaging in medicine. Volumetric three-dimensional (3D) and four-dimensional (4D) USGs are bright examples of such innovations (Fig. 22.1).

The advent of volumetric CT and MRI has inspired the innovation of volumetric USG into reality. There are few limitations in 2D USG which can be overcome by volumetric study. Firstly, the radiological interpretation is dependent on discontinuous, representative images of the complex anatomy. Secondly, there is lack of spatial relationship while reviewing the images. Finally, the volume measurements typically rely on assumptions.

The principle of volumetric USG is to digitally reconstruct a series of 2D slices and reproduce a volumetric 3D image. With 4D USG, the added dimension is the time which makes the 3D image appears in motion with real time. 3D/4D USG uses the same beams as the 2D USG while the processing is mediated by the USG machine with the help of specifically installed software. There has to be an additional 3D/4D probe to make volumetric imaging possible in real time. Nowadays these probes are easily available with machines of varied ranges.

Volumetric USG has been used for three decades now, but it has been in frequent practice only in recent times. Initially, its use was limited to gynecology and obstetrics practice and has now expanded its utility in many other fields of general medicine practice.

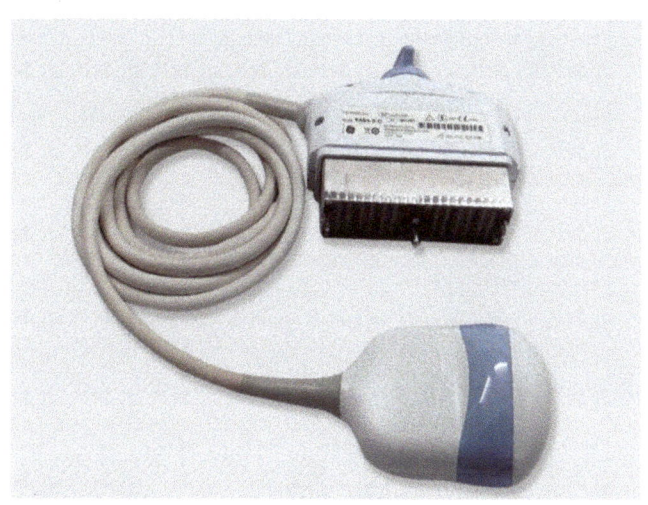

Fig. 22.1: Volumetric USG probe with connector.

APPLICATIONS IN CLINICAL PRACTICE

Application in Abdomen and Pelvis

Liver: 3D USG can be used for accurate calculation of liver volume which has implication in pediatrics and cirrhotic patients. There is increase in specificity of nodular appearance of liver in cirrhosis by 3D image accusation.

Gallbladder: Anatomy can be well studied which can guide in presurgical planning. The calculus volume can also be calculated with ease.

Urological application: It is helpful in both urodynamic studies as well as in anatomical assessment. 3D USG is intrinsically superior in assessing renal anomalies and ureteric configuration in pediatrics. There can be actual assessment of vesicoureteric reflux with grading.

The 4D USG can accurately measure the real time voiding bladder volume on micturition.

Volumetric assessment is superior to 2D USG in diagnosing urinary bladder diverticula, focal wall thickening, and mass lesion.

In the scrotum, 3D increases the diagnostic accuracy of complex epididymal and other extratesticular pathologies.

Application in Cardiovascular System

The 2D USG has a well established application in assessing vascular anatomy and physiology with the help of color and spectral Doppler. With the help of 3D application, the actual volume of blood passing through a specific cross section of blood vessel can be measured.

It also accurately assesses the exact extent of atherosclerotic plaque and vessel stenosis.

The 3D echocardiography enables complete visualization of cardiac anatomy and real time valvular motion.

Application in Breast Imaging

In the assessment of breast masses, role of volumetric scanning has started evolving as a helpful tool. There can be better analysis of the orientation of masses in relation to ductal anatomy. However, there are few studies which state that 3D USG is not very useful in differentiating benign and malignant breast masses.

Application in Gynecology and Obstetrics

Role of USG as imaging tool in obstetrics and gynecology has already proven to have unmatched benefits. 3D estimation of uterine fibroids and polyps (Fig. 22.2) is very useful for presurgical planning and follow-up imaging. The uterine anomalies (Fig. 22.3) can be evaluated with better accuracy. It is also useful in corneal ectopic pregnancy, intrauterine contraceptive device placement and in assessing adnexal lesions.

The 3D/4D USG has proven to be very attractive in evaluating fetus in utero. The fetal structures are easy to assess (Fig. 22.4). There is real time 3D imaging possible without any extra effort. Post imaging review has increased accuracy. The limitation of high accuracy of 2D USG in detecting cleft lip and palate has been overcome by volumetry scanning. It is also more accurate in detecting structural neurological disorders.

Application in Intervention

The 3D USG has provided better spatial guidance for various interventional procedures. There is increased visibility of biopsy needle not only in a single plane but in a volume with resultant better orientation of the target lesion and the needle movement. Smaller target lesions could be more accurately defined with high success rate of the procedure.

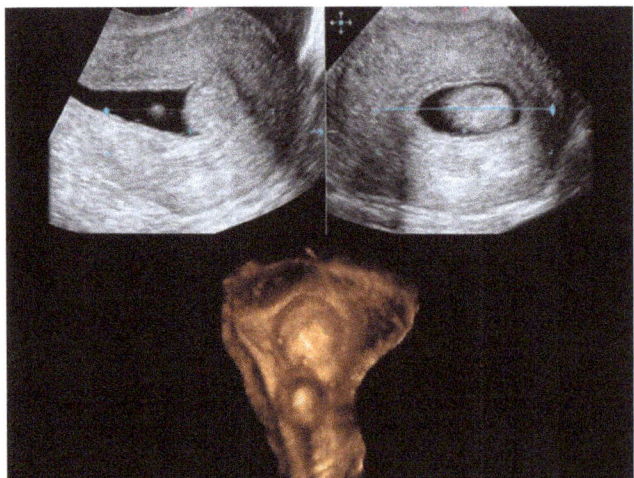

Fig. 22.2: Axial and sagittal images of sonohysterogram demonstrating endometrial polyps which can be seen in a single image in volumetric representation.

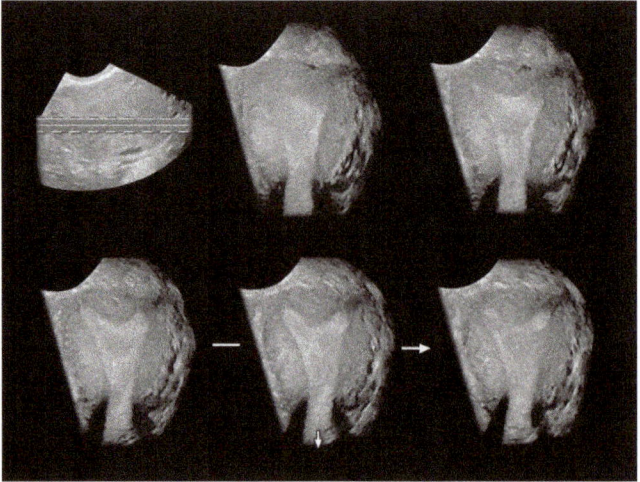

Fig. 22.3: Volumetric reconstructed images of uterus demonstrating the fundal anatomy which is helpful in differentiating arcuate from bicornuate uterus.

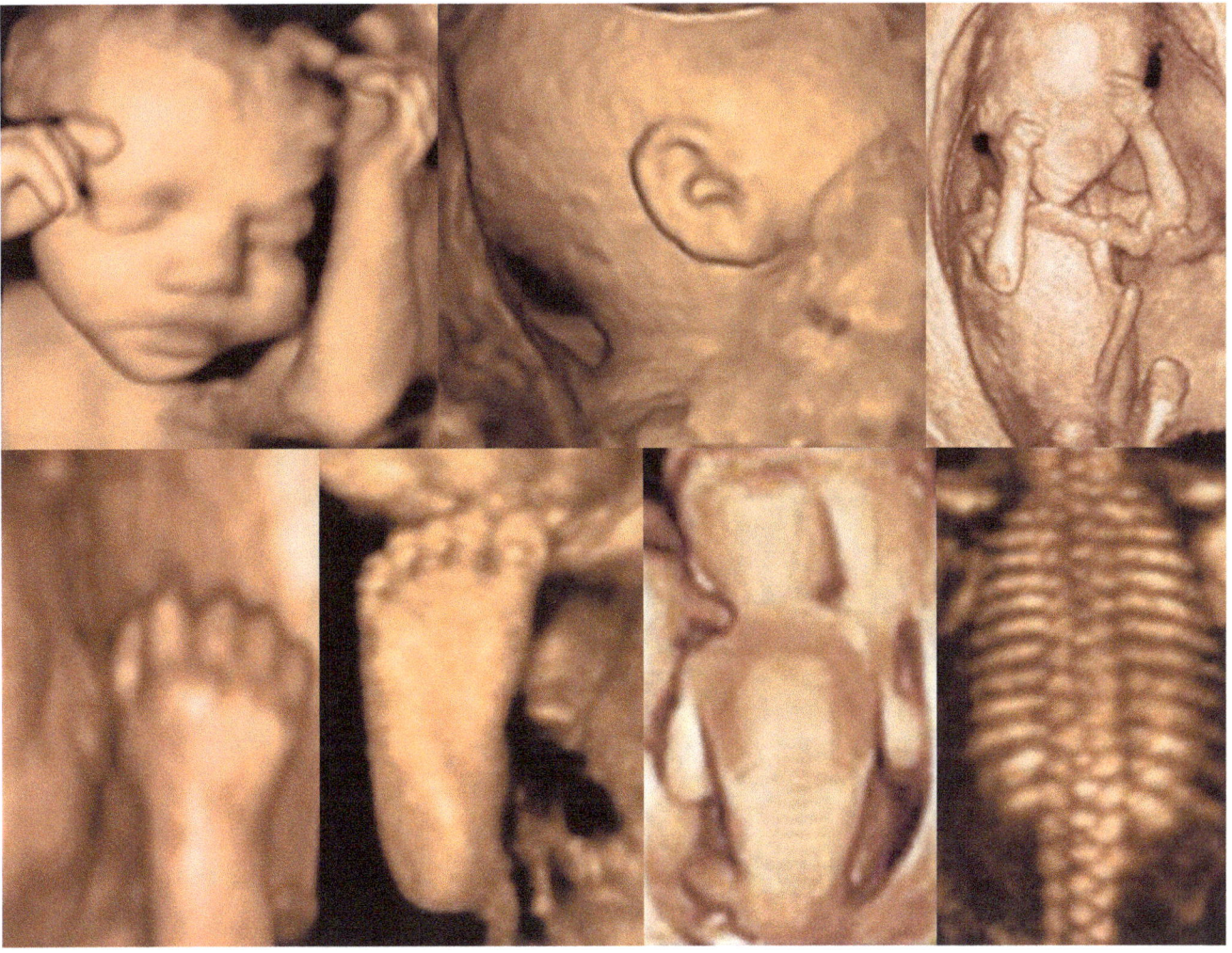

Fig. 22.4: 3D obstetrics USG images demonstrating various parts of fetus in utero.

LIMITATIONS OF VOLUMETRY USG

- It requires special probe and software
- Additional procedural time is required, resulting in prolonging the scan time
- The volumetry probe is heavy which makes it inconvenient for the performer to handle
- Highly dependent upon the operator as it requires a smooth sweep through the area of study.

However, the benefits overweigh these technical limitations which are likely to be solved in near future.

Index

Page numbers followed by *f* refer to figure, and *t* refer to table

A

Abdomen, application in 215
Abortion 202
    complete 202
    incomplete 202
Abscess 107
    testicular 134*f*
Acceleration index 25*f*
Acceleration time 25*f*
Adnexal mass, complex right 189*f*
Adnexal ovarian torsion 187
Adolescent stretch syndrome 64
Alcohol abuse 90
Alpha-fetoprotein, elevated 84
Anechoic lesions, nonspecific 92
Anemia, hemolytic 99
Aneurysms 40, 56, 122, 124, 162, 177
    anterior of 120
    diagnosis of 120
    posterior borders of 120
Angiography 117
    catheter-based 174
    use of 93
Ankle index 158, 158*t*
Antecubital vein 41
Anticancer drug 44
Anticoagulation 67
Antiplatelet therapy 67
Aorta 115, 117, 157
    abdominal 115, 116
    dilated abdominal 118*f*
    distal 117*f*
    longitudinal scans of 118*f*
    proximal 124*f*
    sonography 116
    transverse scans of 118*f*
Aortic aneurysm 119
    abdominal 119
    complication, catastrophic of 120
    dissecting 120
    inflammatory 119
    types of 119*f*
Aortic branches 116, 123
Aortic dissection 120, 121*f*, 122, 179

Aortic graft 122
    distal 122
Aortic pathology 117
Aortic pseudoaneurysm, abdominal 121
Aortic rupture 120
Aortic valve abnormalities 49
Aortic wall 117
Aortoarteritis 178*f*
    nonspecific 177
Aortoenteric fistulas 119
Aortofemoral graft 122
Aortoiliac graft 122
Arcuate artery 125*f*, 185*f*
Arterial anastomosis, types of 105
Arterial anatomy, normal 175
Arterial aneurysm, peripheral 162
Arterial branching 26
Arterial disease
    occlusive 69
    peripheral 158
Arterial Doppler, peripheral 40
Arterial flow
    turbulent 92
    velocity waveform 87*f*
Arterial insufficiency 141
Arterial integrity 93
Arterial obstruction 27
    diagnosis of 26
    effect of 8
Arterial occlusive disease 157
    peripheral 158
Arterial pressure 7
    wave 6
Arterial stenosis 87
    and occlusion 62
    local effects of 28*f*
    severity of 26
    sign of severe 27
Arterial wall 175
Arterial waveform 153*f*, 158
Arterioles, vasoconstriction of 4
Arteriosclerosis 124, 160*f*
Arteriovenous fistulas
    congenital 164
    extrarenal 107
    intrarenal 106

Arteriovenous malformations 68, 125, 146, 147*f*
    renal 128
Artery
    flow disturbance, large 64
    intracranial 57
    intratesticular 131*f*
    muscular 176
    normal 117
    peripheral 156, 157*f*
    popliteal 162*f*
    posterior communicating 57*f*
    pulmonary 176
    stenosis, extremity 27
    subclavian 158
    superficial femoral 160*f*
Atherectomy 178, 179
Atheroma 52
Atheromatous disease 117
Atherosclerosis 176, 177
Atherosclerotic disease 64
Atherosclerotic emboli 106
Atherosclerotic plaques 118*f*, 119
    dissections of 178
Atrial fibrillation 67
Atrophy
    age-related 138
    renal 99
Augmentation 168
Axillary artery 158

B

Balloon angioplasty 178, 179
Basal arteries 68
Basal cell carcinoma 145*f*
Basic Doppler system 16, 18
Basilar artery 58, 62
Bifurcation flow disturbance, normal 26*f*
Biliary atresia 85
Biliary ducts, dilated 76
Biliary obstruction 85
Blood 175
    cell 25
        movement, parallel lines of 25*f*

circulation 5
dynamic circulation of 3
flow 21, 33, 75
    augmentation of 169f
    direction of 76
    Doppler measurement of 183f
    energy 4
    intratumoral 186
    sampling, accurate 182
    splenic 75, 90
    velocity 19, 193
velocity of 36
vessels 148
    Doppler scan of 54
volumetric flow of 15
Blunt splenic trauma 91
Bone fracture 214
Brachial artery 7f
Brachial index 158, 158t
Brain death 68
Breast 146
    carcinoma of 149f
    imaging, application in 216
    lumps
        benign 149t
        malignant 149t
    masses 216
        benign 216
        malignant 216
Budd-Chiari syndrome 81, 82, 85, 87
    primary 81
    secondary 81
Buerger's disease 158
Bulky uterus 202f
Burned-out tumor 137
Bypass graft, evaluation of 159

C

Cadaver kidneys 105
Caliber variations 74
Callus formation, evidence of 213f
Cancer, prostatic 111
Captopril scintigraphy 103
Carcinoma 150
    endometrial 189, 190f
    intraductal 148
    lobular 150
    pancreatic 93
    thyroid 146f
Cardiac cycle, phases of 74f
Cardiac embolic disease 67
Cardiopulmonary bypass 67, 68
Cardiovascular system, application in 216
Carotid 15
    aneurysms 53

angioplasty 67
artery 46, 48f
    external 47-49, 52f, 65f
    internal 7f, 23f, 26f, 47-49, 52, 52f,
        54, 59, 59f, 62, 65f
    normal 47f, 48f
    occlusion 28f, 47
    plaque, internal 67f
    right internal 48f
    stenosis, internal 27f
    terminal 59f
body tumors 53
bulb reverse flow, region of 46
cavernous sinus fistulas 155
dissection 52
Doppler 40, 52
endarterectomy 66, 67
occlusion 52
siphon 60
    stenosis 63
stenosis 64, 67
ultrasound 46
vessel 49
Carrel patch 105
Cavernosa 139, 140
Cavernosal artery 140f
Cavernous transformation 86
Cavity, endometrial 189
Celiac artery 93, 116
Celiac trunk 123, 124f
Central necrosis 145
Cerebral
    artery 63f
        acute middle 63
        anterior 54, 57f, 58, 59f, 60-62, 62f
        dilated posterior 65f
        middle 54, 57f, 58, 58f, 60-62, 63f,
            64t, 66f, 69f
        occlusion, middle 63
        posterior 57f, 58-60, 62, 66f
        stenosis, middle 63, 63f
    autoregulation 69
    blood flow 69
    perfusion 69
        reserve 55
    trauma 68
    venous thrombosis 56
Cerebrovascular Doppler sonography 46
Cerebrum, capillaries of 48
Cervical internal carotid artery 65f, 67f
Cervix, carcinoma of 191
Changing shades method 30
Cholelithiasis 86f
Chorionic sac stage 200
Choroidal melanoma 154f
Circle of Willis 207f

Circumaortic veins 127
Cirrhosis 75
    advanced 77f
Clinical Doppler ultrasound imaging 1
Colonic ischemia 128
Color Doppler 196, 214
    evaluation 143
    flow 86f
        image 76f, 83, 102f, 135f
        images 65f, 67f, 77f, 152
    role of 82, 90
    sonographic criteria 93
    sonography 93, 106, 109, 153f
        accuracy of 93
Color flow images 29, 31
    advantage of 31, 32
    asynchronous 183
    clinical advantages of 31
    limitations of 32
    principle of 29
    quality, optimizing 33
    synchronous 184
    system 18, 29, 182
    technique 30
Color flow
    schemes 29f
    system 30f
Color mode 39f
Common carotid artery 9, 26f, 28f, 47f, 48,
    49, 50f, 51f, 61, 61t
    color doppler images of 47f
    power Doppler image of 50f
    transverse color Doppler image of 52f
Common femoral
    artery 156, 164f
    vein 164f, 167, 169f, 170f, 172
Common iliac artery 116, 117f
    bifurcation 116
Compression 168
Conventional sonography 97
Coronary angiography 67
Coronary vein, dilated 78f
Corpus luteum
    color
        Doppler in 193f
        flow pattern of 186f
Cranial vasculature, power Doppler image
    of 32f
Cryptorchidism 130

D

Deep dorsal artery 139
Deep venous system 166, 172
Deep venous thrombosis 170, 172f
    chronic 171

lower extremity 169
   signs of 170
   symptoms of 170
Diastolic notch 205*f*
Diastolic pressures 7
Diastolic umbilical flow, absent 210
Diastolic velocity 27, 49, 141
Dilated collection system, intrarenal duplex Doppler sonography of 97
Distal common carotid artery, B-mode image of 51*f*
Distal lower limb, compression of 169*f*
Distal ureter, dilated 109
Distal vertebral artery 64
Distant vein 41
Doppler
   analysis of 99
   color imaging 108
   criteria 48
   effect 13
   equation 21
   flow detection 12
   frequency 25
      shift 29
      mixture of 21
      spectrum 21, 22, 23, 24
   imaging 110
   indices 210*t*
   postulate concerning frequency 1
   principle 1
      and instrumentation 13
   shift method 13
   signal 36, 183
   spectral analysis 21, 24
   spectrum
      display 22, 22*f*
      envelope traces of 24
   systems 2, 19*f*, 36
      limitations of 18
      multigated 29
   traces 25
   ultrasonography 94
   ultrasound 3, 182
   waveform 156, 157
Dorsalis pedis
   artery waveform 28*f*
   vein 172
Ductal ectasia 112
Ductus
   abnormal 210
   venosus 208*f*
Duplex Doppler 74*f*, 81, 207*f*
   findings 84
   image 125*f*
   sonography 100, 121
   systems 20

E

Echogenic focal masses 83
Echogenic tumor thrombus 76*f*
Elastic lamina
   external 176
   internal 176*f*
Emboli
   cardiac source of 57
   detection 66
      potential uses of 67*t*
Embolic source, localization of 67
Embryo transfer, optimal conditions for 198
Embryonal cell carcinoma 136, 137
End diastolic
   flow, loss of 207*f*
   frequencies, artifactual loss of 200
   velocity 49, 140
   volume, abnormal 142
Endarterectomy 46
Endocavitary duplex transducers 81
Endometrial evaluation, role of ultrasound and color Doppler in 192
Endometrial polyp, vascularity in 190*f*
Endometrial thickness 190*f*
Endometriosis 187, 195
Endometritis 189
Endometrium 192*f*, 200
   changes in 193
   secretory changes in 192
Endoscopic Doppler ultrasound 81
Epididymis 130, 132, 133*f*, 135*f*
   enlargement of 132
Epididymitis, acute 133*f*
Epididymo-orchitis 132, 134*f*
Erectile dysfunction 139
   duplex ultrasonography of 139
   evaluation of 139
   technique 140
   treatment of complications 142
Erythrocytes 15
Extracranial
   arteries, status of 57
   occlusive disease 64
Extratesticular tumors, majority of 138

F

False lumen 177
Fast Fourier transformation 21
Fatal pulmonary embolism, potentially 12
Fatty tissue 136
Femoral artery, distal superficial 160*f*
Femoral vein, proximal superficial 172

Fetal
   aorta, normal flow pattern in 207*f*
   breathing movements 201
   circulation, normal 202*f*
   death 201
   descending thoracic aorta 205
   distress 208*f*
   echocardiography 208, 209*f*
   heartbeat, detection of 13
   middle cerebral artery 205, 207*f*
   vasculature, normal 207*f*
   venous circulation 208
Fetoplacental circulation 201
Fetus in utero, parts of 217*f*
Fibroadenoma 150
Fibroadenosis 150
Fibroid 186, 187, 195
   pedunculated 186
   peripheral vascularity in 187*f*
Fibromuscular stroma, anterior 110
Fistula
   arteriovenous 163, 164
   extrarenal arteriovenous 105
   traumatic 164
Flank pain 100
Flow disturbance, severe 26, 27
Flow velocity
   measurement of 10*f*
   slight decrease of 61
   waveform 183*f*
Fluids, motion of 3
Foley's catheter 197
Follicles, small peripheral 196*f*
Foramen magnum 57
Fracture treatment 212
Fusiform 120
Fuzzy fracture 212

G

Gallbladder 85, 215
   body of 86*f*
   carcinoma of 85, 86*f*
Gastric artery 123, 124*f*
Gastroduodenal artery 124*f*
Gastroesophageal junction 78*f*
Germ cell layers 137
Gestation, ectopic 203*f*
Gestational sac, empty 204*f*
Gestational trophoblastic
   disease 187
   tumors 188
Glagov effect 176
Glandular
   prostate 110
   tissue, periurethral 110

Graft 106
    implantation, complications of 122
    infection 123
Graves' disease 148
Gray's anatomy 184

H

Harmonic imaging 35
    relies 35
    requires 35
Harmonic mode 38
Head injury, severe 69
Hemangioma 83, 145
    cavernous 146
    intraocular 155f
    superficial 147f
Hematocele 134
Hematoma 107, 121
    intratesticular 134, 135
    small hypoechoic 213
Hemolytic uremic syndrome 99
Hemorrhage
    subarachnoid 56, 60, 62f, 63f
    subcapsular 91
Hepatic abscess 84f
    early stage 84
Hepatic artery 73, 86, 87f, 93, 123
    common 123, 124f
    postoperative occlusion of 86
Hepatic lesions, color Doppler in 83
Hepatic portion, segmental obstruction of 81
Hepatic transplantation 85
Hepatic veins 73, 81, 82, 82f, 87, 127
    major 81
    thrombosis 81
        early 87
Hepatic veno-occlusive diseases 81
Hepatocellular carcinoma 42f, 83, 84
Hepatofugal portal flow 76, 87f, 90
Hepatopetal, monophasic flow 81
Hepatorenal syndrome 100
High frequency arterial signals 76
High graft failure, causes of 93
High intensity focused ultrasound 44
High resolution ultrasonography, current role of 130
High velocity venous flow 77
Hydatiform mole 188f
    high vascularity around 188f
Hydrocele 134, 134f, 135f
    large 135f
Hydronephrosis 119

Hydrosalpinx-contrast agent 39f
Hyperparathyroidism 152f
Hyperplasia
    endometrial 190f
    intimal 106, 175, 176f
Hypertension
    portal 74, 75, 75f, 78f, 79, 80, 90, 90f
    renovascular 102
Hypoechoic
    layer, middle 176f
    lesion, focal 111f
    mass 138f, 191f
    rim 83
    testis 133f
Hypoplasia 53, 54
Hysterosalpingography 198

I

Iliac artery
    external 105, 117f
    internal 117f
Iliac flow 184
Iliac veins 127
In vitro fertilization 196
    color Doppler in 195
Infarction, scar stage of 91
Inferior mesenteric artery, division of 128
Inferior vena cava 40, 81, 82, 82f, 126
    anatomy 126
    pathology 126
    sonography 126
Infertility 130, 195, 199
    color Doppler in 199
    role of color Doppler in 191
Inflammation
    acute 132
    chronic 132
Inflammatory diseases 132
Inguinal ligament, level of 156
Intra-arterial digital subtraction 102
Intracranial disease 62, 69
Intraocular mass 154f
Intraovarian perfusion 196f
Intrarenal artery, normal pulse Doppler waveform of 97f
Intrasplenic arterial branches 91
Intrasplenic pseudoaneurysm, hemostasis of 92
Intrastenotic spectrum 9f
Intrauterine polyp 189
Intravascular ultrasound, limitations of 179
Ischemia, symptomatic 46
Ischemic attacks, transient 63f

K

Kidney 96
    color amplitude image of 32f
    contralateral normal 101
    failure
        cause of 100
        functional 100
    states, subsequent 100
Knee, swelling of 147f

L

Laminar flow 4, 25f
    parabolic profile of 4f
    principle of 4f
Laplace's law 119
Lesions
    malignant 146f, 187
    mural 126
Leydig cell 137
Lienorenal collaterals 78f
    voluminous 91f
Lienorenal shunt, duplex Doppler of 80f
Liver 73, 104, 215
    benign tumor of 83
    disease 100
        recurrent 86
    Doppler in 73
    failure, severe 81
    transplantation 85-87
    tumor 84
        metastatic 83
Low density lipoprotein, levels of 117
Low flow velocity 27
Low pulse repetition frequency 33
Low velocity turbulent flow 80f
Lower limb 156
    arterial doppler technique 157
    pain 117
    veins 166, 167
Lower splenic pole 90
Lumen, partial canalization of 172f
Lumps, malignant 150t
Luteal phase defect 195
Lymphocele 94, 107

M

Main renal artery, thrombosis of 106
Malignancy, prostatic 112
Malignant lesions 84
Marfan's syndrome 119
Median arcuate ligament 116
Mediastinum testis 130
Melanoma, ocular 154f
Menstrual cycle 191, 193f

Mesenteric artery 23
    superior 77
Mesenteric vein 75
    superior 73, 86, 90
Metastasis 146, 146*f*
    subcutaneous 145*f*
Metastatic lesions 127
Microbubbles, liver specific phase of 41
Microemboli 67*f*
Midaorta 125*f*
Middle cerebral artery embolus, detection of 67*f*
Moya-moya disease 64, 65*f*, 66*f*
Multiple portosystemic collaterals, development of 90
Multiple radionuclide techniques 170
Multiple small arterial vessels, development of 144
Musculoskeletal mass lesions 143
Musculoskeletal system 143
    instrumentation 143
    technique 143
Mycobacterium tuberculosis 132
Mycotic aneurysms 121
Myometrium-endometrium border 192

N

Native valve disease 67
Neck, color Doppler in 152*f*
Neoplasia 86
    prostatic epithelial 112
Nephron loss 99
Neurovascular bundles, adjacent 110
Nodular hyperplasia, focal 41, 43*f*, 44, 83
Non-Doppler systems 17
Non-Hodgkin's lymphoma 137
Non-lymphoproliferative diseases, secondary 138

O

Obesity, maternal 201
Obstructed kidneys, acutely 98
Obstruction
    mild 98
    resistive index analysis of 99
Occlusion 125
Occlusive disease 117
Oligohydramnios 201
Omentum 136
Ophthalmic artery 153
Optic nerve 153
Orbit 152
Orbital vessels, normal 153

Organ transplants 93
Ovarian arterial flow pattern 185*f*
Ovarian artery 199
    waveform of 185*f*
Ovarian dermoid 186*f*
Ovarian flow, in-active 187
Ovarian masses 184
Ovarian stimulation 196*f*
Ovarian uterine discordance 194
Ovarian vascularity 192
Ovarian vein 127
    thrombosis 128
Ovarian vessels 184
Ovary
    changes in 192
    corpus luteum 192
    endometrioma of 188*f*
Ovulation stimulation 195

P

Pain 130
Pampiniform plexus, normal 131*f*
Pancreas 94
    color Doppler in 93
    transplant, postoperative evaluation of 94
Pancreatic transplant, first segmental 93
Papilloma, intraductal 148
Parathyroid
    adenoma 151, 152*f*
    glands 148
Paraumbilical veins 77, 81
    flow gradients 77*f*
    patent 77*f*
Parotid
    hemangioma 153*f*
    lesion, benign 153*f*
Peak systolic velocity, abnormal 142
Pelvic
    congestion syndrome 188
    venous plexus 191
Pelvis, application in 215
Penile erection
    anatomy of 139
    physiology of 139
Penis
    dorsal surface of 142*f*
    dorsum of 139
Percent area stenosis 176
Perfluoropropane 37
Perigraft fluid 123
Perinatal mortality 210*t*
Peripheral arteries, Doppler imaging of 156
Peripheral flow resistance, influence of 7*f*
Peritesticular flow 132*f*

Peritoneal cavity 91
Peritransplant fluid collections 94
Peroneal vein
    distal 172
    proximal 172
Peyronie's disease 142, 142*f*
Pharmacopenile duplex ultrasonography 139
Phylloides 150
Plaque morphology, classification of 50
Plug flow 5
Poiseuille's equation 5
Poiseuille's law 5
Polyarteritis nodosa 124
Polycystic ovarian disease 195
Polyp, endometrial 190*f*
Polypoid mass, focal 85
Pons, power border of 54
Porta hepatis 73, 76
Portal cavernoma formation 76*f*
Portal flow
    normalization of 85*f*
    reversal of 84*f*
Portal hypertension
    complications of 80
    extrahepatic 87
    sign of 76, 90
Portal system
    intrasplenic 86
    thrombosis 76
Portal thrombosis, chronic 76
Portal vein 73, 82, 87, 87*f*
    anatomy, abnormal 87
    branches 73, 80*f*
    dilatation of 90
    Doppler 40
        measurements of 79*t*
    duplex Doppler evaluation of 74*f*
    flow pattern 74*f*
    main 93
    normal 81
    occlusion, diagnosis of 86
    patency 85
    stenosis of 87
    system 79, 85
    thrombosis 76*f*, 79
    waveform, normal 74*f*
Portosystemic surgical shunts, evaluation of 80
Posterior fossa ischemia 46
Postmyocardial infarction 67
Poststenotic flow 11*f*
    disturbance 27
Poststenotic segment 106
Poststenotic spectrum 9*f*

Power Doppler
　flow imaging 34
　image 34, 43f, 82f
　sonography 84
　system 34
Pregnancy
　changes in 200
　ectopic 188, 189f, 203
　molar 187, 203
Prostate
　Doppler evaluation of 110
　hypertrophy, benign 110
Prosthetic cardiac valves 67
Proximal renal artery stenosis, severe 28f
Pseudoaneurysm 106, 107, 121, 121f, 122, 162, 163
　develop 92
　extrarenal 107
　gray scale sonography 121
　intrasplenic 91
　post-traumatic 91
　types of 122
Pseudosac, recognition of 203
Pulsatile
　flow 6, 8
　　pattern 8
　masses 46
　neck masses 52
Pulsatility 23f
　index 24f
　measurements 24f
Pulse
　Doppler
　　image femoral vein, longitudinal 169f
　　instruments 17, 57
　　tracing 103f
　pressure 7
　repetition frequency 73, 97
　wave Doppler 17
Pulsed Doppler
　equipment 115
　instrument, principal components of 17f
　interrogation 97
　sonography 84
Pyelocaliectasis 108
Pyogenic granuloma 146, 146f

R

Radial artery 185f
Radial veins 166
Rayleigh Tyndall scattering 15
Renal artery 96, 103f, 120, 124, 178f
　and veins, intraparenchymal 96f
　aneurysms 124
　level of 116
　main 103
　multiple donor 105
　normal 97f
　parenchymal branches of 108
　stenosis 102, 103, 105
　thrombosis 106
Renal cell carcinoma 101f, 105
Renal failure 99
　irreversible chronic 105
Renal function, recovery of 100
Renal mass 100
　evaluation of 100
Renal medical disease 99
Renal obstruction, acute 98
Renal scintigraphy 99
Renal sinus 125f
Renal transplant 104, 108, 112
　dysfunction 108
　rejection 108f
　vascular complication of 105
Renal vascular resistance 98
Renal vein 102, 127
　large 80
　right 127
　stenosis 107
　thrombosis 100, 105, 107, 127
Resistivity index 24f
Respiration, venous effect of 12
Retinal artery, central 153
Retinal vein, central 153
Retinal vessels abnormalities 155
Retrograde inherently laminar flow, zone of 10
Retroperitoneum 115
Reversible ischemic neurological deficit 46
Reynolds number 6
Rhabdomyosarcoma 144f

S

Saccular collection, anechoic 121f
Salivary gland 152
　adenoma, pleomorphic 152
　tumors 152
Saphenofemoral junction 167, 168f, 172, 173f
Saphenous vein
　great 166, 168f
　lesser 166
　mapping, preoperative 173
　small 167
Scrotal
　calcifications 136
　calculus 135f
　diseases, diagnosis of 130
　hernias 136
　mass, palpable 130
　sac and testis, empty right 136f
　trauma 133
　wall 130
Seminoma 136, 137f
Senile testicular atrophy 138f
Sertoli cell 137
Sharp systolic peak 23
Shifting line method 30
Sion procedure 197, 199t
Sion test 198t, 199
Skin
　and subcutaneous tissues 144
　lesions 146t
Snail shell curl 132
Sonosalpingography 191, 197
　technique 197f
Spatial pulse 17
Spectral counter parts 31
Spectral widening, degree of 25
Spermatic cord 133f, 136f
Splanchnic aneurysms 124
Splanchnic arteries 91
Splanchnic system 74
Spleen 104
Splenic artery 93, 124f
　aneurysm 125f
　dilatation of 90
Splenic hilum 73
Splenic infarction 91
　characteristics of 91
　diagnosis of 91
Splenic vein 73, 90, 93
　dilatation of 75
　dilated and tortuous 90f
　flow pattern 90f
Spongiosa 139
Stenosis 8, 10f, 27, 27f, 50f, 104, 125, 178f
　arterial 107
　assessing severity of 8
　degree of 11f
　diagnosis of 64t
　high grade 27
　moderate 27
　proximal subclavian 53
　severity of 9
　suspicion of 106
　various degrees of 49t
　visual measurement of 32
Stenotic internal carotid lumen 27f
Stenotic lumen 27
Stenotic measurements, direct 49
Stenotic zone refers 26

Stent graft placement 179
Stent thrombosis 81
Stimulate micturition 38
Stomach, fundus of 78f
Stroke
    ischemic 56
    mild 46
    risk of 50
Stromal echogenicity 196f
Subclavian arteries, proximal 158
Subclavian steal syndrome 46, 64
Superficial femoral artery, thrombosis of 160f
Superficial temporal artery 47
Superficial venous system 166
Superior mesenteric
    artery 93, 96, 116, 118f, 123, 124f
    vein 93
Systolic peak, early 104
Systolic pressure 7
Systolic slope 103
Systolic velocity, peak 96, 140
Systolic window 24, 25

T

Tardus refers 103
Teratocarcinoma 137
Teratoma 137, 138f
Terminal internal carotid artery 58, 60
Testicular calcifications, isolated 136
Testicular flow, spectral waveforms of 130
Testicular rupture 134
Testicular torsion 131, 132
    late phase of 132f
Testicular tumors 132, 135, 136
    majority of 135
Testicular vascularity, normal 131f
Testicular vessels 132
Testis 130
    enlargement of 132
    neoplasms of 136
    senile atrophy of 138
    torsion of 132f
    undescended 135, 136f
Thrombocytopenia 99
Thrombus 177
Thyroid
    benign lesion of 151f
    gland 148, 150f-152f
    inferno sign 150f
    nodules 148, 151f
    solitary nodule in 151f
Thyrotoxicosis 150f

Tibial vein
    distal
        anterior 172
        posterior 172
    proximal anterior 172
Tiny air embolisms 56
Tissue attenuation 182
Tortuous vessels 15
Transcranial Doppler 39, 55, 69
    clinical applications of 70t
    sonography 57
    ultrasound 53
Transforaminal window 59
Transient ischemia 46
Transjugular intrahepatic portosystemic shunt 80
Transorbital window 54, 59
Transplant rejection 108, 112
    role of Doppler in 94
Transplantation
    complication of 107
    pancreatic 93, 94
Transtemporal window 54, 58
Transvaginal color Doppler sonography, goal of 186
Treponema pallidum 132
Triphasic flow pattern 157
Tubal patency, confirming 198f
Tuberculosis, chronic 136
Tumors 85
    ocular 153
    orbital 153
Tunica vaginalis 130

U

Ulnar veins 166
Umbilical artery 204
    diastolic flow in 206f
    normal 205f
    waveform, limitations of 208
Umbilical flow velocity waveforms 201
Umbilical resistance, high 210
Umbilical vein, normal flow pattern in 208f
Upper limb 158, 168
Ureteral pressure 98
Ureteric drainage 105
Ureterovesical junctions 109
Urethra, proximal 139
Urinary
    bladders 109f
    obstruction 108
    system
        color Doppler in 96
        role of color Doppler in 96

Urinoma 107
Urological application 215
Uterine 185f, 191
    arteriovenous malformation 189
    artery 192, 199, 204, 205f
        flow 193f
        in nonpregnant state 204f
        in pregnancy, flow pattern of 204f
        low velocity, normal 187
        waveform 185f
    biophysical profile 194, 199
        ultrasound technique for 193
    blood flow 195
    factor 195
    fibroid 187f
    perfusion 192
    tumors, malignant 189
    vessels, main 184
    wall, vasculature of 184f
Uteroplacental
    circulation 201
    vasculature, normal 201f
Uterus, bicornuate 216f

V

Vaginal probe 198
Valsalva maneuver 128, 131, 137f, 168, 169f
Variceal bleeding 78f
Varicocele 135, 135f, 136, 136f
Vascular
    bypass graft 31
    calcification, prominent 9
    color flow signals, multiple 153f
    complications 105
    congestion 100
    lesions 145, 153
    phantom 10f
    phenomena 214
    rejection, acute 108
    velocity, peripheral 38
Vasculogenic impotence 139, 142
Veins 105
    perforating 166, 172
    popliteal 172
    superficial 166
        femoral 169f
Vena cava filter 179
Venous compression, lack of 170
Venous Doppler, peripheral 41
Venous flow
    arterialization of 147f
    continuous 153f
Venous integrity 93
Venous obstruction 12

Venous pressure 12
Venous system 166
    instrumentation and technique 166
Venous thrombosis 94
Venous waveform, normal 169*f*
Vertebral artery 47, 53, 58, 62, 65*f*
    course of 47
    junction 59
Vertebral vessels 46
Vesicoureteric junction, color Doppler in 99
Vesicoureteric reflux, detection of 109
Vessels 21
    abdominal 73
    great 115
    identification 58*t*
        criteria 60*t*
    lumen 93, 117
    segments 177
    sudden interruption of 93
    superficial femoral 164*f*
    walls, elasticity of 3
Viral hepatitis, chronic 90
Viscosity 3
Voiding cystourethrogram 109*f*
Volumetric flow 16

W

Waterfall sign 191
Waveforms 22
    interpretations of 208
Wilm's tumor 101*f*

Z

Zygoma 47